AI and IoT-Enhanced Skin Cancer Detection and Care

(Part 1)

Edited by

Akhil Sharma
R.J. College of Pharmacy
Raipur, Uttar Pradesh, India

Shaweta Sharma
School of Medical and Allied Sciences
Galgotias University, Greater Noida
Uttar Pradesh, India

Shivkanya Fuloria
Faculty of Pharmacy, AIMST University
Semeling Campus, Bedong-08100
Kedah, Malaysia

&

Sudhir Kumar
Faculty of Pharmaceutical Sciences
DAV University, Jalandhar
India

AI and IoT-Enhanced Skin Cancer Detection and Care *(Part 1)*

Editors: Akhil Sharma, Shaweta Sharma, Shivkanya Fuloria & Sudhir Kumar

ISBN (Online): 979-8-89881-195-2

ISBN (Print): 979-8-89881-196-9

ISBN (Paperback): 979-8-89881-197-6

Published by Bentham Science Publishers Pte. Ltd. Singapore,

in collaboration with Eureka Conferences, USA.

First published in 2025.

Bentham Science Publishers Pte. Ltd.
No. 9 Raffles Place
Office No. 26-01
Singapore 048619
Singapore
Email: subscriptions@benthamscience.net

BENTHAM SCIENCE

CONTENTS

FOREWORD

Skin cancer remains one of the most prevalent and potentially deadly forms of cancer, yet its prognosis improves significantly with early detection and timely intervention. In the age of rapid technological advancement, traditional diagnostic approaches are being augmented and in some cases transformed by cutting-edge innovations such as Artificial Intelligence (AI), Internet of Things (IoT), and mobile health applications. This book provides a comprehensive examination of how these technologies are revolutionizing dermatological diagnostics, particularly in the context of skin cancer.

Each chapter meticulously outlines a critical area, ranging from digital dermoscopy to teledermatology, wearable UV-monitoring devices, and AI-driven imaging, presented by a collaborative team of researchers and clinicians. The content not only highlights current capabilities but also examines future directions, ethical implications, and challenges still to be addressed.

This volume stands as a timely and essential contribution to the field of digital dermatology. It is especially beneficial for clinicians, biomedical researchers, healthcare technologists, and policy-makers committed to improving patient outcomes through innovation.

The authors are commended for this significant endeavor, and it is hoped this work inspires further research and application in the pursuit of smarter, more accessible skin cancer diagnostics.

Neeraj Kumar Fuloria
Faculty of Pharmacy, AIMST University, Malaysia

PREFACE

The idea for this book originated from a shared recognition of the urgent need to modernize skin cancer diagnostics through technological advancements. With skin cancer cases steadily rising worldwide, the limitations of conventional diagnostic methods manual inspections, delayed biopsy results, and uneven access to specialists, have become increasingly evident. This work aims to bridge that gap by showcasing the integration of AI, IoT, machine learning, and wearable technologies in dermatology.

This volume is a collaborative effort involving experts from diverse disciplines, including clinical dermatology, biomedical engineering, artificial intelligence, and public health. Each chapter delves into a specialized aspect of the evolving diagnostic landscape, including AI-powered lesion detection, remote monitoring, mobile apps, transfer learning models, and digital dermoscopy.

We have structured the book to provide both foundational knowledge and insight into future technologies, challenges, and clinical applicability. Our goal is to inform and inspire researchers, clinicians, and students to leverage these technological advances for early detection, personalized care, and enhanced treatment outcomes.

We hope this book serves not only as an academic resource but also as a call to action for integrating smarter solutions into mainstream dermatological practice.

Akhil Sharma
R.J. College of Pharmacy
Raipur, Uttar Pradesh, India

Shaweta Sharma
School of Medical and Allied Sciences
Galgotias University, Greater Noida
Uttar Pradesh, India

Shivkanya Fuloria
Faculty of Pharmacy, AIMST University
Semeling Campus, Bedong-08100
Kedah, Malaysia

&

Sudhir Kumar
Faculty of Pharmaceutical Sciences
DAV University, Jalandhar
India

List of Contributors

Apoorva Chourey	Ujjain Institute of Pharmaceutical Sciences, Madhya Pradesh, 456664, India
Akhil Sharma	R.J. College of Pharmacy, Raipur, Uttar Pradesh, India
Akanksha Sharma	R. J. College of Pharmacy, Raipur, Uttar Pradesh, India
Ayushi Chourasia	Bhopal Institute of Technology & Science-Pharmacy, Bhopal, 462045, India
Ashish Verma	Mangalmay Pharmacy College, Greater Noida, Uttar Pradesh, 201306, India
E. Keshamma	Department of Biochemistry, Maharani's Science College for Women (Maharani Cluster University), Bangalore, 560001, India
Gourishankar Birtia	Dr C.V. Raman Institute of Pharmacy, Dr C.V. Raman University, Chattisgarh, India
Neeraj Kumar Fuloria	Department of Pharmaceutical Chemistry, Faculty of Pharmacy, AIMST University, Semeling Campus, Bedong, 08100, Malaysia
Raghav Dixit	ICFAI School of Pharmaceutical Sciences, ICFAI University, Dehradun, Uttarakhand, 248011, India
R. Seetharaman	SRM College of Pharmacy, SRM Institute of Science and Technology, Tamil Nadu, 603203, India
Sajeeda Niketh	Department of Chemistry and Biochemistry, Nrupathunga University, Bengaluru, 560001, India
Suraj Mandal	Department of Pharmacy, IIMT College of Medical Sciences, IIMT University, Ganganagar, Meerut, 250001, India
Sonali D. Pawar	MGV's Pharmacy College, Panchavati, Nashik, India
Shaweta Sharma	School of Medical and Allied Sciences, Galgotias University, Uttar Pradesh, 201310, India
Shivkanya Fuloria	Faculty of Pharmacy, AIMST University, Semeling Campus, Bedong, Kedah, 08100, Malaysia
Sunita	R. J. College of Pharmacy, Raipur, Uttar Pradesh, India
Sakshi Aole	Mahakal Institute of Pharmaceutical Studies, Ujjain, Madhya Pradesh, 456664, India
Safiya Bee	Mahakal Institute of Pharmaceutical Studies, Ujjain, Madhya Pradesh, 456664, India
Shilpa Thukral	Dnyan Ganga College of Pharmacy, Thane, Maharashtra, 400615, India
Taru Shrivastava	Mahakal Institute of Pharmaceutical Studies, Ujjain, Madhya Pradesh, 456664, India
T. Naga Aparna	Faculty of Pharmaceutical Sciences, G. Pulla Reddy College of Pharmacy, Hyderabad, India
Zeba Siddiqui	Amity Institute of Pharmacy, Amity University, Madhya Pradesh, 474005, India

CHAPTER 1

The Evolving Landscape of Skin Cancer Diagnostics

T. Naga Aparna[1], **Sajeeda Niketh**[2], **E. Keshamma**[3], **Suraj Mandal**[4] and **Akhil Sharma**[5,*]

[1] *Faculty of Pharmaceutical Sciences, G. Pulla Reddy College of Pharmacy, Hyderabad, India*

[2] *Department of Chemistry and Biochemistry, Nrupathunga University, Bengaluru-560001, India*

[3] *Department of Biochemistry, Maharani's Science College for Women (Maharani Cluster University), Bangalore-560001, India*

[4] *Department of Pharmacy, IIMT College of Medical Sciences, IIMT University, Ganganagar, Meerut-250001, India*

[5] *R.J. College of Pharmacy, Raipur, Uttar Pradesh, India*

Abstract: Recent discoveries in skin cancer and technological advances making accurate diagnostics far more practical are rapidly changing how skin cancer is diagnosed. Imaging skin tumors or relevant skin pathology with high-resolution, non-invasive anatomical methods have increased the diagnostic precision for these very difficult-to-diagnose entities. The advent of imaging technologies such as Reflectance Confocal Microscopy (RCM) correlative Optical Coherence Tomography (OCT) now allows a high-resolution visualization of skin lesions, subsequently allowing for increased diagnostic accuracy. Novel molecular diagnostics, including gene expression profiling and mutational analysis, reveal the underlying genetic changes associated with skin cancers and pave the way for personalized therapy. Integrating artificial intelligence (AI) into dermatology may yield numerous advantages, including but not limited to improved clinical accuracy, the ability to detect skin cancers at early stages, recommendations for skin lesion and eruption treatments, and enhanced continuity of care. AI-driven diagnostic tools can diagnose skin diseases faster and more accurately than human dermatologists, which could augment the abilities of dermatologists. Non-invasive methodologies, including molecular imaging, liquid biopsies, and Raman spectroscopy, have recently become promising diagnostic methods for skin cancer biomarkers without tissue samples. Wearable diagnostics and nanotechnology advances provide a valuable opportunity for point-of-care testing and continuous monitoring. Despite these developments, challenges remain regarding their cost, accessibility, and integration into clinical practice. This chapter will elaborate on the ultimate transformative effect of these technological advancements, the remaining challenges, and the future of skin cancer diagnosis, pointing out the importance of continued innovation in improving patient outcomes and facilitating clinical procedures.

* **Corresponding author Akhil Sharma:** R.J. College of Pharmacy, Raipur, Uttar Pradesh, India; E-mail: xs2akhil@gmail.com

Akhil Sharma, Shaweta Sharma, Shivkanya Fuloria & Sudhir Kumar (Eds.)

Keywords: Artificial intelligence, biopsy, Computer-aided diagnosis systems, Diagnosis, Fluorescence *in situ* hybridization, Machine learning, Melanoma, Next-generation sequencing, Non-melanoma, Polymerase chain reaction, Skin cancer.

INTRODUCTION

Skin cancer is currently a major global public health concern, and its prevalence is steadily increasing. This might have a significant impact on both the world's labor force and economy. The epidermis and dermis are the two main layers of skin. The outermost layer of skin, known as the epidermis, comprises Langerhans, Merkel, melanocyte, and keratinocyte cells. Cancer is one type of skin injury that can result from any aberration in this layer. In different parts of the world, skin cancer incidence, morbidity, and death rates are on the rise. In the United States, 5.4 million new cases of skin cancer are recorded annually. Generally speaking, there are two main types of skin cancer: melanoma, which is caused by malfunctioning melanocytes, and non-melanoma skin cancers, which are formed from epidermal cells [1 - 3].

Human melanocytes, pigment-containing cells that makeup 90%, 5%, and 1% of the skin, eyes, and gut, respectively, increase abnormally and cause melanoma. Melanoma makes up only 1% of skin malignant tumors, a small percentage compared to other skin injuries. Even with recent improvements in treatment methods, melanoma remains the most severe type of skin cancer, with just 15-20% of cases ending in a five-year survival. Roughly 95% of skin cancer cases are non-melanoma skin cancer (NMSC), which is brought on by a combination of environmental and hereditary causes. Non-melanoma skin cancer (NMSC) is a broad term that includes a wide variety of malignant skin cancer types.

However, 99% of NMSCs are classified into two primary subtypes: basal cell carcinoma (BCC) and cutaneous squamous cell carcinoma (SCC). According to several studies, the incidence rate of non-melanoma skin cancer (NMSC) has risen globally every year by 3-8% since 1960 and is 18–20 times higher than that of melanoma. NMSC is more common in men than women, and environmental, phenotypic, and genetic factors affect how likely NMSC is to advance. Given the increasing incidence of skin malignancies and the difficulties in developing effective medication delivery methods, it is imperative to explore all available avenues for disease prevention and treatment [4 - 7].

Several variables influence the genesis of cancer. However, biological (non-modifiable) and non-biological (adjustable) are two important risk factors linked to the pathogenesis of many cutaneous malignancies, and they are depicted in Fig. (**1**) [8].

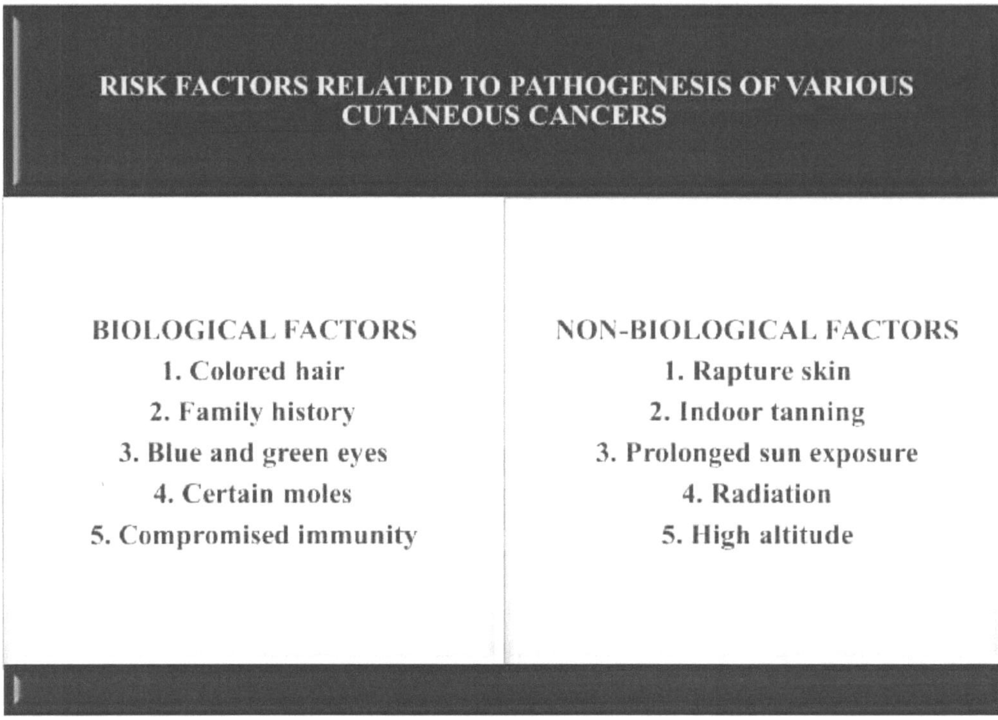

Fig. (1). Risk factors related to the pathogenesis of various cutaneous cancers.

Importance of Early Detection

The goal of population-based cancer screening is to lower the overall cancer death rate in the general population by utilizing an early neoplasm detection method. This approach also includes the long-term surveillance of individuals who have already received a neoplasm diagnosis to detect any relapses, recurrences, or related neoplasms that may manifest over the patient's lifetime and diagnose them early. As many cases of malignant melanoma (MM) as possible can be identified early in life thanks to the use of dermatoscopy, video dermatoscopy, and the "ugly duckling" sign for population screening and self-examination, respectively [9].

To aid in the clinical diagnosis of MM, Friedman *et al.* first defined the ABCD criteria, which include asymmetry, border irregularity, color variegation, and a diameter of at least 6 mm. The ABCDE criteria, where E stands for evolutionary change, were added to the ABCD criteria to increase the diagnostic sensitivity. However, the ABCDE criteria overlook that MMs with a diameter of less than 6 mm exist and that their frequency has grown. Additionally, *in situ* or very early MMs might not meet these requirements. Dermoscopy can enhance the shortcomings of the clinical examination and the ABCDE criteria, irrespective of the diagnosis algorithm employed. By using dermoscopy, the sensitivity of the assessment with the unaided eye was raised by 18% (95% CI 9–27%; p = 0.002) to 90% (95% CI 80–95%). The early detection of skin malignancies would be positively impacted by optimal screening, further lowering morbidity, mortality, and related expenses [10 - 13].

Overview of Traditional Diagnostic Methods

Dermatologists have historically diagnosed skin cancer by manual evaluation and techniques, such as BIOPSY and visual inspection by dermatologists or general practitioners. However, these approaches have several drawbacks and restrictions. BIOPSY is an intrusive diagnostic technique that can be uncomfortable, time-consuming, and even lead to the disease spreading. When a lesion seems suspicious, a biopsy is necessary for a conclusive diagnosis; however, this procedure can be costly and leave the patient with scars, infections, and discomfort. The naked eye is another way doctors utilize their expertise and senses to assess whether or not a patient has cancer. Visual inspection significantly depends on the healthcare provider's experience and subjective assessment [14 - 16].

Various practitioners may have various interpretations of the same lesion, which could result in variations in diagnosis. Even when highly qualified physicians detect skin lesions, mistakes might happen. The eye inspection method is unreliable since it can lead to overdiagnosis (identifying benign lesions as malignant) and underdiagnosis (missing malignant lesions). One of the drawbacks of older approaches is their inability to distinguish between lesions accurately. It might be difficult to distinguish benign from malignant tumors only by visual inspection, particularly when the lesions are young or have unusual characteristics [17, 18].

Another drawback is that dermatologists and other specialists in skin cancer diagnostics are not always easily accessible in many areas, particularly in underserved or rural areas. Treatment and diagnosis delays may result from this restriction. To get around these restrictions, technologies, including teledermatology, dermoscopy, and computer-aided diagnosis systems, are being researched and developed to increase the accessibility, efficacy, and accuracy of skin cancer detection. The non-invasive skin imaging method, dermoscopy, is used to diagnose skin cancer. It obtains an enlarged picture of a specific area of skin. Compared to visual evaluation, it is more accurate [19 - 21].

Overview of Artificial Intelligence

The technology that allows computers and other devices to mimic human learning, comprehension, problem-solving, decision-making, creativity, and autonomy is known as artificial intelligence (AI). The fundamental branch of AI is Machine Learning (ML), which allows computers to learn patterns from data without explicit programming. ML algorithms can be classified into supervised learning, where models learn from labeled data using techniques like linear regression and decision trees; unsupervised learning, which finds hidden patterns in data through clustering and dimensionality reduction; and reinforcement learning, where agents learn optimal behaviors through trial and error using techniques like Q-learning and deep Q-networks. At the core of ML is neural networks, which mimic the human brain by using interconnected layers of nodes to process information. Deep learning, a subset of ML, employs multi-layered neural networks to extract complex patterns from vast datasets, with its performance largely dependent on the quality and quantity of data available [22 - 24].

Another critical AI domain is Natural Language Processing (NLP), which enables computers to understand and process human language. NLP techniques include text analysis, which involves breaking text into words (tokenization), identifying grammatical roles (part-of-speech tagging), recognizing named entities (*e.g.*, people and organizations), and determining the emotional tone of text (sentiment analysis). Advanced language models predict the next word in a sequence, powering applications such as text generation, translation, and intelligent virtual assistants [25, 26].

In the realm of Computer Vision, AI algorithms empower computers to interpret and analyze images. This includes image recognition tasks like object detection (identifying objects within an image), image classification (categorizing images), and image segmentation (dividing images into meaningful regions). Convolutional Neural Networks (CNNs), a specialized type of neural network, are particularly effective in image processing, enabling breakthroughs in fields such as medical imaging and autonomous vehicles [27, 28].

AI is also making significant advancements in robotics, where machines interact with the physical world using sensors (*e.g.*, cameras, lidar, and sonar) to perceive their environment and actuators (*e.g.*, motors and robotic arms) to perform actions. AI-driven control algorithms allow robots to navigate spaces, manipulate objects, and perform complex tasks autonomously, finding applications in industries such as healthcare, manufacturing, and space exploration.

Another crucial aspect of AI is knowledge representation and reasoning, which involves structuring information so that machines can reason and make decisions. This is achieved using ontologies, which define concepts and relationships in a domain, and logic-based reasoning, which enables AI systems to infer new information from existing knowledge [29, 30].

Beyond these technical foundations, AI research also addresses important challenges such as AI ethics, ensuring that AI systems remain fair, unbiased, and aligned with human values. Specialized AI hardware, such as Graphics Processing Units (GPUs) and Tensor Processing Units (TPUs), accelerates AI computations, while powerful AI software frameworks, like TensorFlow and PyTorch, provide tools for developing sophisticated AI applications.

AI is revolutionizing numerous industries, particularly healthcare, where it aids in disease diagnosis, drug discovery, and personalized treatment plans. From autonomous vehicles and smart assistants to medical imaging and predictive analytics, AI continues to redefine the way humans interact with technology, making it one of the most transformative fields in modern science and engineering [31, 32].

ADVANCEMENTS IN DIAGNOSTIC TECHNOLOGIES

Imaging Techniques

Imaging techniques have advanced significantly, providing a noninvasive method for detecting skin cancer. These techniques include dermoscopy, reflectance confocal microscopy (RCM), Optical Coherence Tomography (OCT), and high-frequency ultrasound (HFUS). Fig. (**2**) summarises the various imaging techniques used in skin cancer detection.

Dermoscopy

Through improved imaging of cutaneous features not visible to the unaided eye, dermoscopy, a non-invasive technique, has transformed the diagnosis of skin lesions and greatly increased the precision of dermatologic examinations. Several algorithms have been devised in the context of skin cancer, using dermoscopy to help in diagnosis. These algorithms are based mostly on the recognition of particular dermoscopic characteristics, such as the presence of ulceration, pigmented structures like blue-grey ovoid nests, and vascular structures like arborizing vessels. Further aiding in the differentiation of skin cancer is the lack of structures linked to melanocytic lesions, such as network patches. Clinicians can identify skin cancer more accurately and dependably using these dermoscopic criteria, allowing prompt intervention and better patient care [33 - 36].

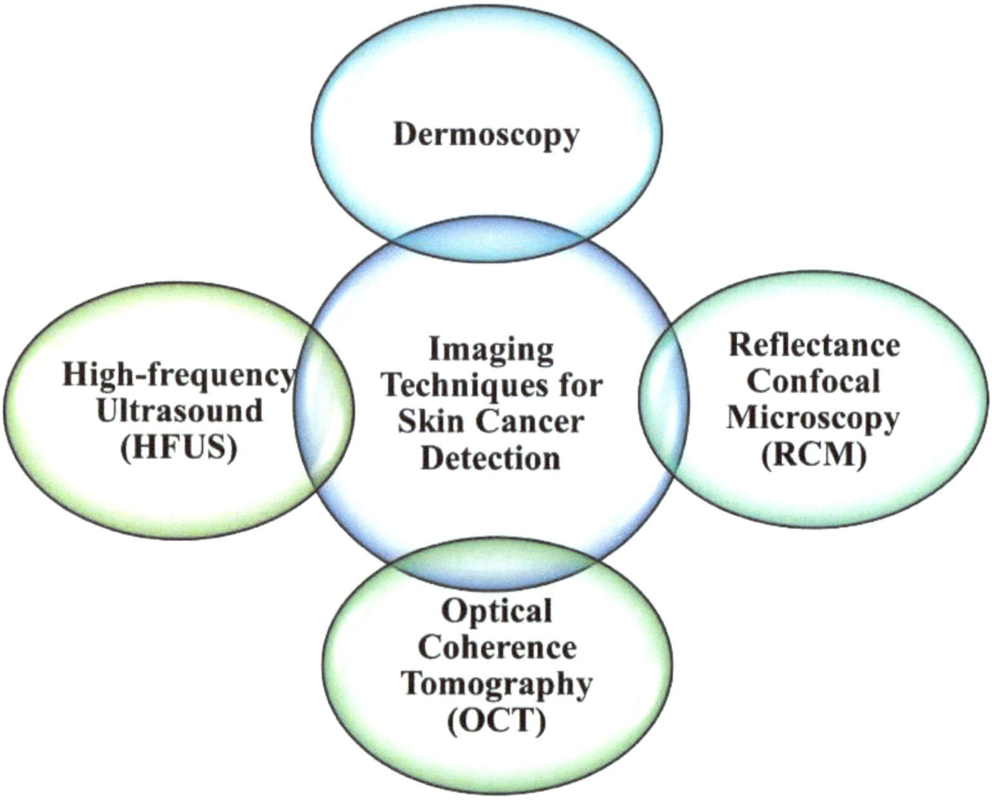

Fig. (2). Various imaging techniques used in skin cancer detection.

Reflectance Confocal Microscopy (RCM)

An innovative optical imaging method called reflectance confocal microscopy (RCM) allows for the noninvasive, *in-vivo* assessment of skin lesions in real-time. Its high-resolution imaging capabilities allow for observing tissue architecture in great detail. Remarkably, RCM has been utilized to directly define the histopathologic aspects of Basal Cell Carcinoma (BCC) *in vivo*, and a good correlation has been found between the detected confocal features and histological findings. This demonstrates how RCM can offer insightful information about the microscopic features of skin cancer lesions [37 - 39].

Optical Coherence Tomography (OCT)

OCT is the most advanced imaging modality that provides efficient tissue penetration and high resolution. It allows for observing several cutaneous features, including appendages, the complete epidermis, and part of the dermis. OCT technology has more applications now that it has advanced. When evaluating the treatment of vascular lesions, optical Doppler tomography uses Doppler sensitivity, whereas polarization-sensitive OCT uses the polarization information provided by light to detect tissue birefringence. When it comes to skin, birefringence is mostly caused by the way collagen fibers are arranged in the dermis.

Recent studies employing line-field confocal optical coherence tomography (LC-OCT) have shown promise for the early identification and subtype classification of skin cancer. By combining the technological benefits of OCT with reflectance confocal microscopy, LC-OCT makes it possible to distinguish accurately between skin cancer and its clinical imitators. Furthermore, it has been determined that LC-OCT criteria may serve as predictors for different subtypes of skin cancer.

For instance, superficial skin cancer frequently manifests as epidermal bulges intruding into the upper part of the dermis, surrounded by a darker rim, and infiltrative skin cancer appears as ill-defined, narrow, dark, longish structures in the dermis, surrounded by brighter tissue. Nodular skin cancer, on the other hand, is characterized by a poorly defined dermo-epidermal junction and dark ovoid structures (often with bright centers). When combined with LC-OCT criteria, these developments in OCT technology can potentially improve noninvasive skin cancer diagnosis and subtype categorization, providing important information for treating the condition [40 - 43].

High-frequency Ultrasound (HFUS)

Using sound waves with frequencies higher than 20 megahertz (MHz), HFUS imaging is a noninvasive diagnostic method that creates images of tissue features. HFUS can quantify tumor depth, define margins, and find hypoechoic skin cancer nests within hyperechoic collagen fibers. The primary determinants of skin cancer risk are the tumor's size, location, and histological subtype (HST). Currently, invasive biopsies are used to establish the HST, even if location and size are obvious at diagnosis. Typically, nodular-shaped hypoechoic lesions with distinct borders, such as several hyperechoic spots and cystic degeneration zones, are called nodular HSTs.

These lesions frequently exhibit a posterior acoustic shadowing and a hyperechoic surface. The homogenous hypoechoic lesions that crawl and are well-defined are the hallmarks of superficial HSTs. Their surfaces are flat and devoid of aberrant keratinization, unlike nodular HSTs. Like nodular HSTs, pigmented HSTs have raised surfaces, irregular or oval shapes, a clearly defined edge, and hyperechoic areas inside the lesion. Morphea forms skin cancer lesions that primarily penetrate the dermis and are irregular, hypoechoic-heterogenous lesions. Increased fibrosis and edema around the tumor frequently increase echogenicity [44 - 47].

Molecular Diagnostics

Molecular diagnostics play an important role in diagnosing and managing skin cancer. The key approaches of molecular diagnostics are gene expression profiling and mutational analysis.

Gene Expression Profiling

The number of non-FDA-approved molecular skin cancer biomarker tests is increasing. Many of these assays are commercially accessible based on the characterization of gene expression profiles (GEPs). Cells express a portion of their genes at any given time through mRNA transcription. Genes that are differently expressed are found using gene expression profiling, which measures and compares cell mRNA levels under various experimental or disease-state scenarios.

Gene expression profiles are distinct signatures for different cell types or disease states and offer insights into cellular processes. Using microarray analysis, which involves converting sample mRNA to cDNA, fluorescently labeling it, and hybridizing it with a reference sample onto an oligo-covered array, each oligo denoting a distinct mRNA transcript, many of the current melanoma GEPs were discovered. To create a gene expression profile, the fold-change genes in a sample are identified using the sample/reference fluorescence ratio at each oligo [48].

An epidermal genetic information retrieval kit consisting of a non-invasive adhesive sticker (Smart sticker) that gathers surface keratinocytes for gene expression analysis of a two-gene signature is provided by DermTech (La Jolla, CA) as a minimally invasive melanoma diagnostic. Patients self-administer the four 17-mm adhesive tape discs with a polyurethane backing, two for each two-gene test and two controls that come with the epidermal genetic information retrieval kit onto worrisome lesions.

After that, the stickers are shipped to DermTech laboratories for processing and enclosed in return packaging. Every sticker usually lifts enough cells to yield three pgs of RNA. This RNA is then extracted for real-time PCR using a small-molecule RNAse inhibitor, a proprietary blend of catabolic enzymes, and a multi-enzymatic liquefaction of tissue total nucleic acid isolation system (Ambion, Austin, TX) [49].

Rather than DermTech, more skin cancer Gene Expression Profile (GEP) tests are undergoing trials. MelaGenix (8-GEP), Neracare, which utilizes real-time Polymerase Chain Reaction (PCR), prognosis prediction (low- and high-risk score), and DecisionDx (31-GEP), Castle Biosciences, which utilizes real-time PCR, and risk of metastasis with low risk (class 1A/1B) and high risk (2A/2B) [50, 51].

Mutational Analysis

The key cellular signaling mechanisms for transforming melanocytes include prolonged activation of the RAS/RAF/MAPK and PI3K pathways. These mutations cause the overactivation of the intracellular network of downstream signaling cascades, which promotes the abnormal growth of melanocytes [52]. Mutually exclusive mutations in the BRAF, NRAS, C-KIT, and NF-1 genes have been associated in various studies with melanoma development. A meta-analysis carried out in 2010 by Lee *et al.* found that the NRAS gene had an 18% mutation frequency while the BRAF gene had a 41% mutation frequency. 28 and 36% of mucosal melanoma and acral lentiginous melanoma cases have mutations in the C-KIT gene [53].

With a frequency of 60–80%, V600E (T1799A; substitution of valine for glutamic acid) is the most prevalent mutation in the BRAF gene. V600K and V600R have estimated frequencies of 20% and 20%, respectively, after them. Three to five percent of melanomas have non-V600 BRAF mutations. The V600K mutation is associated with UVR exposure, is more common in persons over 65, and influences demographic differences in prevalence. With a frequency ranging from 20 to 30%, the most prevalent mutations in the NRAS gene are p.G12D and p.Q61K in exons 1 and 2, respectively [54].

About 15% of Malignant Melanomas (MM) cases have mutations in various exons of the C-KIT gene. Melanomas can be categorized into four genomic groups based on these mutations, combined with information released by The Cancer Genome Atlas (TCGA) from a complete exome sequence analysis of samples from patients with primary and metastatic melanoma: BRAF mutants, NRAS mutants, NF1 mutants (gene for neurofibromatosis type 1), and triple wild-type mutants. Given that specific therapy is available for cancers with these molecular changes, these subtypes might have prognostic utility [55, 56].

Artificial Intelligence and Machine Learning

In dermatology, mainly in skin cancer diagnosis, Artificial Intelligence (AI) and Machine Learning (ML) play a revolutionizing role, which is discussed below:

AI-Based Dermoscopy

AI-based diagnostic technologies directed towards dermatological diagnostics transform diagnostic ease, exactness, and efficiency. In this context, developing advanced diagnostic tools, such as artificial intelligence models, can increase dermatopathology accuracy and efficiency. Though it might delay the dermatological examination process by a few minutes to take good-quality images for AI study, the benefits of optimal treatment results and diagnostic accuracy will outweigh this time commitment. AI can be used to analyze images of skin lesions and provide automated diagnosis or aid dermatologists in decision-making.

On the other hand, these algorithms may recognize patterns and features of skin disorders, including skin cancer, psoriasis, eczema, and acne. Dermatology practices have already utilized AI techniques. AI algorithms can analyze clinical and genetic information to develop personalized treatment plans for dermatology patients. By incorporating individual patient features such as genetic susceptibility, medical history, and prior treatment response, AI-powered algorithms can better predict treatment outcomes and deliver personalized therapy. Patients can upload pictures of skin lesions, which dermatologists or AI diagnostic systems can then evaluate *via* telemedicine. Image analysis and triage in telemedicine powered by image-based AI algorithms.

AI is also driving the development of innovative medicines for skin issues through molecular modeling and virtual screening. These algorithms can identify viable medication candidates by analyzing large datasets of chemical compounds and biological targets and help us optimize their properties to ensure their safety and efficacy. With real-time examination of patient data, AI-driven decision support systems can provide dermatologists with real-time suggestions. They can be beneficial for faster and more accurate diagnosis and treatment planning. AI can enhance patient care and outcomes by streamlining complete skin exams in dermatology and reducing the time required for physical examination and results interpretation [57, 58].

Deep Learning Algorithms

Deep learning is typically a sub-field of machine learning that uses networks of neurons to examine more complicated data types, *e.g.*, dermoscopic imagery. The concept of artificial neural network (ANN) mimics the functioning of brain nerve cells and is inspired by biological neural networks. The simplest type of ANN is the feedforward neural network. It has three layers: hidden, output, and input. The output node receives data from the hidden layer, and the input layer passes data through the hidden layer and into the output node. CNNs are a modified version of deep feedforward ANNs commonly used to analyze visual images. This is mainly due to the network's convolution layer and pooling layer not being able to encrypt image attributes [59, 60].

Mobile Apps and Teledermatology

Mobile applications have revolutionized skin cancer diagnostics and enabled early detection and continuous monitoring since they facilitate access to advanced diagnostic systems in the hands of individuals. The main innovations include accessing an AI-powered app (SkinVision and MoleScope are popular examples) to take a picture of suspicious moles or skin lesions using a smartphone with the app. These apps process the photos with sophisticated AIs trained on vast skin disease libraries [61].

The app analyses photos of lesions to determine risk levels. These apps are utilized to indicate early warning signs of skin cancers (*e.g.*, changes in mole size, shape, and color). In this regard, AI serves as an initial screening tool, giving customers information about them that can make them visit a healthcare professional. Such AI attachment aids in early detection and treatment, especially in areas with limited dermatologists [62].

In addition to initial diagnostics, mobile applications that allow remote monitoring provide capabilities like tracking the history of images taken of the skin over time. This is particularly helpful when tracking changes in moles and lesions that might be malignant. In addition to skin check reminders, these kinds of apps promote self-monitoring and give power to the patients. In addition, a few apps also connect the users to dermatologists who will assess the images sent by the users if the chatbot cannot interpret the analysis from AI. It is a faster and more convenient process because it leverages mobile technology, and in this case, there is instant access to medical professionals, thereby improving the diagnostic process [63, 64].

Teledermatology has changed the landscape of skin cancer diagnostics by utilizing technology to bridge the distance between patients and dermatologists, allowing quicker and more convenient access to expert assessments. With teledermatology, patients can have a virtual skin examination through a video call without a face-to-face visit. This can be particularly harmonious for patients in remote or underserved areas, where access to dermatologists may be limited. The introduction of the 5G connection has enhanced teledermatology by permitting faster data transmission and better image quality, so dermatologists receive sharp, high-definition pictures essential for high-fidelity diagnoses [65].

Besides real-time consultations, teledermatology also employs store-and-forward systems, with patients uploading images of their skin conditions to secure portals for dermatologists to review later. In this asynchronous consultation model, dermatologists can diagnose conditions at their convenience without having to be present during image capture. This also provides flexibility in diagnosis and decreases patients' waiting time while increasing healthcare providers' throughput [66].

Teledermatology overcomes geographical barriers by eliminating the barrier for patients in rural or remote locations, solving the problem of restricted access to skin cancer screenings and consultations limited to urban centers. This enhanced accessibility promotes wider equity in healthcare, as more patients can obtain timely skin cancer assessments, regardless of location. Teledermatology can also be a more affordable option than traditional in-person visits. It can provide a more cost-effective solution for patients with inadequate access to traditional healthcare services [67].

While some advancements have been made, some challenges and concerns need to be addressed. With the use of mobile apps and teledermatology platforms, data privacy and security have become major concerns regarding the safe transmission and storage of sensitive medical images. Data privacy is critical to maintaining trust and compliance with regulations like HIPAA and needs to be secured. Moreover, despite the promise that AI-powered apps have demonstrated, they are not error-free [68].

AI diagnoses are not always accurate; they depend on dermatologists to prevent false positives or negatives. To improve their accuracy and avoid possible errors, efforts will be made to refine AI algorithms. Wider utilization of teledermatology will also necessitate additional infrastructure investment, provider training, and updated practice policies to integrate these technologies into practice. Adopting teledermatology

and mobile diagnostic tools for widespread use hinge on ensuring comfort among patients and dermatologists alike [69].

NON-INVASIVE DIAGNOSTIC METHODS

Changing skin cancer diagnostics with non-invasive methods that make it comfortable and fast to provide an alternative to the often-painful biopsy pathways. These cutting-edge methods allow for non-invasive differentiation of skin cancer with high sensitivity and specificity, facilitating a better patient experience and aiding in diagnostic accuracy.

Liquid Biopsies

Liquid biopsies are an exciting non-invasive technology that analyses body fluids, primarily blood, to identify circulating tumor cells or molecules released into the circulation, such as circulating tumor DNA (ctDNA). Liquid biopsies require no physical removal of skin tissue, making them far less invasive for the patient than traditional tissue biopsies. Liquid biopsies are based on circulating tumor DNA (ctDNA). The ability to identify specific tumor-derived DNA in circulation means that using ctDNA, melanoma or other skin cancers can be diagnosed or discovered for the first time without the need for biopsy [70].

Although these tests are more often related to other cancers, such as lung or breast cancer, liquid biopsies are becoming more important for the diagnosis of skin cancer. These provide different approaches to classical methods for melanoma detection, especially for progression, metastasis, and recurrence monitoring. They thus have considerable utility not just for diagnosis but for the long-term management of skin cancer. Marked by their complementing importance in personalized skin cancer management, these include the option of a non-invasive cancer detection method, such as liquid biopsies, and providing real-time information on tumor evolution [71].

Non-Invasive Imaging

Non-invasive imaging techniques, like multiphoton microscopy (MPM), provide relatively high-resolution, in-depth information about skin architecture without surgical incision of the skin or excision of tissue. MPM is an advanced imaging method that utilizes many photons to penetrate deeper into the skin layers compared to standard imaging techniques. It produces cellular-level three-dimensional images, enabling dermatologists to assess the skin's architecture better. MPM provides high-resolution imaging of the tissue without physically disrupting the skin, making it an excellent tool for early cancer detection [72, 73].

MPM is especially useful for detecting abnormal cellular structures associated with melanocytic pathologies of melanoma and other skin cancers. It allows us to assess suspicious lesions *in vivo* and follow the evolution of these lesions over time. Potentially, this technique can reduce the requirement of standard biopsies, as it facilitates the specific localization of possible cancers without breaking the skin. Despite remaining in the early implementation phase into clinical practice, MPM offers a non-invasive and efficient method with high diagnostic potential, providing rapid and detailed information on the status of skin lesions, which may have a larger role in future developments of skin cancer diagnostics [74].

Raman Spectroscopy

Another potential non-invasive diagnostic tool is Raman spectroscopy, which uses light scattering to characterize the molecular composition of skin cells. Raman spectroscopy is a technique that gives rise to a molecular 'fingerprint' of tissues, analyzing the interaction of light with molecules within the skin. However, Raman spectroscopy is based on the principle of interaction between skin and laser rays, and the scattered light after the interaction is collected and measured to identify the molecular level composition of skin tissue. Every single molecule scatters in a certain manner, and each has a specific spectral signature that is scattered, which can be used to identify cancerous cells [75].

Such a technique is also very useful for early melanoma and other skin cancer detection. Raman spectroscopy provides an opportunity to overcome this limitation through the noninvasive detection of early lesions by identifying subtle molecular changes that are invisible to the naked eye and by conventional imaging examination and require no tissue removal or other invasive procedures. Raman Spectroscopy can become a convenient and non-invasive detection method for skin cancer, facilitating examination of skin malignancies at the molecular level before any physical or visual presentation [76].

Such techniques not only help to avoid the need for invasive biopsies but also enable us to get as much information as possible, cellular and molecular, regarding the skin unit in the targeted area, with extreme accuracy. As these technologies advance and become more integrated into clinical practice, they will play a critical role in early detection, better patient outcomes, and enhancing the overall diagnostic process. Non-invasive methods could change the future of skin cancer care by offering an appropriate, speedy, and secure approach to traditional biopsy techniques [77].

BIOMARKERS IN SKIN CANCER

Biomarkers are becoming increasingly important for diagnosing, prognosis, and treating skin cancer as they provide a better molecular characterization. Biomarkers are biological molecules, genes, or processes that provide a measurable reflection of a biological state, normal or abnormal, such as the presence or progression of cancer. Biomarkers are essential for clinicians' decision-making processes in skin cancer for early detection, personalized treatment planning, and disease progression follow-up or recurrence [78]. Biomarkers used in skin cancer are summarised in Fig. (**3**).

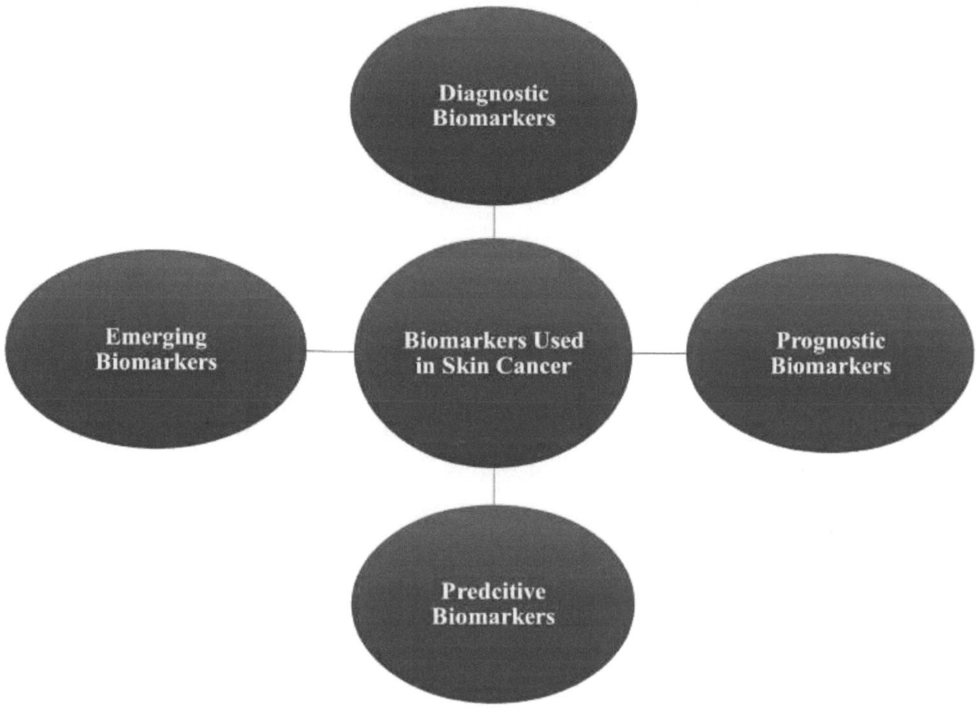

Fig. (3). Biomarkers used in skin cancer.

Diagnostic Biomarkers

Diagnostic biomarkers play a role in early skin cancer detection by signaling that cancerous cells or tumors are present in the body. Lactate Dehydrogenase (LDH) – LDH is an enzyme involved in energy production and is frequently elevated in patients with metastatic melanoma. In blood testing, elevated LDH may serve as a biomarker for more aggressive forms of skin cancer and has been associated with poorer prognoses. This biomarker can be useful in monitoring the disease process of skin cancer. Melanoma Inhibitory Activity (MIA) is an adhesive protein secreted by melanoma. Higher MIA levels in blood tests may indicate melanoma, potentially even before there are visible signs of metastatic disease. It can also be used for treatment response monitoring and is indicated for early detection [79, 80].

Prognostic Biomarkers

Prognostic biomarkers provide information about the likely progression of the disease, essentially, how aggressive the cancer is likely to behave and the chance of recovery for the patient. The BRAF gene is often mutated in melanoma, particularly the V600E mutation of BRAF is very common. This mutation plays a major role in melanoma diagnosis and acts as a prognostic biomarker as well. While BRAF mutations can imply a more aggressive form of melanoma, it is also important to recognize that answers exist in the form of targeted therapies that often improve outcomes in patients with these mutations. NRAS mutations are also linked to melanoma and occur in some patients [81].

NRAS mutations, like BRAF mutations, are concordant with a more aggressive cancer and are frequently associated with adverse outcomes. Nevertheless, NRAS mutations can guide treatment approaches and eligibility for clinical trials. The MITF (Microphthalmia-associated transcription factor) is also a master melanocyte survival and development regulator. Changes in the expression of MITF are linked with melanoma progression and survival, highlighting its role as a potential prognostic marker of tumor behavior [82].

Predictive Biomarkers

Predictive biomarkers assess a patient's probability of response to a given treatment; thus, they are an important part of personalized medicine with critical implications for treatment efficacy. Pd-L1 is a biomarker often expressed on the surface of melanoma cells. PD-L1 binds to the PD-1 receptor found on T-cells, suppressing the immune response and enabling the tumor to escape immune surveillance.

High expression of PD-L1 correlates with a favorable response to immune checkpoint inhibitors like pembrolizumab and nivolumab, which block this interaction and permit immune-based attack of tumor cells. One more immune checkpoint protein is cytotoxic T-lymphocyte-associated protein 4 (CTLA-4); therefore, patients with high-level expression of CTLA-4 may benefit from immunotherapies targeting this pathway, such as ipilimumab. CTLA-4 expression testing is used to determine treatment options and improve melanoma survival [83, 84].

Emerging Biomarkers

Circulating tumor DNA (ctDNA) is an exciting new melanoma biomarker. It will help to analyze small pieces of tumor DNA inside the blood to monitor cancer progression, treatment response, and recurrence without invasive methods. Analyzing ctDNA is less invasive and real-time compared with traditional tissue biopsies [85].

MicroRNAs (miRNAs) are a small, non-coding RNA molecule class that regulates gene expression. For example, dysregulated expression of some miRNAs in melanoma, such as miR-211 and miR-203, might be useful in predicting disease progression or response to treatment. They are emerging as a point of interest because of their potential for diagnostics and targeted therapies [86].

Tumor-infiltrating lymphocytes (TILs) are immune cells inside the tumor microenvironment. Skin melanomas with high TIL levels in patients have been associated with better clinical outcomes and response to immunotherapy. TILs are an emerging biomarker for response to immune checkpoint inhibitors, as their presence indicates the development of an immune response towards that tumor [87].

Therapeutic Implications of Biomarkers

The identification and validation of skin cancer biomarkers enable the arrival of personalized medicine. This allows for treatment to be personalized based on a patient's cancer genetic and biomarker profile. Targeted therapies such as BRAF inhibitors (*e.g.*, vemurafenib) or MEK inhibitors (*e.g.*, trametinib) can be most highly used in conditions with mutations of BRAF or NRAS. For instance, PD-L1 expression level is associated with the use of drugs targeting the PD-1/PD-L1 pathway [88].

In addition, biomarkers such as ctDNA and TILs can indicate how a patient responds to therapy in real time, helping modify treatment plans if necessary. Such an adaptive treatment approach not only increases the effectiveness of treatment but also prevents patients from being exposed to ineffective treatment and its side effects [89].

GENETIC AND GENOMIC APPROACHES

Role of Genetic Testing in Skin Cancer

In the case of skin cancer, genetic testing is especially important in looking for mutations or variations in a person`s DNA that are associated with the possibility of developing the disease. It is particularly useful in identifying hereditary traits and predispositions for high-risk groups, for example, carriers of genes such as CDKN2A, MC1R, and BRAF highly related to melanoma/skin cancer susceptibility. Knowledge of an individual's genetic phenotype can lead to individualized prevention strategies, such as more frequent screening and behavioral changes [90].

Genetic testing facilitates the detection of familial melanoma syndromes where members of the family have inherited genes (like CDKN2A) that increase the probability of developing skin cancer. Genetic markers could help identify high-risk individuals early, screening their family members for life-saving treatment in some cases. Genetic testing provides a predictive benefit for families with a history of skin cancer, allowing for preventive measures like increased sun protection, more frequent skin examinations, and surveillance of skin lesions, which in turn aid in early detection and a better outlook for patients [91].

Genomic Sequencing

Genomic sequencing, which sequences an entire genome, captures a wider array of mutations and abnormalities related to cancer than targeted genetic testing, provides a richer portrait of genetic abnormalities relevant to tumorigenesis, and is a useful approach for examining complex genetic traits like those for skin cancer. Methods such as whole genome sequencing (WGS) and whole exon sequencing (WES) are commonly performed to identify skin cancer-associated mutations using whole or exome-specific information. This enables researchers to identify rare or novel mutations, expanding our knowledge of the genetic basis of skin cancer [92, 93]. Genomic sequencing of skin cancer, mainly melanomas, aids in identifying mutations driving cancer progression [94].

Personalized Medicine

In skin cancer, personalized medicine involves using genetic and genomic information to inform personalized treatment and prevention strategies, resulting in more effective, less toxic therapies and improved outcomes. In this respect, personalized medicine directly addresses those genetic mutations that govern the growth of a patient-specific tumor with targeted therapies; for instance, BRAF inhibitors work well in patients whose tumors have BRAF mutations, whereas NRAS or KIT mutations promise to be challenging [95].

However, immunotherapy, which has proven especially effective for melanoma, is enhanced by genomic profiling that can find and determine biomarkers predicted to be responsive to specific therapies, such as PD-1 inhibitors. Targeted therapies based on an individual genetic signature minimize the impact of treatment on normal cells and greatly improve efficacy; thus, personalizing treatment plans similarly reduces toxicity. They also work as prognostic markers, identifying the risk of recurrent disease and survival, such as patients with genetic signatures that correlate to a greater risk of metastasis, and adjusting treatment intensity and follow-up accordingly [96].

EMERGING TECHNOLOGIES AND FUTURE DIRECTIONS

The new methods will change the landscape of skin cancer diagnostics and patient care, allowing for more accessible, accurate, and timely treatment. The following discusses the potential of wearable diagnostic devices alongside point-of-care testing, nanotechnology innovations, and a preview of future technologies for skin cancer detection and management.

Wearable Diagnostic Devices

Wearable diagnostic devices are becoming important in skin cancer diagnostics and prevention, enabling continuous monitoring and data collection through sensors, AI, and wireless connectivity. Wearable devices with UV sensors will track daily sun exposure and alert users when exposed to too much sun and risk damage to their skin, which could eventually lead to skin cancer. Personalization features can adjust feedback based on a user's skin type, location, and exposure history [97].

Advanced wearables, such as smartwatches with dermoscopy ability, can have imaging sensors that use image analysis to photograph moles and lesions. If necessary, AI algorithms search for unusual changes and alert the user to a medical evaluation. Also, most wearables connect with health apps or platforms, which allow users to store, track, and easily share data with healthcare providers. This connectivity facilitates remote monitoring, which lets dermatologists analyze patient data and spot signs of skin cancer early, especially in those at high risk [98, 99].

Point-of-Care Testing

Point-of-care testing (POCT) facilitates skin cancer diagnostics by placing new tools at the patient's side, reducing workup time by skipping laboratory-based assessments, and providing immediate results in nonlaboratory settings. Hence, this is more advantageous where POCT solutions make skin cancer diagnosis easily accessible in remote/underserved areas. AI-based algorithms within handheld or smartphone-integrated scanners allow clinicians to examine suspicious lesions directly on the spot with portable dermatoscopes that rapidly identify skin abnormalities and proceed to further testing if necessary [100].

POCT devices have been developed that additionally employ AI algorithms trained to detect patterns associated with skin cancer to provide preliminary diagnostic analyses as an adjunct to skin examination by non-specialist clinicians to guide decision-making and expand access to care in areas with few dermatologists. Finally, an emerging POCT ability involves rapid biomarker testing, particularly for skin cancer, employing minimally invasive devices to identify skin cancer biomarkers in sweat or saliva, thus potentially allowing for non-invasive melanoma screening that may complement standard visual screening [101].

Innovations in Nanotechnology for Diagnostics

The most important role of nanotechnology is developing ultra-sensitive diagnostic tools for skin cancer, which enable the molecular-level detection of skin cancer. Advances in this field are pushing the boundaries of early-stage diagnosis and targeted therapeutic delivery. Table **1** summarises the innovations in nanotechnology for diagnostics, focusing on the advancements and applications in skin cancer detection and monitoring.

Table 1. Innovations in nanotechnology for diagnostics, with their advancements and applications in skin cancer detection and monitoring.

Innovation	Applications in Skin Cancer Diagnostics	Benefits
Nanosensors for Biomarker Detection	Identifying markers of skin cancer in blood, sweat, or saliva in advance of evidence of physical disease.	Allow for highly sensitive, non-invasive, and early detection [102].
Gold Nanoparticles for Enhanced Imaging	Better monitoring of skin cancer lesions with easy detection of tumor cells.	Improved imaging quality and better identification of malignant tissue [103].
Quantum Dots for Fluorescence Imaging	Redirect detection of cancer cells in biopsy tissues and *in vivo* imaging.	High sensitivity and specificity help detect small or early-stage tumors [104].
Nanoparticle-Enhanced Liquid Biopsies	Early detection of skin cancer through ctDNA or exosome analysis, avoiding invasive biopsies.	Non-invasive; allow monitoring of disease progression and response to treatment [105].
Magnetic Nanoparticles for Targeted MRI	Targeted MRI imaging is used for melanoma detection and tracking of the spread.	Enhance the resolution of images and enable tracking of metastasis [106].
Nanocarriers for Targeted Drug Delivery with Diagnostics	Dual-use in treating skin cancer and monitoring the therapeutic response.	Decrease adverse effects; allow for real-time assessment of treatment effectiveness [107].
Carbon Nanotubes in Biosensing	Faster detection of skin cancer biomarkers in a highly sensitive manner.	High sensitivity and rapid response; potential for portable diagnostic devices [108].

Potential Impact of Future Technologies

New technologies are poised to improve skin cancer diagnosis and treatment by making care more available, precise, and tailored. Among a range of other benefits, wearables, as well as POCT devices, may also reduce health disparities by giving people the choice to obtain low-cost, accessible, remote diagnostics, especially in those in rural or underserved communities, which helps capture cases that otherwise would go undiagnosed. In addition, wearable devices and nanotechnology will provide personalized assessments of skin cancer risk for prevention and enable patients to act as early as possible in skin cancer prevention tailored to their individualized risk profile [109].

Data from these devices can easily be integrated into the telemedicine platform so that dermatologists can monitor and evaluate patients and even guide them remotely. This allows continuity of care, particularly for patients at increased risk or treatment. In addition, AI and machine learning algorithms will also enable predictive models to use vast data sets from wearables, genomic profiles, and imaging, further refining risk prediction models and allowing personalized screening interval recommendations in high-risk patients, ultimately improving screening accuracy for skin cancer [110].

CHALLENGES AND LIMITATIONS

Despite their great potential for better skin cancer care, the high cost of many emerging technologies, particularly wearable diagnostic devices, advanced imaging tools, and nanotechnology-based diagnostics, is a major limiting factor for wide adoption. These technologies often have high costs related to specialized materials, distinct manufacturing processes, and ongoing development costs, which make them relatively expensive to bring to healthcare professionals and patients. Increasing the cost, the case is even worse in low-resource or rural regions with low access to these innovations. Not everyone has access to the advantages of early diagnosis and tailor-made treatment choices. Subsidizing costs or finding cheaper alternatives is necessary to guarantee that efficiency gains can be translated to more populations [111, 112].

Implementing new technologies into established clinical workflows can be logistically and operationally difficult. Healthcare providers must adjust to a world with tools like wearables, point-of-care testing devices, and more, running provider-frequented tests on patients, likely requiring training, protocols, and resources. It may take time for clinicians to be experienced in using these tools accurately, analyzing resulting data, and interpreting results in the context of conventional diagnostics. To best utilize these technologies in skin cancer care, it is important to develop standard guidelines and workflows for their implementation into routine practice [113, 114].

Wearable and digital diagnostic devices are more common today, but with this improvement in health data gathering, data privacy and security have become part of the conversation. They gather sensitive health information, including genetic data and biometric information, which, in the wrong hands, can inflict severe ethical challenges and privacy complications. Patients might fear that third parties, such as insurers, employers, and even hackers, will access or abuse their health data. Data protection measures must weigh these considerations seriously, and transparency about how and where data are used is paramount to sustaining public trust in technology-driven health care [115, 116].

Potentially useful methodologies for diagnostic discovery will magnify the consequences for skin cancer patients if subject to false positive or negative results. While false positives can cause undue stress, further diagnostics, and even invasive procedures, false negatives can postpone diagnosis and treatment and worsen patient outcomes. Inconsistency in device precision, especially in AI-driven devices, which are dependent on data quality and algorithms that train machine learning systems, may affect the trustworthiness of these technologies. Diagnostic algorithms must continue to be refined, validated, and improved to reduce errors so patients and clinicians can obtain reliable assessments [117, 118].

CONCLUSION

Emerging technologies, including portable diagnostic devices, point-of-care testing, and nanotechnology, have incredible potential to revolutionize skin cancer diagnostics, enabling earlier disease detection, continuous monitoring, and personalized treatment. Although facing issues such as cost, implementation into the clinical environment, ethical dilemmas, and problems with sensitivity and specificity, these advances represent important steps for the future of humanity and the quality of care patients receive. This always-on innovation will be critical because refining these technologies to overcome the limitations in accessibility and reliability in real-world applications is what will take precedence. Future skin cancer diagnostics will probably rely further on AI-driven models, mobile health platforms, and non-invasive biomarker assessment, providing healthcare professionals with tailored care. As research continues and technology advances through partnerships between technology providers, healthcare institutions, and public policymakers, these innovations will become increasingly accessible and user-friendly. This type of progression will enable a new standard of skin cancer care by making early intervention, remote monitoring, and personalized prevention plans available to everyone, thus greatly alleviating the skin cancer burden globally.

REFERENCES

[1] Losquadro WD. Anatomy of the skin and the pathogenesis of nonmelanoma skin cancer. Facial Plast Surg Clin North Am 2017; 25(3): 283-9.
[http://dx.doi.org/10.1016/j.fsc.2017.03.001] [PMID: 28676156]

[2] Urban K, Mehrmal S, Uppal P, Giesey RL, Delost GR. The global burden of skin cancer: A longitudinal analysis from the Global Burden of Disease Study, 1990–2017. JAAD Int 2021; 2: 98-108.
[http://dx.doi.org/10.1016/j.jdin.2020.10.013] [PMID: 34409358]

[3] Esteva A, Kuprel B, Novoa RA, *et al.* Dermatologist-level classification of skin cancer with deep neural networks. Nature 2017; 542(7639): 115-8.
[http://dx.doi.org/10.1038/nature21056] [PMID: 28117445]

[4] Davids LM, Kleemann B. The menace of melanoma: a photodynamic approach to adjunctive cancer therapy. In Melanoma-From Early Detection to Treatment. IntechOpen. 2013.
[http://dx.doi.org/10.5772/53676]

[5] Didona D, Paolino G, Bottoni U, Cantisani C. Non-melanoma skin cancer pathogenesis overview. Biomedicines 2018; 6(1): 6.
[http://dx.doi.org/10.3390/biomedicines6010006] [PMID: 29301290]

[6] Barton V, Armeson K, Hampras S, *et al.* Nonmelanoma skin cancer and risk of all-cause and cancer-related mortality: a systematic review. Arch Dermatol Res 2017; 309(4): 243-51.
[http://dx.doi.org/10.1007/s00403-017-1724-5] [PMID: 28285366]

[7] Apalla Z, Lallas A, Sotiriou E, Lazaridou E, Ioannides D. Epidemiological trends in skin cancer. Dermatol Pract Concept 2017; 7(2): 1-6.
[http://dx.doi.org/10.5826/dpc.0702a01] [PMID: 28515985]

[8] Khan NH, Mir M, Qian L, *et al.* Skin cancer biology and barriers to treatment: Recent polymeric micro/nanostructures applications. J Adv Res 2022; 36: 223-47.
[http://dx.doi.org/10.1016/j.jare.2021.06.014] [PMID: 35127174]

[9] Stătescu L, Cojocaru E, Trandafir LM, *et al.* Catching Cancer Early: The Importance of Dermato-Oncology Screening. Cancers (Basel) 2023; 15(12): 3066.
[http://dx.doi.org/10.3390/cancers15123066] [PMID: 37370677]

[10] Gaudy-Marqueste C, Wazaefi Y, Bruneu Y, *et al.* Ugly duckling sign as a major factor of efficiency in melanoma detection. JAMA Dermatol 2017; 153(4): 279-84.
[http://dx.doi.org/10.1001/jamadermatol.2016.5500] [PMID: 28196213]

[11] Hazen BP, Bhatia AC, Zaim T, Brodell RT. The clinical diagnosis of early malignant melanoma: expansion of the ABCD criteria to improve diagnostic sensitivity. Dermatol Online J 1999; 5(2): 3.
[http://dx.doi.org/10.5070/D366X188MB] [PMID: 10673456]

[12] Nazzaro G, Passoni E, Pozzessere F, Maronese CA, Marzano AV. Dermoscopy use leads to earlier cutaneous melanoma diagnosis in terms of invasiveness and size. A single-center, retrospective experience. J Clin Med 2022; 11(16): 4912.
[http://dx.doi.org/10.3390/jcm11164912] [PMID: 36013151]

[13] Vestergaard ME, Macaskill P, Holt PE, Menzies SW. Dermoscopy compared with naked eye examination for the diagnosis of primary melanoma: a meta-analysis of studies performed in a clinical setting. Br J Dermatol 2008; 159(3): 669-76.
[http://dx.doi.org/10.1111/j.1365-2133.2008.08713.x] [PMID: 18616769]

[14] Mahmoud NM, Soliman AM. Early automated detection system for skin cancer diagnosis using artificial intelligent techniques. Sci Rep 2024; 14(1): 9749.
[http://dx.doi.org/10.1038/s41598-024-59783-0] [PMID: 38679633]

[15] Heibel HD, Hooey L, Cockerell CJ. A review of noninvasive techniques for skin cancer detection in dermatology. Am J Clin Dermatol 2020; 21(4): 513-24.
[http://dx.doi.org/10.1007/s40257-020-00517-z] [PMID: 32383142]

[16] Greenwood JD, Merry SP, Boswell CL. Skin biopsy techniques. Prim Care 2022; 49(1): 1-22.
[http://dx.doi.org/10.1016/j.pop.2021.10.001] [PMID: 35125151]

[17] Jiyad Z, Plasmeijer EI, Keegan S, Samarasinghe V, Green AC, Akhras V. Defining the validity of skin self-examination as a screening test for detecting suspicious pigmented lesions: a meta-analysis of diagnostic test accuracy. Dermatology 2022; 238(4): 640-8.
[http://dx.doi.org/10.1159/000520592] [PMID: 34979506]

[18] Ferrante di Ruffano L, Takwoingi Y, Dinnes J, *et al.* Computer-assisted diagnosis techniques (dermoscopy and spectroscopy-based) for diagnosing skin cancer in adults. Cochrane Libr 2018; 2018(12).
[http://dx.doi.org/10.1002/14651858.CD013186]

[19] Adelson P, Eckert M. Skin cancer in regional, rural and remote Australia; opportunities for service improvement through technological advances and interdisciplinary care. Aust J Adv Nurs 2020; 37(2): 25-30.
[http://dx.doi.org/10.37464/2020.372.74]

[20] Wei ML, Tada M, So A, Torres R. Artificial intelligence and skin cancer. Front Med (Lausanne) 2024; 11: 1331895.
[http://dx.doi.org/10.3389/fmed.2024.1331895] [PMID: 38566925]

[21] Narayanamurthy V, Padmapriya P, Noorasafrin A, *et al.* Skin cancer detection using non-invasive techniques. RSC Advances 2018; 8(49): 28095-130.
[http://dx.doi.org/10.1039/C8RA04164D] [PMID: 35542700]

[22] Sarker IH. Deep learning: a comprehensive overview of techniques, taxonomy, applications, and research directions. SN Comput Sci 2021; 2(6): 420.
[http://dx.doi.org/10.1007/s42979-021-00815-1] [PMID: 34426802]

[23] Ibrahim R, Al-Haija QA. Fundamentals of machine learning models. Adv AI Simul Optim Energy Syst. CRC Press. ; pp. 1-17.
[http://dx.doi.org/10.1201/9781003520498-1]

[24] Bilal U. Understanding neural networks: A comprehensive overview of AI techniques. Frontiers in Artificial Intelligence Research 2024; 1(02): 172-208.

[25] Chowdhary K, Chowdhary KR. Natural language processing. Fundam Artif Intell 2020; 603-49.
[http://dx.doi.org/10.1007/978-81-322-3972-7_19]

[26] Veeramachaneni V. Large Language Models: A comprehensive survey on architectures, applications, and challenges. Advanced Innovations in Computer Programming Languages 2025; 7(1): 20-39.

[27] Manakitsa N, Maraslidis GS, Moysis L, Fragulis GF. A review of machine learning and deep learning for object detection, semantic segmentation, and human action recognition in machine and robotic vision. Technologies (Basel) 2024; 12(2): 15.
[http://dx.doi.org/10.3390/technologies12020015]

[28] Sarvamangala DR, Kulkarni RV. Convolutional neural networks in medical image understanding: a survey. Evol Intell 2022; 15(1): 1-22.
[http://dx.doi.org/10.1007/s12065-020-00540-3] [PMID: 33425040]

[29] Neupane S, Mitra S, Fernandez IA, *et al.* Security Considerations in AI-Robotics: A Survey of Current Methods, Challenges, and Opportunities. IEEE Access 2024; 12: 22072-97.

[http://dx.doi.org/10.1109/ACCESS.2024.3363657]

[30] Duan Y, Edwards JS, Dwivedi YK. Artificial intelligence for decision making in the era of Big Data – evolution, challenges and research agenda. Int J Inf Manage 2019; 48: 63-71. [http://dx.doi.org/10.1016/j.ijinfomgt.2019.01.021]

[31] Nagarajan R, Kondo M, Salas F, *et al.* Economics and equity of large language models: health care perspective. J Med Internet Res 2024; 26: 64226. [http://dx.doi.org/10.2196/64226] [PMID: 39541580]

[32] Alowais SA, Alghamdi SS, Alsuhebany N, *et al.* Revolutionizing healthcare: the role of artificial intelligence in clinical practice. BMC Med Educ 2023; 23(1): 689. [http://dx.doi.org/10.1186/s12909-023-04698-z] [PMID: 37740191]

[33] Bozsányi S, Boostani M, Farkas K, *et al.* Optically guided high-frequency ultrasound to differentiate high-risk basal cell carcinoma subtypes: A single-centre prospective study. J Clin Med 2023; 12(21): 6910. [http://dx.doi.org/10.3390/jcm12216910] [PMID: 37959375]

[34] Jones OT, Jurascheck LC, Van Melle MA, Hickman S, Burrows NP, Hall PN, Emery J, Walter FM. Dermoscopy for melanoma detection and triage in primary care: a systematic review. BMJ open. 2019 Aug 1;9(8):e027529.

[35] Álvarez-Salafranca M, Ara M, Zaballos P. Dermoscopy in basal cell carcinoma: an updated review. Actas Dermosifiliogr 2021; 112(4): 330-8. [http://dx.doi.org/10.1016/j.adengl.2021.01.023] [PMID: 33259816]

[36] Zalaudek I, Kreusch J, Giacomel J, Ferrara G, Catricalà C, Argenziano G. How to diagnose nonpigmented skin tumors: A review of vascular structures seen with dermoscopy. J Am Acad Dermatol 2010; 63(3): 361-74. [http://dx.doi.org/10.1016/j.jaad.2009.11.698] [PMID: 20708469]

[37] Ilie MA, Caruntu C, Lixandru D, *et al. in vivo* confocal laser scanning microscopy imaging of skin inflammation: Clinical applications and research directions. Exp Ther Med 2019; 17(2): 1004-11. [PMID: 30679966]

[38] Guida S, Arginelli F, Farnetani F, *et al.* Clinical applications of *in vivo* and *ex vivo* confocal microscopy. Appl Sci (Basel) 2021; 11(5): 1979. [http://dx.doi.org/10.3390/app11051979]

[39] Niculet E, Craescu M, Rebegea L, *et al.* Basal cell carcinoma: Comprehensive clinical and histopathological aspects, novel imaging tools and therapeutic approaches (Review). Exp Ther Med 2021; 23(1): 60. [http://dx.doi.org/10.3892/etm.2021.10982] [PMID: 34917186]

[40] Holmes J, von Braunmühl T, Berking C, *et al.* Optical coherence tomography of basal cell carcinoma: influence of location, subtype, observer variability and image quality on diagnostic performance. Br J Dermatol 2018; 178(5): 1102-10. [http://dx.doi.org/10.1111/bjd.16154] [PMID: 29193003]

[41] Suppa M, Fontaine M, Dejonckheere G, *et al.* Line-field confocal optical coherence tomography of basal cell carcinoma: a descriptive study. J Eur Acad Dermatol Venereol 2021; 35(5): 1099-110. [http://dx.doi.org/10.1111/jdv.17078] [PMID: 33398911]

[42] Latriglia F, Ogien J, Tavernier C, *et al.* Line-field confocal optical coherence tomography (LC-OCT) for skin imaging in dermatology. Life (Basel) 2023; 13(12): 2268. [http://dx.doi.org/10.3390/life13122268] [PMID: 38137869]

[43] Khan R, Ahmed A, Khachemoune A. Ultrasound features of high-risk basal cell carcinoma: A systematic review. Archives of Dermatological Research. 2024;316(6):210.

[44] Halip IA, Vâţă D, Statescu L, *et al.* Assessment of basal cell carcinoma using dermoscopy and high-frequency ultrasound examination. Diagnostics (Basel) 2022; 12(3): 735.

[http://dx.doi.org/10.3390/diagnostics12030735] [PMID: 35328289]

[45] Kim DP, Kus KJ, Ruiz E. Basal cell carcinoma review. Hematol Oncol Clin 2019; 33(1): 13-24. [http://dx.doi.org/10.1016/j.hoc.2018.09.004]

[46] Xu H, Guo L, Wang Q, Eds. Diagnostic ultrasound in dermatology. Berlin/Heidelberg, Germany: Springer 2022. [http://dx.doi.org/10.1007/978-981-16-7345-0]

[47] Zhang LW, Shen X, Fu LX, *et al.* Dermoscopy, reflectance confocal microscopy, and high-frequency ultrasound for noninvasive morphea-form basal cell carcinoma diagnosis. Skin Res Technol 2022; 28(5): 766. [http://dx.doi.org/10.1111/srt.13197] [PMID: 35871487]

[48] Nataren N, Yamada M, Prow T. Molecular skin cancer diagnosis: Promise and limitations. J Mol Diagn 2023; 25(1): 17-35. [http://dx.doi.org/10.1016/j.jmoldx.2022.09.008] [PMID: 36243291]

[49] Gerami P, Yao Z, Polsky D, *et al.* Development and validation of a noninvasive 2-gene molecular assay for cutaneous melanoma. J Am Acad Dermatol 2017; 76(1): 114-120.e2. [http://dx.doi.org/10.1016/j.jaad.2016.07.038] [PMID: 27707590]

[50] Brunner G, Heinecke A, Falk TM, *et al.* A prognostic gene signature expressed in primary cutaneous melanoma: synergism with conventional staging. JNCI Cancer Spectr 2018; 2(3): pky032. [http://dx.doi.org/10.1093/jncics/pky032] [PMID: 31360859]

[51] Kangas-Dick AW, Greenbaum A, Gall V, *et al.* Evaluation of a gene expression profiling assay in primary cutaneous melanoma. Ann Surg Oncol 2021; 28(8): 4582-9. [http://dx.doi.org/10.1245/s10434-020-09563-7] [PMID: 33486642]

[52] Gutiérrez-Castañeda LD, Gamboa M, Nova JA, Pulido L, Tovar-Parra JD. Mutations in the BRAF, NRAS, and C-KIT genes of patients diagnosed with melanoma in Colombia population. BioMed Res Int 2020; 2020(1): 2046947. [http://dx.doi.org/10.1155/2020/2046947] [PMID: 32775409]

[53] Lee JH, Choi JW, Kim YS. Frequencies of BRAF and NRAS mutations are different in histological types and sites of origin of cutaneous melanoma: a meta-analysis. Br J Dermatol 2011; 164(4): 776-84. [http://dx.doi.org/10.1111/j.1365-2133.2010.10185.x] [PMID: 21166657]

[54] Johnson DB, Dahlman KB. Class matters: sensitivity of BRAF-mutant melanoma to MAPK inhibition. Clin Cancer Res 2018; 24(24): 6107-9. [http://dx.doi.org/10.1158/1078-0432.CCR-18-1795] [PMID: 30042206]

[55] Dietel M, Jöhrens K, Laffert MV, *et al.* A 2015 update on predictive molecular pathology and its role in targeted cancer therapy: a review focussing on clinical relevance. Cancer Gene Ther 2015; 22(9): 417-30. [http://dx.doi.org/10.1038/cgt.2015.39] [PMID: 26358176]

[56] Akbani R, Akdemir KC, Aksoy BA, *et al.* Genomic classification of cutaneous melanoma. Cell 2015; 161(7): 1681-96. [http://dx.doi.org/10.1016/j.cell.2015.05.044] [PMID: 26091043]

[57] Veeramani N, Jayaraman P, Krishankumar R, Ravichandran KS, Gandomi AH. DDCNN-F: double decker convolutional neural network 'F' feature fusion as a medical image classification framework. Sci Rep 2024; 14(1): 676. [http://dx.doi.org/10.1038/s41598-023-49721-x] [PMID: 38182607]

[58] Reddy S, Shaheed A, Patel R. Artificial intelligence in dermoscopy: enhancing diagnosis to distinguish benign and malignant skin lesions. Cureus 2024; 16(2): 54656. [http://dx.doi.org/10.7759/cureus.54656] [PMID: 38523958]

[59] Adegun A, Viriri S. Deep learning techniques for skin lesion analysis and melanoma cancer detection: a survey of state-of-the-art. Artif Intell Rev 2021; 54(2): 811-41.

[http://dx.doi.org/10.1007/s10462-020-09865-y]

[60] Hasan M, Barman SD, Islam S, Reza AW. Skin cancer detection using convolutional neural network. Proceedings of the. 254-8.
[http://dx.doi.org/10.1145/3330482.3330525]

[61] Fitzgerald RC, Antoniou AC, Fruk L, Rosenfeld N. The future of early cancer detection. Nat Med 2022; 28(4): 666-77.
[http://dx.doi.org/10.1038/s41591-022-01746-x] [PMID: 35440720]

[62] Kumar P, Chauhan R, Shankar A, Stephan T. Role of artificial intelligence for skin cancer detection. Evol Role AI IoMT Healthc Mark 2021; 141-74.
[http://dx.doi.org/10.1007/978-3-030-82079-4_7]

[63] Jin JQ, Hong J, Elhage KG, *et al.* Development of SkinTracker, an integrated dermatology mobile app and web portal enabling remote clinical research studies. Front Digit Health 2023; 5: 1228503.
[http://dx.doi.org/10.3389/fdgth.2023.1228503] [PMID: 37744686]

[64] Kang HS, Exworthy M. Wearing the future—wearables to empower users to take greater responsibility for their health and care: a scoping review. JMIR Mhealth Uhealth 2022; 10(7): 35684.
[http://dx.doi.org/10.2196/35684] [PMID: 35830222]

[65] Foltz EA, Ludzik J, Leachman S, *et al.* Revolutionizing Skin Cancer Triage: The Role of Patient-Initiated Teledermoscopy in Remote Diagnosis. Cancers (Basel) 2024; 16(14): 2565.
[http://dx.doi.org/10.3390/cancers16142565] [PMID: 39061204]

[66] Dobry A, Almanza J, Stavert R. Teledermatology: platforms. Teledermatol Compr Overv 2023; 1-8.
[http://dx.doi.org/10.1007/978-3-031-27276-9_1]

[67] Glenister K, Witherspoon S, Crouch A. A qualitative descriptive study of a novel nurse-led skin cancer screening model in rural Australia. BMC Health Serv Res 2022; 22(1): 1019.
[http://dx.doi.org/10.1186/s12913-022-08411-6] [PMID: 35948920]

[68] Manikandan A, Sanjay T, Menon G, *et al.* Issues and challenges in security and privacy with e-healthcare: a thorough literature analysis. Internet Things Enable Mach Learn Biomed Appl 2025; 222-47.

[69] Karalis VD. The integration of artificial intelligence into clinical practice. Applied Biosciences 2024; 3(1): 14-44.
[http://dx.doi.org/10.3390/applbiosci3010002]

[70] Allen TA. The role of circulating tumor cells as a liquid biopsy for cancer: Advances, biology, technical challenges, and clinical relevance. Cancers (Basel) 2024; 16(7): 1377.
[http://dx.doi.org/10.3390/cancers16071377] [PMID: 38611055]

[71] Dobre eg, Surcel M, Constantin C, *et al.* Skin cancer pathobiology at a glance: a focus on imaging techniques and their potential for improved diagnosis and surveillance in clinical cohorts. Int J Mol Sci 2023; 24(2): 1079.
[http://dx.doi.org/10.3390/ijms24021079] [PMID: 36674595]

[72] Zhao J, Zhao Y, Wu Z, Tian Y, Zeng H. Nonlinear optical microscopy for skin *in vivo* : Basics, development and applications. J Innov Opt Health Sci 2023; 16(1): 2230018.
[http://dx.doi.org/10.1142/S179354582230018X]

[73] Csuka EA, Ward SC, Ekelem C, Csuka DA, Ardigò M, Mesinkovska NA. Reflectance confocal microscopy, optical coherence tomography, and multiphoton microscopy in inflammatory skin disease diagnosis. Lasers Surg Med 2021; 53(6): 776-97.
[http://dx.doi.org/10.1002/lsm.23386] [PMID: 33527483]

[74] Myslicka M, Kawala-Sterniuk A, Bryniarska A, *et al.* Review of the application of the most current sophisticated image processing methods for the skin cancer diagnostics purposes. Arch Dermatol Res 2024; 316(4): 99.
[http://dx.doi.org/10.1007/s00403-024-02828-1] [PMID: 38446274]

[75] Zhang S, Qi Y, Tan SPH, Bi R, Olivo M. Molecular fingerprint detection using Raman and infrared spectroscopy technologies for cancer detection: a progress review. Biosensors (Basel) 2023; 13(5): 557.
[http://dx.doi.org/10.3390/bios13050557] [PMID: 37232918]

[76] Gaba F, Tipping WJ, Salji M, Faulds K, Graham D, Leung HY. Raman spectroscopy in prostate cancer: techniques, applications, and advancements. Cancers (Basel) 2022; 14(6): 1535.
[http://dx.doi.org/10.3390/cancers14061535] [PMID: 35326686]

[77] El-Shafai W, El-Fattah IA, Taha TE. Advancements in non-invasive optical imaging techniques for precise diagnosis of skin disorders. Opt Quantum Electron 2024; 56(7): 1112.
[http://dx.doi.org/10.1007/s11082-024-06823-8]

[78] Das S, Dey MK, Devireddy R, Gartia MR. Biomarkers in cancer detection, diagnosis, and prognosis. Sensors (Basel) 2023; 24(1): 37.
[http://dx.doi.org/10.3390/s24010037] [PMID: 38202898]

[79] Desai AD, Chinta S, Yeh C, *et al.* An analysis of lactate dehydrogenase (LDH) levels in advanced stage IV melanoma of the skin: prognostic capabilities and demographic variability. Arch Dermatol Res 2022; 315(4): 799-806.
[http://dx.doi.org/10.1007/s00403-022-02425-0] [PMID: 36318305]

[80] Chatzilakou E, Hu Y, Jiang N, Yetisen AK. Biosensors for melanoma skin cancer diagnostics. Biosens Bioelectron 2024; 250: 116045.
[http://dx.doi.org/10.1016/j.bios.2024.116045] [PMID: 38301546]

[81] Castellani G, Buccarelli M, Arasi MB, *et al.* BRAF mutations in melanoma: biological aspects, therapeutic implications, and circulating biomarkers. Cancers (Basel) 2023; 15(16): 4026.
[http://dx.doi.org/10.3390/cancers15164026] [PMID: 37627054]

[82] Grothey A, Fakih M, Tabernero J. Management of BRAF-mutant metastatic colorectal cancer: a review of treatment options and evidence-based guidelines. Ann Oncol 2021; 32(8): 959-67.
[http://dx.doi.org/10.1016/j.annonc.2021.03.206] [PMID: 33836264]

[83] Koulis C, Yap R, Engel R, *et al.* Personalized medicine—current and emerging predictive and prognostic biomarkers in colorectal cancer. Cancers (Basel) 2020; 12(4): 812.
[http://dx.doi.org/10.3390/cancers12040812] [PMID: 32231042]

[84] Paver EC, Cooper WA, Colebatch AJ, *et al.* Programmed death ligand-1 (PD-L1) as a predictive marker for immunotherapy in solid tumours: a guide to immunohistochemistry implementation and interpretation. Pathology 2021; 53(2): 141-56.
[http://dx.doi.org/10.1016/j.pathol.2020.10.007] [PMID: 33388161]

[85] Prasanth BK, Alkhowaiter S, Sawarkar G, Dharshini BD, R Baskaran A. Unlocking Early Cancer Detection: Exploring Biomarkers, Circulating DNA, and Innovative Technological Approaches. Cureus 2023; 15(12): 51090.
[http://dx.doi.org/10.7759/cureus.51090] [PMID: 38274938]

[86] Durante G, Broseghini E, Comito F, *et al.* Circulating microRNA biomarkers in melanoma and non-melanoma skin cancer. Expert Rev Mol Diagn 2022; 22(3): 305-18.
[http://dx.doi.org/10.1080/14737159.2022.2049243] [PMID: 35235479]

[87] Maibach F, Sadozai H, Seyed Jafari SM, Hunger RE, Schenk M. Tumor-infiltrating lymphocytes and their prognostic value in cutaneous melanoma. Front Immunol 2020; 11: 2105.
[http://dx.doi.org/10.3389/fimmu.2020.02105] [PMID: 33013886]

[88] Tsamis I, Gomatou G, Chachali SP, *et al.* BRAF/MEK inhibition in NSCLC: mechanisms of resistance and how to overcome it. Clin Transl Oncol 2022; 25(1): 10-20.
[http://dx.doi.org/10.1007/s12094-022-02849-0] [PMID: 35729451]

[89] Passaro A, Al Bakir M, Hamilton eg, *et al.* Cancer biomarkers: Emerging trends and clinical implications for personalized treatment. Cell 2024; 187(7): 1617-35.

[http://dx.doi.org/10.1016/j.cell.2024.02.041] [PMID: 38552610]

[90] Hartmane I. Study of genetic mutations and their association with the development of atopic dermatitis and other skin diseases. Plast Aesthet Nurs (Phila) 2024; 44(3): 200-9. [http://dx.doi.org/10.1097/PSN.0000000000000564] [PMID: 39028474]

[91] Wunderlich K, Suppa M, Gandini S, Lipski J, White JM, Del Marmol V. Risk factors and innovations in risk assessment for melanoma, basal cell carcinoma, and squamous cell carcinoma. Cancers (Basel) 2024; 16(5): 1016. [http://dx.doi.org/10.3390/cancers16051016] [PMID: 38473375]

[92] Chakravarty D, Solit DB. Clinical cancer genomic profiling. Nat Rev Genet 2021; 22(8): 483-501. [http://dx.doi.org/10.1038/s41576-021-00338-8] [PMID: 33762738]

[93] Rotunno M, Barajas R, Clyne M, *et al.* A systematic literature review of whole exome and genome sequencing population studies of genetic susceptibility to cancer. Cancer Epidemiol Biomarkers Prev 2020; 29(8): 1519-34. [http://dx.doi.org/10.1158/1055-9965.EPI-19-1551] [PMID: 32467344]

[94] Kim HJ, Kim YH. Molecular frontiers in melanoma: Pathogenesis, diagnosis, and therapeutic advances. Int J Mol Sci 2024; 25(5): 2984. [http://dx.doi.org/10.3390/ijms25052984] [PMID: 38474231]

[95] Wang JY, Sarin KY. Dermatology advances into an era of precision medicine. JAMA Dermatol 2021; 157(7): 770-2. [http://dx.doi.org/10.1001/jamadermatol.2021.0024] [PMID: 34076667]

[96] Puglisi R, Bellenghi M, Pontecorvi G, Pallante G, Carè A, Mattia G. Biomarkers for diagnosis, prognosis, and response to immunotherapy in melanoma. Cancers (Basel) 2021; 13(12): 2875. [http://dx.doi.org/10.3390/cancers13122875] [PMID: 34207514]

[97] Beg S, Handa M, Shukla R, *et al.* Wearable smart devices in cancer diagnosis and remote clinical trial monitoring: Transforming the healthcare applications. Drug Discov Today 2022; 27(10): 103314. [http://dx.doi.org/10.1016/j.drudis.2022.06.014] [PMID: 35798227]

[98] Brault N, Duchemann B, Saxena M. Epistemological issues and challenges with artificial intelligence in healthcare. Big Data Artif Intell Healthc Appl 2021; 235-70. [http://dx.doi.org/10.1201/9781003093770-14]

[99] Muzny M, Henriksen A, Giordanengo A, *et al.* Wearable sensors with possibilities for data exchange: Analyzing status and needs of different actors in mobile health monitoring systems. Int J Med Inform 2020; 133: 104017. [http://dx.doi.org/10.1016/j.ijmedinf.2019.104017] [PMID: 31778885]

[100] Harpaldas H, Arumugam S, Campillo Rodriguez C, Kumar BA, Shi V, Sia SK. Point-of-care diagnostics: recent developments in a pandemic age. Lab Chip 2021; 21(23): 4517-48. [http://dx.doi.org/10.1039/D1LC00627D] [PMID: 34778896]

[101] Mollarasouli F, Bahrani S. Low-molecular-weight biomarkers: types and detection strategies. Detect Biomarkers 2022; 23-69.

[102] Ahmad A, Imran M, Ahsan H. Biomarkers as biomedical bioindicators: approaches and techniques for the detection, analysis, and validation of novel Biomarkers of diseases. Pharmaceutics 2023; 15(6): 1630. [http://dx.doi.org/10.3390/pharmaceutics15061630] [PMID: 37376078]

[103] Luo D, Wang X, Burda C, Basilion JP. Recent development of gold nanoparticles as contrast agents for cancer diagnosis. Cancers (Basel) 2021; 13(8): 1825. [http://dx.doi.org/10.3390/cancers13081825] [PMID: 33920453]

[104] Mohammadi R, Naderi-Manesh H, Farzin L, *et al.* Fluorescence sensing and imaging with carbon-based quantum dots for early diagnosis of cancer: A review. J Pharm Biomed Anal 2022; 212: 114628. [http://dx.doi.org/10.1016/j.jpba.2022.114628] [PMID: 35151068]

[105] Fu L, Lin CT, Karimi-Maleh H, Chen F, Zhao S. Plasmonic Nanoparticle-Enhanced Optical Techniques for Cancer Biomarker Sensing. Biosensors (Basel) 2023; 13(11): 977. [http://dx.doi.org/10.3390/bios13110977] [PMID: 37998152]

[106] Shevtsov M, Kaesler S, Posch C, Multhoff G, Biedermann T. Magnetic nanoparticles in theranostics of malignant melanoma. EJNMMI Res 2021; 11(1): 127. [http://dx.doi.org/10.1186/s13550-021-00868-6] [PMID: 34905138]

[107] Domiński A, Konieczny T, Duale K, Krawczyk M, Pastuch-Gawołek G, Kurcok P. Stimuli-responsive aliphatic polycarbonate nanocarriers for tumour-targeted drug delivery. Polymers (Basel) 2020; 12(12): 2890. [http://dx.doi.org/10.3390/polym12122890] [PMID: 33276597]

[108] Sengupta J, Hussain CM. CNT and graphene-based transistor biosensors for cancer detection: a review. Biomolecules 2023; 13(7): 1024. [http://dx.doi.org/10.3390/biom13071024] [PMID: 37509060]

[109] Shrivastava S, Trung TQ, Lee NE. Recent progress, challenges, and prospects of fully integrated mobile and wearable point-of-care testing systems for self-testing. Chem Soc Rev 2020; 49(6): 1812-66. [http://dx.doi.org/10.1039/C9CS00319C] [PMID: 32100760]

[110] Rasool S, Husnain A, Saeed A, Gill AY, Hussain HK. Harnessing predictive power: exploring the crucial role of machine learning in early disease detection. Jurihum J Inov Hum 2023; 1(2): 302-15.

[111] Sharma PK. Innovative biomedical equipment for diagnosis of cancer. Target Cancer Ther Biomed Eng. Singapore: Springer Nature Singapore. 2023; pp. 405-36.

[112] Haleem A, Javaid M, Pratap Singh R, Suman R. Medical 4.0 technologies for healthcare: Features, capabilities, and applications. Internet of Things and Cyber-Physical Systems 2022; 2: 12-30. [http://dx.doi.org/10.1016/j.iotcps.2022.04.001]

[113] Rasheed S, Kanwal T, Ahmad N, Fatima B, Najam-ul-Haq M, Hussain D. Advances and challenges in portable optical biosensors for onsite detection and point-of-care diagnostics. Trends Analyt Chem 2024; 173: 117640. [http://dx.doi.org/10.1016/j.trac.2024.117640]

[114] Zeb S, Fnu N, Abbasi N, Fahad M. AI in Healthcare: Revolutionizing Diagnosis and Therapy. International Journal of Multidisciplinary Sciences and Arts 2024; 3(3): 118-28. [http://dx.doi.org/10.47709/ijmdsa.v3i3.4546]

[115] Sivakumar CLV, Mone V, Abdumukhtor R. Addressing privacy concerns with wearable health monitoring technology. Wiley Interdiscip Rev Data Min Knowl Discov 2024; 14(3): 1535. [http://dx.doi.org/10.1002/widm.1535]

[116] Layode O, Naiho HN, Adeleke GS, Udeh EO, Labake TT. Data privacy and security challenges in environmental research: Approaches to safeguarding sensitive information. International Journal of Applied Research in Social Sciences 2024; 6(6): 1193-214. [http://dx.doi.org/10.51594/ijarss.v6i6.1210]

[117] Zhang J, Zhong F, He K, Ji M, Li S, Li C. Recent advancements and perspectives in the diagnosis of skin diseases using machine learning and deep learning: A review. Diagnostics (Basel) 2023; 13(23): 3506. [http://dx.doi.org/10.3390/diagnostics13233506] [PMID: 38066747]

[118] Avula R, Tummala S. Assessing the impact of data quality on predictive analytics in healthcare: Strategies, tools, and techniques for ensuring accuracy, completeness, and timeliness in electronic health records. Sage Science Review of Applied Machine Learning 2021; 4(2): 31-47.

CHAPTER 2

Transformation of Skin Cancer Diagnosis with the Utilization of IoT

R. Seetharaman[1], **Sonali D. Pawar**[2], **Raghav Dixit**[3], **Zeba Siddiqui**[4], **Gourishankar Birtia**[5] and **Shaweta Sharma**[6,*]

[1] *SRM College of Pharmacy, SRM Institute of Science and Technology, Tamil Nadu - 603203, India*

[2] *MGV's Pharmacy College, Panchavati, Nashik, India*

[3] *ICFAI School of Pharmaceutical Sciences, ICFAI University, Dehradun, Uttarakhand-248011, India*

[4] *Amity Institute of Pharmacy, Amity University, Madhya Pradesh-474005, India*

[5] *Dr C.V. Raman Institute of Pharmacy, Dr C.V. Raman University, Chattisgarh, India*

[6] *School of Medical and Allied Sciences, Galgotias University, Uttar Pradesh-201310, India*

Abstract: Skin cancer is a serious health threat that affects almost 125,000 new people diagnosed with melanoma each year. Among the various types of cancer, skin cancer is one of the most vicious ones. Skin cancer is known for the fact that it often spreads (moves to other parts of the body over time), and thus, it is harder to treat when diagnosed later; therefore, early detection is paramount. Dermatoscopy, clinical assessment, and other visual techniques were some of the primary methods used to identify skin lesions. The study says that the performance of first-time and inexperienced physicians could lead to bias in skin lesion diagnosis. Skin cancer can be life-threatening, but the sooner it is detected, the lesser its chance of killing people. Much research has shown that IoT does better than the best professional in various vision-based tasks. This chapter explores the technologies of IoT, for example, wearable devices, smartwatches, and fitness trackers with UV sensors, skin patches with sensors for monitoring changes, mobile applications for tracking moles and skin changes, smart dermatoscopy, and cloud computing approaches for the diagnosis of skin cancer. The chapter concludes by discussing the role of IoT role in the enhancement of skin cancer diagnosis and also assists in controlling the general health of the skin. Besides the advancement of IoT, challenges such as system integration and patient data privacy have remained critical.

Keywords: Dermatoscopy, Diagnosis, IoT, Skin cancer, Smartwatches.

* **Corresponding author Shaweta Sharma:** School of Medical and Allied Sciences, Galgotias University, Uttar Pradesh-201310, India; E-mail: shawetasharma@galgotiasuniversity.edu.in

Akhil Sharma, Shaweta Sharma, Shivkanya Fuloria & Sudhir Kumar (Eds.)

INTRODUCTION

Skin cancer is one of the most common cancers in the world and the U.S. and its incidence has increased. It is estimated that one in five Americans will develop skin cancer in their lifetime, so by the time they reach 70 years old [1]. Non-melanomatous skin cancer (NMSC) is the most common form, such as squamous cell carcinoma (SCC) and basal cell carcinoma (BCC). Melanoma is among the types of skin cancer with a higher mortality rate, while Merkel cell carcinoma (MCC) is less common [2]. Neoplastic transformation of skin cells occurs when DNA is damaged by UV radiation from the sun or artificial sources like tanning beds and sunlamps. Besides damaging DNA, ultraviolet radiation (UVR) creates an inflammatory and immunosuppressive environment that promotes the progression of premalignant cells into tumors [3]. Fig. (**1**) depicts the stages of skin cancer progression.

Skin Cancer

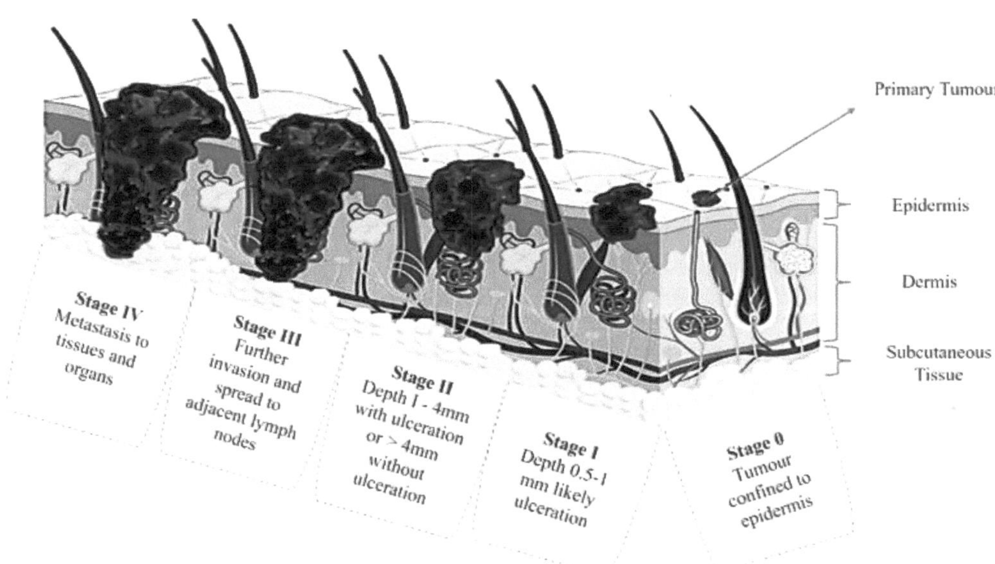

Fig. (1). Stages of skin cancer progression.

Basal cell carcinoma (BCC) is the most common form of skin cancer, with about 3.6 million occurring in the United States each year. The basal cell layer of the skin becomes abnormal and grows uncontrollably in this most superficial layer of skin. Most of the time, BCCs develop on the skin in sun-exposed areas like the face, neck, ears, scalp, shoulders, and back. Apart from UV exposure, other risk factors for BCC are male gender, fair skin, age, and outdoor workplace.

Aberrations of hedgehog pathway genes are responsible for most BCCs. BCCs rarely spread and grow very slowly; they cause minimal harm if they are quickly identified and treated. Some lesions can, however, cause severe morbidity [4] if they are not treated.

Squamous cell carcinoma (SCC) is the second most common type of skin cancer, with approximately 1.8 million cases diagnosed each year in the United States. SCC, or Squamous cell carcinoma, is a cancer of the epidermis characterized by uncontrolled and aberrant growth of squamous cells. Unsurprisingly, SCC is also noticed on sun-exposed skin of the body [5]. Other SCC risk factors are similar to those for BCCs and include a compromised immune system, sun-sensitive diseases such as Xeroderma pigmentosum, skin precancers such as actinic keratosis (AK), and a history of human papillomavirus infections. In particular, they explain that people who have undergone organ transplants and are subjected to long-term immunosuppressive drug therapy are more likely to develop skin cancer: the risk of developing basal cell carcinoma (BCC) is ten times higher, but squamous cell carcinoma (SCC) is increased 65–250 times higher. Compared to BCC, SCC can metastasize more readily and at a faster rate if not recognized early and treated [6].

Malignant melanoma is skin cancer originating from pigment-containing cells called melanocytes. Melanoma is a skin cancer that can be deadly [7]. Over the past several decades, more people in the United States have developed melanoma than any other cancer. Unlike other types of skin cancer, melanoma may spread to an already existing mole or develop in an area of the skin that has not been exposed to sunlight [8]. Melanoma risk factors include atypical moles, pale skin, exposure to ultraviolet (UV) radiation, a weakened immune system, and a history of skin cancer and melanoma in the family [9].

Merkel cell carcinoma (MCC) is a rare type of skin cancer with high aggressiveness characterized by neuroendocrine differentiation [10]. MCC has potential risk factors, including older age, light skin, history of a variety of skin cancers, history of prolonged ultraviolet exposure, and long-term immunosuppression (related to solid organ donation or HIV). About 80% of MCC (Merkel Cell Carcinoma) cases can be attributed to Merkel Cell Polyomavirus infection, while the remaining 20% are caused by skin damage mediated by UV radiation [11].

Besides immunosuppressants, more concerns were raised in recent years regarding the risk of skin cancer associated with some other commonly prescribed medications such as angiotensin-receptor blockers (ARBs), phosphodiesterase type 5 inhibitors, 3-hydroxy-3-methylglutaryl coenzyme A (HMG-CoA)–

reductase inhibitors, and tumor necrosis factor-alpha (TNF-α) antagonists. Such drugs have effects on UV light and may come with photosensitivity reactions in susceptible individuals [12].

Skin cancers, in contrast to many other tumors, are usually seen on the top of the skin and can easily be detected by self-examination of the skin and by dermatologists [13]. Although many NMSCs are curable by surgical excision, the high prevalence of these disorders poses a significant burden on healthcare systems [14]. Along with earlier detection, we must control the established skin cancer risk factors, particularly through UV protective measures like using sunscreen and avoiding solar exposure. However, limited data exists to measure whether the use of sunscreens reduces the risk of skin cancer, and UV-protective practices are also highly variable [15].

Internet of Things

The Internet of Things (IoT) is an expansive and rapidly evolving network of interconnected devices embedded with sensors, software, and network connectivity, enabling seamless data collection and exchange. This interconnectivity has transformed numerous industries, from smart homes and wearable technology to industrial automation and smart cities, enhancing efficiency, automation, and real-time decision-making. At the core of IoT are sensors, which detect and measure physical parameters such as temperature, motion, and pressure, converting them into electrical signals for processing [16, 17].

IoT devices rely on diverse connectivity protocols, including Wi-Fi, Bluetooth, Zigbee, cellular networks, and LPWANs (Low Power Wide Area Networks), ensuring seamless communication across devices. Data processing occurs either locally using edge computing, which minimizes latency and bandwidth usage, or in the cloud, which provides scalable storage, processing, and analytics. Machine learning and AI play a crucial role in IoT by analyzing vast datasets, identifying patterns, and enabling predictive automation. However, with this connectivity comes the need for robust security measures to protect sensitive data and prevent vulnerabilities [18, 19].

Despite its advantages, IoT faces several technical challenges, including scalability issues in managing billions of devices, interoperability difficulties due to varying communication standards, and security concerns arising from resource-constrained devices lacking strong protective features. Data management remains a significant challenge, requiring efficient techniques for storage, processing, and real-time analytics, while privacy issues demand stringent data protection measures [20].

Emerging technical trends are addressing these challenges, with edge computing reducing latency, AI and machine learning enhancing predictive capabilities, and 5G and LPWANs providing high-speed and low-power connectivity. Blockchain technology is being explored for its potential to secure decentralized IoT networks and ensure tamper-proof data management, while digital twins offer virtual simulations for system optimization [21].

IoT applications span multiple sectors, significantly enhancing daily life and industry operations. In smart homes, connected appliances, lighting, and security systems provide automation and energy efficiency. Wearable technology, such as smartwatches and fitness trackers, continuously monitor health metrics, improving personal wellness. Industrial IoT (IIoT) enables predictive maintenance, supply chain management, and operational efficiency in manufacturing [22].

Smart cities leverage IoT to optimize traffic flow, waste management, energy consumption, and public safety, creating sustainable urban environments. In healthcare, remote patient monitoring, connected medical devices, and smart hospital systems enhance patient care and medical efficiency. As IoT continues to evolve, fueled by advancements in connectivity and data analytics, its potential for innovation across industries remains immense, paving the way for a highly interconnected and intelligent world [23].

ROLE OF BIOMARKERS FOR DIAGNOSIS OF SKIN CANCER

The origin of cutaneous melanoma is the mutations in pigment-producing cells located at the base of the epidermis that lead to uncontrollable cell proliferation and, ultimately, malignant tumors [24]. This is the deadliest and most aggressive type of skin cancer, as it can infiltrate other organs if not treated immediately [25]. Histologically, cutaneous melanoma can be classified into four major subtypes: superficial spreading (70% of cases), nodular (5%), lentigo maligna (4 −15%), and acral lentiginous melanoma (2-5%) [26].

The most commonly used profile of melanoma staging is based on that created by the "American Joint Committee on Cancer (AJCC)," which covers five stages and is based primarily on tumors, nodes, and metastases [27]. A prognostic biomarker gives information about the expected prognosis if the patient has developed enumerated lesions in later stages (II-IV) after confirming the diagnosis. In contrast, diagnostic biomarkers are used from stages 0-II to confirm the disease and its type [28].

Predictive biomarkers are evaluated before treatment and provide generally relevant information that helps determine the genetic or histologic features of a tumor. The overall diagnosis is influenced by all the clinically significant factors, including thickness, ulceration, mitotic rate, serum levels of lactate dehydrogenase (LDH), tumor-infiltrating lymphocytes, vertical growth phase, and regression. Based on these factors, the aggressive behavior of tumors, their metastatic potential, and the effectiveness of immune response can be assessed [29].

Biosensors for Diagnostics

The second most common cause of malpractice and misdiagnosis claims after breast cancer is melanoma misdiagnosis; early misdiagnosis significantly lowers a patient's chance of survival. The insufficiency of the current methods to significantly lower the death rate from skin cancer and improve early, verified diagnosis emphasizes the significance of developing accurate, quantitative, early, and decisive skin cancer diagnostic techniques. To this end, the indicative tools that are currently on the market could be combined with biosensing technologies to locate trouble spots and detect biomarkers using appropriate novel receptors [30].

Such approaches have the potential to enable specific, sensitive, and low-cost point-of-care (POC) diagnostic modalities. In biosensors designed for skin cancer detection, the physical transduction element and a recognition element are located very closely to each other. Thus, biosensors compose an analytical tool for skin cancer diagnosis. These consist of three main concepts: (i) the detector, which detects the biological component associated with skin cancer or trigger (biorecognition); (ii) the transducer, which transforms the stimulus addressed to skin cancer into the signal (signalization); and (iii) the signal processing system that quantifies the output signal [31 - 34].

Skin Cancer Biomarkers

Biosensors can be used to diagnose skin cancer. However, access to fluids that are appropriate for biomarker detection is a required initial step. Other non-invasive or minimally invasive fluids such as saliva, sweat, blood, and urine are more accessible; they make it easy to extract samples because of their availability and provide important warnings/diagnostics [35]. Biomarkers detectable in serum have attracted further attention in the quest for optimal biomolecules to induce and propagate melanoma. Nonetheless, most indicators of skin melanoma have been localized to the extracellular fluid adjacent to melanocytes, in ISF, or intracellularly within melanocytes. The fraction of ISF volume is approximately 15–35%, 40%, and 20% in the epidermis, dermis, and subcutaneous tissue [36].

Almost all analytes in blood, such as circulatory proteins and species of RNA, are also present in ISF, with >90% of the protein being common between ISF and blood. Furthermore, approximately 83% of serum proteins are found in skin ISF. Still, approximately 50% of ISF proteins are not present in serum, which demonstrates that ISF is a potential resource for the discovery of both common and unique biomarkers. ISF can be obtained with minimal invasiveness and does not require any prior treatment in order for blood to be free of contamination for biological marker measurement [37, 38].

For skin cancer, three types of biomarkers are defined: prognosis markers that follow patients for their progression after diagnosis, predictive markers that predict treatment outcomes, and diagnostic markers for early screening [39]. This classification is tenuous because the profiles and utility of these biomarkers have not yet been comprehensively studied. These include tyrosinase, MITF, s100, Melan-A (also called MART-1), Premelanosome protein (PMEL) (referred to as gp100), and several recently described new biomarkers suitable for melanoma identification [40].

Furthermore, established immunohistochemical assays are complemented by new biosensing-based approaches in the identification of diagnostic and prognostic biomarkers. Such tools comprise activating enzymatic functions, antigen-antibody mechanism on the location [41], and *in situ* fluorescent hybridization of ribonucleic acids. Since melanoma can acquire multiple mutations as it progresses to malignancy, a combination of biomarkers may be required to distinguish them from melanocytic nevi. From this perspective, it would be more consistent with a specific diagnosis for combinations of mutations to up or down-regulate certain genes [42]. As cell surface markers can yield accurate and reliable information about the characteristics of melanoma cells and may assist in detecting circulating tumor cells (CTCs), they are amenable to biosensing technologies for cutaneous melanoma detection.

IOT IN HEALTHCARE

The surge in health problems and the soaring cost of healthcare have prompted more people (including elderly and disabled individuals) to adopt computer-aided technology for long-distance health management. In recent years, an IoT has emerged as a comprehensive network that interconnects various devices and plays a crucial role in automating different activities across many disciplines, including intelligent and remote healthcare systems [43]. The benefits of IoT with the help of some kind are majorly used technological features such as Wireless body area networks (WBAN), wireless sensor networks (WSNs), and radio frequency identification (RFID) [44]. They help transfer the data to the cloud for analysis and extract important information, which helps make timely and correct decisions. The Internet of Things (IoT) may be viewed as a prominent technology where the integration into health management systems (*e.g.*, mental health and skin disease) could support ever-increasing demands for healthcare personalization, prevention, and affordability [45].

Thus, IoT applications in healthcare are divided into three categories, namely automatic data sensing and capturing, people authentication and identity, and people and other items tracing (*e.g.*, personnel, medical teams, and patients) [46]. WBAN technology, the Internet of Things, provides health monitoring and treatment from anywhere a patient is located. It also deals with emergencies, post-discharge care, and hospital infections. Hence, the Internet of Things completely restructures people, devices, and applications in the healthcare business [47].

Hereafter, the assimilation of Internet of Things (IoT) potentials similar to the Internet of Medical Things (IoMT) technology will radically transform healthcare environments by incorporating associated medical sensors or targeting unique medical equipment with a smart and intended way for patient-centric provisioning [48]. IoMT predominantly finds its use in healthcare systems known as the Healthcare Internet of Things (IoT), where it connects medical devices to any accessible internet infrastructure and provides a solid base for telehealth services that include elder care supervision, telemonitoring, teleconsultations, and computer-assisted rehabilitation which help develop suitable therapeutic strategies for patients [49, 50].

In most studies, IoMT and HIoT are used interchangeably, which refers to medical devices and app integrations that can be connected in an IoT-based environment with healthcare information technology systems [51]. However, big data and IoT are relatively new concepts within hygienic systems that allow for efficient process monitoring solutions in the healthcare sector. Big data analytics has now allowed for prescriptive, autonomous, and predictive analysis of healthcare strategies. As a result, personalized health care particularly enables remote patient monitoring, diagnosis, early detection, and disease prevention for chronic conditions such as diabetes, obstructive lung disease, cancer, arthritis, and heart diseases [52].

The term "Internet of Things" (IoT) was first used with respect to supply management by Ashton in 1999 [53]. These days, the Internet of Things can mean many things, for instance, a complex system of uniquely assailable and identifiable objects. These devices connect to servers so that they can send out their data and receive the necessary information, which effectively provides relevant services. In other words, the Internet of Things is composed of a vast number of entities and devices (like different types of sensors and actuators) that are connected through the Internet [54]. Mainly, it includes sensors, complex algorithms, an interface to the cloud, and interfaces for communication in a typical IoT setup. Sensors collect data from various sources. In addition, WSN and RFID technologies are the communication and network infrastructures; furthermore, complex algorithms are used for processing and analysis [55]. In a cloud environment, huge numbers of client/server requests can be dispatched, which offers us a chance to access numerous amenities together. Fog computing was designed to overcome the limitations of cloud computing, such as latency, reliability, resource constraints, *etc*., by allowing users to run the same applications they have anywhere around them and enabling real-time analysis and efficient decision-making tools [56].

Even after all the above improvements, IoT is still in the infant stage, and many research issues can be addressed related to standards, device heterogeneity, scalability security, privacy, *etc*. From this perspective, it is clear that one particular concern comes to light: the interoperability of smart devices, which links one device or the other with heterogeneous devices and systems belonging to different vendors in an economical and easy-to-install manner. One key feature of IoT is the low-cost interoperation between objects, which will allow customers to continue interacting with several providers in the future [57]. Finally, the Internet of Things helps reduce costs for building structures themselves, clears out layers from existing organizational infrastructures, and facilitates infrastructure diversity [58].

Nowadays, the IoT perspective includes wide applications such as monitoring, smart cities, transportation, health care, and much more. Even though there is a wide range of IoT devices, data from IoT applications (*e.g*., smart homes and cities) can be easily compared, correlated, and aggregated to meet user needs [59]. As an example, the opportunity of the IoT paradigm to improve sanitary systems in the healthcare field through its technology is presented. This is especially useful for telemonitoring patients in the hospital and elderly patients who have chronic diseases and stay at home [60]. This technology will prove to be a boon for future healthcare systems as it is expected to minimize the response time of anomaly detection and deliver high-quality care at lower hospitalization costs with an increased life span.

IoT has improved the prediction capability of the sanitary system by analyzing large amounts of data and connecting various IoT devices to obtain real-time physiological data from patients, such as blood glucose levels or temperature monitors [61]. The main goal is to provide advanced medical services to individuals, such as continuous tracking of chronic diseases and early detection of disease. In fact, IoT can aid the healthcare industry in remote clinical monitoring, assisted living, disease management, and preventive care. Furthermore, the most popular IoT applications in the healthcare field are limited to several domains, including hospital management, e-healthcare, home healthcare, and mobile healthcare [62]. Finally, increasing alignment of the Internet of Things with health care systems has paved the way for intelligent self-management of health care processes, self-care, and syncing for particular events like seizures, falls that may assist with Parkinson's gait disturbance, stroke rehabilitation, neurologic monitoring and cardiac problems in a bid to reduce medication and human error [63]. However, more challenges remain before the development of safe and effective healthcare applications can occur. These include deficiencies in self-improvement, self-learning, hardware (such as wearables and implantable sensors), privacy, security, and standardization. Nowadays, data is secured under different security protocols against threats/attacks, such as public-key cryptosystems, k-anonymity, encryption techniques, and authentication [64].

By connecting devices to the Internet using modern communication technology, IoT is based and designed for data sharing. The Internet of Things is a new phenomenon that accesses different devices, *e.g.*, body sensor networks, smart grids, and homes, as well as smart cities and automobile ad hoc networks [65]. Information sensing, cloud computing, and wireless sensor networks (WSNs) are some of the key technologies that are evolving along with the Internet of Things. Iota is generally implemented to enhance and expand medical systems because of its functionality for integrating with substructure resources, which permits current structures to get recommendation information from users. On behalf of providing diverse e-health services, including electronic health records, and checking patients remotely, medical platforms exchange a lot of data through WSNs [66].

Skin cancer, the sixth most common type of cancer in the world, still has work to be done. The skin layer consists of melanocytes, basal cells, and squamous cells, which are the cells where the cancerous tissue is found. Consequently, there are some dangerous types of skin tumors, such as melanoma, squamous cell carcinoma (SCC), and basal cell carcinoma (BCC). In the United States and Australia, skin cancer is the most prevalent. The professionals of skincare struggle with cancer diagnosis (mostly at an early stage). Thus, scientists are working on an automated and easy calculator for cancer detection [67].

IOT TECHNOLOGIES FOR SKIN CANCER DIAGNOSIS

Fig. (**2**) summarizes the various IoT technologies used in the diagnosis of skin cancer.

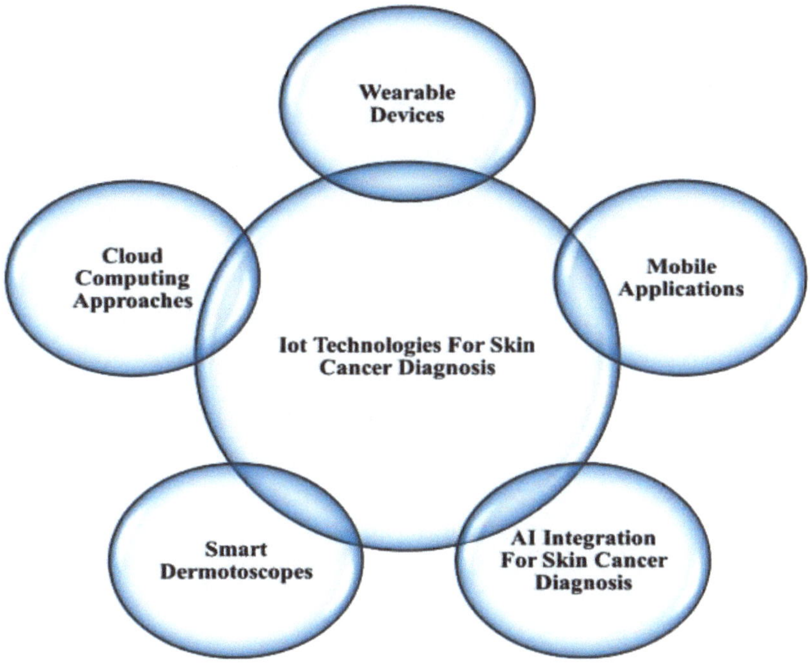

Fig. (2). IoT technologies for skin cancer diagnosis.

Wearable Devices

Smartwatches and Fitness Trackers with UV Sensors

Sensors embedded in smartwatches have made monitoring various aspects of a person's health easier. According to data from the global wristwatch market, shipments in 2021 rose by 24% year-on-year and exceeded 40 million units in the fourth quarter for the first time. This increase is related to the public's growing interest in monitoring their health [68].

Smartwatches have been proven useful and accurate in tracking multiple medical conditions, including epilepsy, falls, chronic disease self-management, medication adherence, and cardiovascular disorders. To illustrate, in research assessing the capability of smartwatches for reporting correct alerts to the users of atrial fibrillation (AF), irregular pulse warnings ended up being consistent with AF in 84% of the cases. It is a fact that these devices save lives treating atrial fibrillation, which, if undiagnosed, may lead to heart failure or stroke. With the increase in popularity of wearable devices like smartwatches, the number and range of sensors and features are continuously increasing [69].

However, existing smartwatches currently only track a small number of dermatological health data points, and none are available for alerts. The acute, chronic, and psychosocial problems of dermatological health, for the most part, are inadequately represented. As such, it seems that smartwatches are not very smart when it comes to dermatology [70].

One in every three cancers diagnosed worldwide is skin cancer, according to estimates from the World Health Organization (WHO). Although there have been efforts conducted to address the risk factors for skin cancer, skin cancer has constantly increased all over the world. For non-melanoma skin cancer, it is estimated that between 37.6% and 64.5% of persons have at least one other skin disorder [71]. Because smartwatches are worn on the skin, they are exposed to a broader and more extreme range of environmental conditions. In reality, any cumulative lifetime exposure to ultraviolet radiation potentially represents a significant threat to the development of skin cancers and also awareness of risk thresholds in patients. Given the startlingly high incidence of skin cancer, lowering morbidity and death requires early identification. Smartwatches have now become an excellent tool to help us identify such abnormalities, particularly for more regular monitoring. These, too, can be adapted for tracking exposures to allergens, irritants, and high or low humidity [72, 73].

Notifications about the UV index on smartwatches might help individuals with xeroderma pigmentosum, porphyrias, photoallergy, lupus erythematosus, and other photosensitivity disorders take suitable sun precautions or avoid the sun during 'danger hours.' And while a number of smartwatches now can measure the UV index, no device uses this kind of alarm. Alerts that may include a one-sentence message regarding the risk of UV exposure (high risk of cancer or photoaging) would be intended to inform users while reducing tanning if applicable. Public awareness of the negative effects of UV radiation may promote sun safety practices, including using sunscreen, looking for shade, and visiting dermatologists for routine skin examinations [74].

Moreover, a strong association exists between cumulative UV exposure and the risk for melanoma, basal cell carcinoma, and squamous cell carcinoma, especially in younger people. Currently, very few smartwatches with UV exposure tracking capability are available on the market because they are equipped with UV and light intensity sensors. In conjunction with UV index data, wearables with integrated UV sensors could potentially provide users with a collective, objective measure of their overall UV exposure over the years. Providing an estimate of how people's own skin cancer risk compares to that of the population, a quantitative summary of the life course of UV exposure can be a wake-up call and guide to healthy behavior [75].

Swim-tracking smartwatches differentiate swimming from washing hands by integrating accelerometer data with water sound detection sensors. Such watches could potentially track the duration of immersion in water and suggest when to reapply sunscreen, especially after moderate to high-intensity exercise when sunscreen may be washed off [76]. Half of beachgoers reported applying sunscreen while they were out and about in the area, according to one study. Even that was left open-ended, with only half of the 50% saying they'd applied a second coat. Sunscreen, in general, has to be reapplied every 2 hours, and some sources say that this requirement does not even count. While correct sunscreen application is an established issue, it can mitigate sunburn and UV-induced skin lesions. Studies giving participants a physical reminder to reapply sunscreen have demonstrated higher reapplication rates than those without a reminder. Users may receive timely reminders from smartwatches to reapply sunscreen [77].

The drive to itch and scratch is important for sustaining symptoms in atopic dermatitis, a type I IgE-mediated hypersensitivity reaction, among other pruritic disorders. They can also strongly influence the lives of affected individuals. Even worse, many patients do not even know that they have a compulsive habit of scratching [78]. Since smartwatches already know when users are moving, the current technology may alert wearers when they make a scratching-like movement that prompts whoever to put their hand down. The device may also monitor how often these individuals scratch and offer the ability for data to be shared with their doctor. The duration of itch has a value that can provide important information to help determine the severity of a patient's disease and how to manage it best [79].

Skin Patches with Sensors for Monitoring Changes

Due to these rapid technological advances in medical, electronics, and digital technologies, next-generation biocompatible health monitoring patches have been developed at a large size incorporated with skin-adhesive patches, E-skin patches, wearable sensors, blood pressure monitors, optoelectronic devices, fitness trackers and transdermal patches. Those patches not only assist with monitoring patients but also deliver expert advice, local treatment, or both to address patients' problems [80].

Smart patches with multiple integrated components like drug reservoirs, drug carriers, a transdermal delivery device, and sensors can achieve the functionalities. In particular, the e-skin devices associated with small biosensors might be able to talk to skin tissues to sense the physiological and biomechanical conditions of our bodies. Hence, they can serve as an *in situ* diagnostic measure that could be translated to tailored clinical applications [81, 82].

Furthermore, wearable transdermal drug delivery systems (TDDS) have been extensively investigated for non-invasive and on-demand stimuli-responsive transport of drugs across the skin barrier into the bloodstream for targeted therapy (auto-medication). Recent studies have reviewed various applications of these devices in areas such as tissue engineering, drug delivery, wound healing, and myocardial infarction [83].

Transcutaneous diagnosis and therapy (theragnostic) based on biomolecule assays, impedance detection, medication delivery, and electrical biostimulation have been widely used in clinical applications. Yet certain common electronic devices, such as wearable electronics, which often come with large, bulky electrochemical biosensing equipment or drug delivery systems that need to carry a large reservoir of liquid electrolytes, may not be best suited for point-of-care (POC) theragnostic deployment. These limitations increase the impracticality of POC and real-time transcutaneous thermometry, therefore omitting its use for a number of disorders. Recent developments in ultrathin and micro-flexible electronics have witnessed the usage of polymeric devices over inorganic ones for their better flexibility and conductivity. However, typical wearable polymer-based devices cannot fit the skin because of the irregularities of the skin surface in length scales, such as microscale wrinkles that result in large air gaps between the device and the skin. This interferes with proper electrical and physical contact, which is essential for true biosignal measurement and monitoring of health conditions [84].

In addition, these kinds of devices cannot effectively store the liquid state ionic molecules for local delivery, particularly electrolytes and drugs. Due to their robust and lasting adhesion, E-skin patches assist in biosensing or electrical stimulation at the interface between the skin surface and the ambient environment [85].

The e-skin is composed of a flexible and elastic substrate material (that mimics the skin) and conductive materials. The electrode of E-skin is usually composed of graphene, carbon nanotubes, poly (3,4-ethylenedioxythiophene) polystyrene sulfonate (PEDOT: PSS), metal nanoparticles, and hydrogel, whereas the substrate is typically made up of elastomers such as silicone rubber or PDMS [86].

Amongst these, polydimethylsiloxane (PDMS) is a widely used substrate material that is appreciated for its impressive biocompatibility, elasticity, and transparent properties. The combination of a rapidly growing population and limited medical resources has triggered an excessive demand for biomedical devices capable of real-time and non-invasive human body monitoring. Such technologies can be very useful for personalized treatment [87].

Mobile Applications

Apps for Tracking Moles and Skin Changes

Self-triaged e-health tools are a relatively new way for patients to evaluate their health status and receive information. In addition, e-health technologies are available and low-cost for skin monitoring. Nowadays, some apps that facilitate skin self-examination (SSE) can also assist in the secondary prevention of melanoma. It illustrates through a few examples of secondary melanoma prevention currently available *via* e-health. The main target of these tools is to aid specialists in detecting melanoma in the most precise stage by an automatic evaluation of a lesion using some characteristics advised by the professional group [88].

An early diagnosis of melanoma can be achieved through secondary prevention (screening) and skin surveillance. The current boom of e-health tools for melanoma detection enables skin self-examination and may facilitate screening patients outside the clinical setting. One just has to search through stores such as the Play Store to find an increasing number of applications in the medical part.

Unsurprisingly, it would appear that there is a strong interest in self-diagnosis applications to help avoid skin cancer and track moles (allowing morphological changes over time). Actually, pointing to the clinical process experts use, surviving melanoma and the avoidability of new incidents each year are often associated with increased scrutiny and widespread knowledge of skin cancer. Despite this encouraging premise, the scientific data to support that apps function as expected in the health industry remains controversial. Recent research has suggested that users need to be careful when they want to use applications for health purposes [89].

ApreSkin You

The latest medical app that caught our attention is the ApreSkin You, which recently launched on the App Store. App development company Creative Intersection and dermatologist Brad Jones developed it. The ApreSkin allows for active patient-doctor communication due to its ease of use, which means the modern EMR software can be utilized effortlessly. In the visual interface, a realistic 3D model shows the lesion automatically located for easier data entry during skin consultations; images can be enclosed directly. To maintain patient privacy and protection, the information uploaded to the above-said app is encrypted and accessible only by using a PIN.

Using a mobile device, physicians can rapidly generate a skin consultation report accompanied by a patient record. The specialist maps specific skin diseases or lesions using realistic 3D models, automatically storing position data to allow for precise future identification of the lesion. Another reason the customizability of the data entry technique is beneficial to doctors is that they can use common terminology and phrases for diagnosis [90].

CompariSkin™

The CompariSkin smartphone app allows patients to obtain consistent photographs across various skin lesion types. Being able to compare and even superimpose photographs of the same lesion taken at different times is a great help in analyzing evolution over time. These are crucial possibilities for the segments of the population who are most vulnerable because of age groupings or genetic considerations.

The CompariSkin App (formerly known as MoleMapper Plus) is a tool to facilitate the detection of change in skin lesions using comparative and registered 3D photographs. The 3D model of participation takes a picture of the skin accurately, including rashes, jaundice, and birthmarks, through CompariSkin, which creates a library of skin changes. It also allows users to create their maps to compare time differences in various body parts. For biopsies and follow-ups, notes from routine medical appointments might be bunched in the patient history. CompariSkin users can reduce unnecessary biopsies by enabling their doctor to have a portable copy of their skin record, making it easy to identify any skin cancer in its initial stages. Having a visual record (essentially a snapshot of how the skin looks at some time point) allows physicians to choose an appropriate course of management and objectively assess the improvements or worsening of the skin or surrounding areas. This app has been instrumental in some interesting applications, such as the monitoring of Spitz nevi [91].

Spitz nevus, a subclass of nevus mainly seen in younger people, is also known as juvenile melanoma. It's pale red, fast-growing but short-lived. It includes large, non-pigmented cells extending to the reticular dermis, such as spindle and epithelioid cells with enlarged nuclei and prominent nucleoli. Although distinguishing melanoma from Spitz nevi can be difficult, the fact that at least some younger children with Spitz nevi are being monitored by means of dermatoscopy and clinical imaging is commendable. When a concerning pigmented lesion is identified, surgical excision is often chosen as the first-line approach due to concern for melanoma. However, when given the opportunity, most patients and their parents choose to observe with pictures in order to avoid excision and subsequent scarring. Spitz nevi were seen every six months, and atypical nevi every three months. A more extensive follow-up allows for a more proper evaluation of the lesion, which facilitates avoiding unnecessary excisions or allowing for the excisation of less of the possible tissue [92].

Miiskin

The Skin Health Alliance has approved Miiskin. It is crucial to emphasize that Miiskin is a skin-tracking app that helps you record the visual skin changes between your regular examinations rather than an image-based lesion diagnostic tool. In the knowledge base section on skin cancer, the user has a range of interesting readings, including articles with specific references to photos of skin cancer, melanoma, and normal & atypical moles. In the premium version of Miiskin, one can save their skin maps and check them out using the Web Compare tool on any big screen. The Miiskin App improves the skin exam monitoring process by allowing users to snap and save images of unusual lesions and normal areas for extended periods. Photographs can be compared over time, allowing differences such as the appearance of a new mole or change to an existing atypical mole to be recognized through concurrent viewing and simultaneous processing of photographs [93].

Due to the challenge of distinguishing between melanoma and skin cancer, the advancement features offered by mobile apps allow both early and accurate detection that helps specialists perform their work. Plus, it opens the door for a low-cost tool for effective self-diagnosis. These include reminders for tracking injuries, as well as help with taking and storing pictures of skin lesions to enable patients to monitor their development over time [94]. Different apps used for tracking moles and skin changes are summarized in Table **1**.

AI Integration for Skin Cancer Diagnosis

Early detection is paramount to better outcomes, as the skin cancer survival rate of 99% is associated with an early diagnosis. But if the disease penetrates beyond the epidermis, survival rates are poor. The current practice is for dermatologists to evaluate patients visually, although with the use of dermoscopy using polarized light magnification to facilitate examination. Commonly, a patient's clinical history, ethnicity, social habits, and sun exposure have played key influential roles in forming a medical diagnosis. For diagnosis, suspicious lesions are biopsied in the office setting, sent to a laboratory, processed as permanent paraffin sections, and viewed as representative glass slides by a pathologist [102].

Table 1. Apps for tracking moles and skin changes.

Name of App	Platform	Function
SkinVision	iOS, Android	Mole analysis, risk indication, usual skin checks, and Al technology [95].
MoleScope	iOS, Android	Mole tracking, high-resolution imaging, teleconsultations with dermatologists [96].
UMSkinCheck	iOS	Step-by-step self-investigation guidelines, image storage, and reminder alerts for self-exams Developed by the University of Michigan Health System, comprehensive self-exam guidance [97].
DermaCompare	iOS, Android	Automated mole comparison, cloud storage for images, and dermatologist consultation [98].
FotoFinder mySkin	iOS, Android	Mole imaging, risk assessment, regular follow-ups, and AI Technology Developed by a leading provider of skin imaging systems integrated with professional systems [99].
MoleMonitor	iOS, Android	Mole mapping, image comparison, mole change Notifications, and a simple interface for tracking changes, integrate with HealthKit on iOS [100].
SkinVision Check	iOS, Android	Skin cancer risk assessment, Personalized advice, regular skin checks, High accuracy of Al-based risk assessments, and easy-to-use interface [101].

AI-powered computer-aided diagnostics (CAD) systems have the potential to completely transform healthcare and medicine, particularly in the field of medical imaging. Medical imaging techniques, including computed tomography (CT), magnetic resonance imaging (MRI), and ultrasound, are widely used in clinical practice. In dermatology, dermatoscopy and, less often, confocal microscopy greatly enhance the ability to visualize characteristics of lesions *in vivo* and classify risks [103]. In many trials, AI systems for illness identification in medical imaging either match or exceed clinician performance. Since the advent of deep learning, several end-to-end solutions for anomaly detection have been proposed in different medical imaging modalities, such as skin lesions, foot ulcers, lung cancer, brain tumors, breast cancer, and oesophageal cancer image datasets [104].

Over the last decade, technology has greatly improved access to advanced imaging techniques, including 3D whole-body photoimaging/scanning/digital image mapping, dermoscopy, high-resolution cameras, and unique wide field-of - view whole-slide digital scanners. These techniques provide high-quality skin cancer image data from patients across the globe. ISIC (International Skin Imaging Collaboration) is the main contributor to digital datasets of skin lesion images with expert annotations that enable automated computer-assisted diagnosis (CAD) solutions for melanoma and other skin malignancies. Inexpensive, rapidly available internet, processing power, and secure cloud storage for organizing and distributing skin cancer datasets are all factors underpinning a widespread interest in applying AI technologies to skin cancer diagnosis. The algorithms can easily be scaled across platforms, devices, and operating systems, turning them into state-of-the-art medical equipment [105].

Feature of AI in Skin Cancer Diagnosis

One unique use case of Artificial Intelligence (AI) in image-based diagnostic medicine is to identify skin cancer. By analyzing large datasets, Artificial Intelligence (AI) algorithms can classify clinical or dermoscopic images with near-perfect accuracy. Though such AI-driven systems can operate independently of humans and with human oversight, the best results are achieved through an integrated process that harnesses the expertise of both AI and human experts. However, researchers often measure how accurately AI technologies can diagnose when placed in artificial environments but not real-world settings, which is an important distinction to keep track of. Therefore, the utility of AI-assisted diagnosis in clinical practice is not yet fully explored [106].

Skin cancer diagnosis depends on the subjective visual reading of clinical and dermoscopy images, making it a clear target for artificial intelligence. The shortage of dermatologists is a serious problem in many parts of the world and often leads to long waiting times for specialist consultations. There is an increasing belief that AI-based systems can be more accurate and consistent than human specialists. A study has indicated that convolutional neural networks (CNNs) can work well for the dermatological classification of photographs. Convolution Neural Networks (CNNs) are specialized types of neural networks that are developed based mainly on supervised learned processes. Hence, they work perfectly with image-processing tasks. This requires labeling the photos from the training dataset with diagnoses, which serves as the ground truth. The system requires this label to understand how input data and related diagnoses correlate [107].

AI is utilized in a wide range of instruments used in dermatology, including tools implemented for the detection of skin cancer *via* dermoscopy and through total body photography (TBP). Dermatologists who use market-approved AI-privileged software, like MoleAnalyzer Pro (FotoFinder ATMB) or DEXI (Vectra WB360), typically have it embedded with specialist hardware. AI assists dermatologists by serving as a support tool when paired with total body photography (TBP) for patients presenting with multiple nevi. In these situations, AI assists in categorizing and visualizing nevi to allow dermatologists to compare images and identify changes or abnormalities quickly. AI uses computational algorithms to compare total body photos taken during a current visit with those taken during prior visits in order to expedite the detection of new or evolving lesions [108].

The total nevi count, which is a risk factor for melanoma development, has yet to be assessed with artificial intelligence. In an Australian study, AI was shown to accurately measure the total number of nevi, with 97% agreement between AI-based counts and those made by senior dermatologists. Alternatively, AI-based nevi count and operative count by experienced dermatologists differed significantly, as a recent study from Switzerland shows. AI-based lesion detection from 3-dimensional (3D) pictures was superior to that from 2-dimensional images; the tendency of both algorithms to overcount lesions made them unsuitable for practical usage in clinical routine [109].

In a prospective diagnostic trial, dermatologists received AI malignancy scores and used the results to change their initial diagnosis. However, there were significant increases in sensitivity and specificity when AI-support outcomes were used for decision-making. Improvement was negligible in more experienced dermatologists but was far greater among less dermoscopy-experienced dermatologists [110].

Smart Dermotoscopes

Dermatoscopes have become widely adopted tools for dermatologists to supplement examinations and aid the visualization of sub-surface structures, allowing for specific patterns that may guide the diagnosis of a number of skin diseases. In the beginning, the early adopters of dermatoscopy among experts in pigmented lesions advocated it to enhance accuracy in diagnosing early melanomas and diminish harvesting of benign lesions. Dermatoscopy is an investigative tool that has formed the basis of some dermatologic diagnostic techniques. Still, it is now in widespread use by most dermatologists to assist in identifying a diverse set of inflammatory, infectious, and vascular conditions involving skin, hair, and nails, giving rise to several branches of dermatoscopy-inflammoscopy, trichoscopy, bronchoscopy, and entodermoscopy. In the future, dermatologoscopy will largely involve the deployment of artificial intelligence, such that the assessment process should become more objective, precise, and global [111].

The dermatoscope has seen a meteoric rise in popularity since the beginning of the new millennium, even being termed the dermatologist's stethoscope. The problem is that the diagnostic utility, initially directed at differentiating between common melanomas and less common melanocytic nevi, has now evolved to include numerous skin diseases in both benign and malignant nonmelanocytic proliferations, infections, and inflammatory processes. In the current age of dermatologic practice, dermatoscopy is quickly reaching its status as the standard of care. In a survey, almost 98% of dermatologists with 5 years or less in dermatology practice employ dermatoscopy, and all have had training in the use of dermatoscopy [112].

A Cochrane review of computer-assisted diagnosis (CAD) techniques included 42 studies consisting of both dermatoscopy-based studies and spectroscopy-based studies. CAD systems achieved a pooled sensitivity of greater than 90% for melanoma detection, making them at least as sensitive as dermatoscopic images across all CAD systems. These preliminary data imply that CAD might be helpful in decreasing the number of missed melanomas; however, these studies did not take into account real-world clinical decision-making. The evidence base most urgently needs randomized controlled trials testing CAD systems *versus* classic dermatoscopy in real-world populations that resemble the ones to which these technologies would be applied [113].

Deep neural networks can now be integrated into mobiles, taking dermatologists out of the clinic. This interesting development has gained impressive speed in the last few years, and it is estimated that 6.3 billion smartphone users will exist by the year 2024, potentially heralding an opportunity for a new device for many physicians around the world. Smartphone applications are proving to be a new frontier in dermatologic diagnosis, with one study showing a 95.1% sensitivity in detecting malignant conditions (93% for malignant melanomas and 97% for keratinocyte carcinomas and precursors) and 78.3% specificity [114]. The various features of smart dermatoscopy are mentioned in Fig. (**3**).

Sequential Digital Monitoring

The process of taking and storing dermoscopic pictures of questionable lesions with the intention of tracking any changes over time is known as sequential digital dermoscopy imaging or SDDI. Research has demonstrated that SDDI reduces the frequency of needless excisions and enables the early diagnosis of melanomas. According to a meta-analysis of SDDI, the length of monitoring increased the likelihood of finding melanoma, indicating the importance of ongoing follow-up, particularly in high-risk groups [115].

Teledermoscopy

Teledermatology, or telederm for short, is an expanding part of the dermatology landscape in the US, with an increasing number of programs and consultations offered annually. Over the last five years, the number of telederm programs has increased by 48%, according to an indexed survey. When it comes to telecom skin cancer screenings, studies have shown that the inclusion of digital dermoscopic images improves diagnostic accuracy over clinical images alone. The two most common telecom modalities currently practiced are store and forward (which focuses on the archive of images for later consultation) and live, interactive video consultation [116].

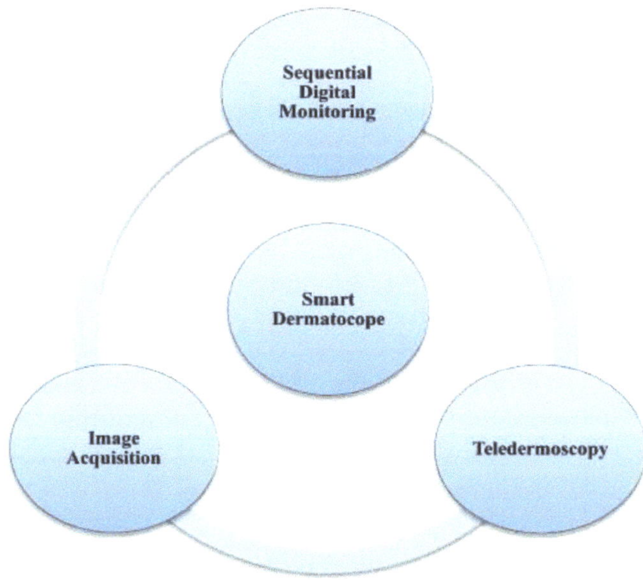

Fig. (3). Smart dermatoscopy features.

Medicaid does provide reimbursement for store-and-forward telederm in some states. At the same time, Medicare reimburses only live-interactive teledermatology for patients located outside of nonmetropolitan areas - as well as store-and-forward telederm pilot programs run in Alaska and Hawaii. Just as dermatoscopy use is not covered in clinical assessments, teledermoscopy is also within the realm of supplementary insurance and cannot be used for coverage. Notably, 214 students from a southern university health center participated in a willingness-to-pay survey, and the results indicated that they would be prepared to spend $55.27 (SD) on average ($39.11) out of pocket for a teledermoscopy/telederm assessment, citing convenience as one of the reasons. Direct-to-consumer telederm provides patients with an alternative method of therapy. In order to promote direct-to-patient teledermoscopy, some dermatoscopes (such as DermLite HÜD [3Gen] and Molescope/Molescope II [Metaoptima Technology Inc]) are presently marketed directly to customers in conjunction with telederm services [117].

Image Acquisition

There are different types of devices, including all-in-one systems and dermatoscopes, that can be connected to digital cameras or smartphones to obtain digital dermoscopic images. A system that balances these factors is utilized depending on the needs of the practitioner (cost, size/portability, speed, image quality, and software). Digital single-lens reflex (DSLR) cameras yield the best image quality, but for video, dermoscopy details are usually recorded at low resolution. Video dermoscopy, or simply with a video camera as an image collector for macroscopic images obtained by other imaging equipment (spectrum imaging devices and reflectance confocal microscopy), yields stored images of relatively lower quality.

Smartphone clinical imaging in dermatology is an emerging field. While DSLR cameras might still be able to deliver the best pictures, modern smartphones now shoot images that compete with digital camera quality. Using the processing power within your computer, computational photography enhances image quality and may bring smartphone image quality closer to that of DSLR cameras. More recent dual-lens cameras in smartphones provide even better images, it has been claimed. Current smartphones have an option called high-dynamic-range imaging (HDRI), which produces a composite image of increased dynamic range of luminosity by combining several photographs in any given scene taken at different exposures. High-dynamic-range imaging has even been shown to improve dermoscopic characteristics of more difficult hypopigmented skin malignancies [118].

A concentrated effort has been made to standardize the acquisition of digital dermatologic images. Standardization holds the potential to enhance data analysis, collaborate better, safeguard patient privacy, and enhance health care. The ISIC group is leading the way in image standardization; it has released its Delphi consensus guidelines on standards for lesion imaging, including dermoscopy [119].

Cloud Computing Approaches

The healthcare research industry requires hardware that can quickly process large volumes of data and mathematical models to provide timely solutions supporting the highest level of medical diagnosis. Automated medical picture diagnosis is one of the widespread applications of artificial intelligence (AI) in healthcare. Image-based diagnosis is a key area of artificial intelligence within the industry that will eventually augment radiology, ophthalmology, dermatology, and beyond. The biggest drawback of this method is that it needs a lot of computing power, both for performing the inference and for training these models. However, below it, the fundamentally parallel vector and matrix operations lay the groundwork for AI systems. As a result, most of the time, they run on parallel architectures for training and inference. Here, HPC (High-performance computing) technologies, such as multi- and many-core processors, play a crucial role. As stated previously, HPC is a general term that includes various solutions from edge and cloud computing approaches [120].

Cloud Computing is a computing model in which one can get access to the available virtualized and dynamically scalable resources as a service *via* the Internet. However, this usually does not always refer to everything from cloud computing power, data storage, and service that is outsourced to outside parties for businesses and consumers. However, edge computing is a paradigm where resources are located at the edge of the Internet (closest edge or off closest to data-generating devices, such as IoT and mobile devices, sensors, and end users). This enables the computation of cloud services and downstream data on behalf of upstream IoT services. They are auxiliary to the data center, classically the heart of cloud computing [121].

The selection of a classification technique is critical in the identification of melanoma, and CNN (Convolutional Neural Network) has been shown to be the most suitable architecture for image recognition. CNN contains fully linked, convolutional, and nonlinear pooling hidden layers. Tons of convolutions happen in the convolutional layers, and the fully connected layers are attached to them. However, due to the overfitting problem, especially when the lesion images have overlapping characteristics, the deeply connected layer is not suitable for melanoma detection. A Convolutional Neural Network (CNN) is used to identify and classify images into different classes in order to deal with the overfitting problem [122].

CHALLENGES IN THE DIAGNOSIS OF SKIN CANCER

The challenges that occur in the diagnosis of skin cancer are summarized in Fig. (**4**).

The Barrier to Communication between Dermatologists and AI

Artificial intelligence for skin cancer diagnosis means it may have found its way to thethe dermatology landscape for years to come; however, it still has been unsuccessful in closing that communication gap between dermatologists and AI. Expanding the role of dermatologists to fully embrace AI applications across multiple settings, both clinical and research-based, is advised. The dominant view on the potential implications of AI on cancer diagnosis that advances in technology may reduce the workforce size sets an undesirable backdrop and engenders fears about its use in this space. AI has evolved with time, and as better tools presumably come into the hands of doctors, it is undeniable that they would still outperform in tracking mimetics and patterns outside of those mapped from the training datasets. Dermatologists not only have to identify and categorize skin abnormalities but also have to make insightful conclusions and actionable data from their observations [123].

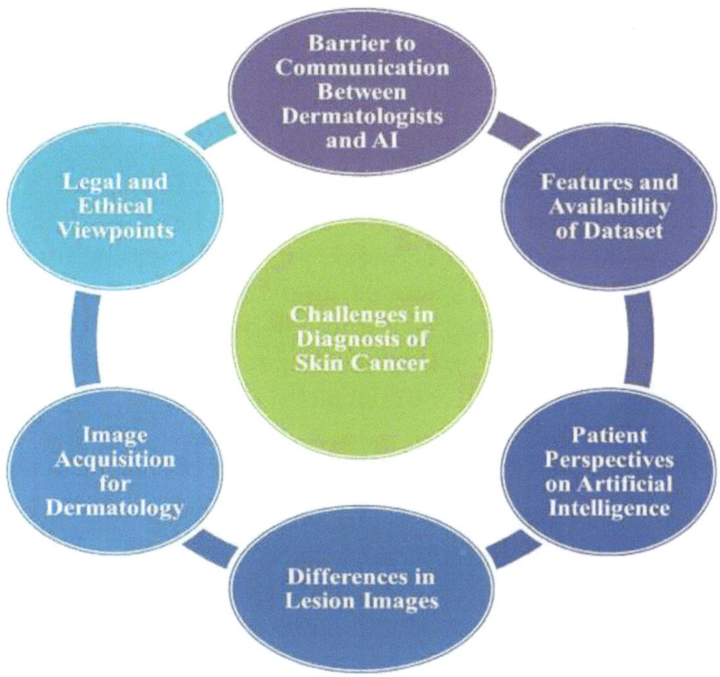

Fig. (4). Challenges in diagnosis of skin cancer.

In an evaluation of Chinese dermatologists, the majority of respondents felt AI was beneficial in the occupational routine of diagnosis or treatment. A study report used survey results to find that only 3 percent of dermatologists believed AI could and would replace facets of their day-to-day jobs. In another survey study, dermatologists using AI to guide their diagnosis had higher accuracy and positive diagnoses than traditional methods. It is imperative that the communication gap between dermatologists and AI be closed, and workplace engagement with the diverse functions provided by AIs must be pursued [124].

Features and Availability of the Dataset

The limited availability of datasets is one of the most serious impediments to deep learning in real-world usages, such as cancer diagnosis. Without huge datasets for machine learning and deep learning, these models would inevitably fall flat. For example, while some databases may exclude certain benign lesions from the everyday diagnosis list, like blisters and warts, these are actually part of our normal diagnostics. But dermatologists see these lesions all the time. Since these lesions are not included in the datasets, this may lead to undiagnosed skin cancer within benign lesions [125].

Most of the datasets available on the internet are mostly raw photos. This essentially means most of the advancements have to come from the researchers themselves. To overcome the general issue of imbalance in the datasets, researchers have been using data augmentation techniques such as cropping, rotation, and filtering. This increases the number of training images that the models can use. While the datasets provide extensive information to researchers, they cannot optimally utilize clinical photographs as key metadata, including skin type and ethnicity, are unclear. Clinical decision support for screening and diagnosis is a precursor of open science initiatives, which have already begun to influence the future of datasets and the development of data-driven diagnostic techniques. To a larger extent, open science has to gain momentum in tackling the problems related to the accessibility of datasets [126].

Patient Perspectives on Artificial Intelligence

While patients' opinions and perceptions regarding the role of artificial intelligence in healthcare remain unchanged yet, there is no doubt AI will change how these activities are executed. Patients response to artificial intelligence in health care, this creates a mutually beneficial relationship between patients and AI use. Although almost 75% of the patients were eager to encourage family members to use AI in healthcare, 25% who expressed anxiety are worth noting [127].

One way to tackle this is by ensuring that the conflict response can be resolved by acquiring a biopsy for the Artificial Intelligence decision process. Within the dataset itself, too, there are worries about misdiagnoses and knowledge of their clinical and medical history being available. Without a proper label, an AI cannot train correctly, which will give wrong diagnosis results. Such labels are then used to create data analytics and make use of AI models to diagnose skin cancer as a way to get further observations by inferring. The withholding or invention of data totally defeats the objective of training an AI. This can be mitigated by ensuring that organizations collecting data maintain confidentiality policies [128].

Differences in Lesion Images

Skin lesion segmentation is the first step when using machine learning and deep learning to diagnose skin cancers, which is a multi-step sequential process. While it sounds trivial, sometimes roadblocks prevent this task from being completed correctly, such as skin color, loose and fuzzy boundaries, and lesion size. The photo pixel values vary within different photos due to variations, *i.e.*, illumination changes provide shadows and lights unevenly in the patches; hence, it becomes difficult for skin lesions segmentation. Traditional algorithms such as CNNs and CNN-based methods are better in terms of labels, but these techniques can still generate images with low contrast for lesions *versus* normal skin. This is due to the dataset irregularities, which derive abnormalities in skin color, *etc* [129].

The datasets are so diverse that little inference can be drawn from the data. Because the established standard, an expert diagnosis, differs from the methodology quality that relates to validity and reliability (*i.e.*, with nontrivial specificity and sensitivity compared to both), this makes the application of AI-in - healthcare utility less advantageous. A review of optical coherence in the diagnosis of adult skin cancer has reviewed the respective diagnostic criteria and qualifications for a specialist. In order to counter the variability of properties shown by skin lesions, the AI models need to increase the diversification and intensification of their samples. Such methods enable the models to overcome stagnation induced by increased diversity. In addition, due to skin colors, the variation in pictures of lesions leads to delayed recognition of skin cancer in patients with other colors until they progress more [130].

Furthermore, models are rarely trained on a range of skin tones because of socioeconomic issues, including care constraints. The model's training on dominant skin tones and lesion colors causes them to acquire an innate bias that eventually lowers the accuracy of the skin cancer diagnosis [131].

Image Acquisition for Dermatology

In dermatology, the most common way to obtain photos has been by taking photographs of lesions or dermatosis in close proximity. The image has the lesion as its main aspect, excluding the surrounding structures, thus losing the anatomical context in this picture. In addition, the use of photographs taken with a smartphone camera in dermatology has grown in step with the increasing adoption of digital skin imaging apps. Although many studies propose methods for detecting melanomas based on uneven dermoscopy images, most have localized results that are not generalizable to a global setting due to training them on isolated data sets with specified lighting conditions, *etc* [132].

Besides, more problems arise due to these variable illumination conditions during the acquisition phase, such as a specular reflection, which deteriorates the quality of the images acquired even more. A GAN (Generative Adversarial Neural Network) [MSM20] is recommended to solve the persistent problems of color inconsistency. We should encourage more people to use these techniques and devise new ideas to solve variability issues in dermoscopy image acquisition [133].

Legal and Ethical Viewpoints

While the benefits of employing AI in clinical practice and health care are innumerable, many ethical considerations remain to be addressed. While health AI is changing the interaction between patients and physicians, there remains a lack of clarity on how informed consent works in this specific context. When clinicians should or should not tell a patient that AI has an opportunity to be part of the relationship is ambiguous to them [134].

AI judgments are extremely notable, and they lead to transparency and safety problems. It is widely accepted that no AI model can be perfect all the time, but choosing the wrong alternative could have catastrophic consequences and make the right decision seem like a risky one. This brings into question the algorithms in terms of bias and fairness model. Models that are trained on a dataset will tend to have the attributes that the underlying data indicates due to the way they fit against it.

Since it is practically difficult for any dataset to sample the whole world's population accurately, there is reason for concern. AI can greatly threaten patient preferences. At the same time, legal questions will always be raised by the use of AI in the healthcare sector. As of now, there is no agreement on the assignment of responsibility after harmful and malefic treatment [135].

Similarly, bias in AI against historically marginalized groups may even result in legal action concerning human rights and anti-discrimination. It remains to be seen whether such patients when AI powers their care, would benefit from the privacy rules in place right now. It is essential to note that the entire system cannot be developed without addressing the ethical and legal aspects of artificial intelligence (AI) in health care despite all possible benefits [136].

FUTURE PROSPECTS

Collaborations between dermatologists and AI will still be important in the near future. For reasons that will become clear, the unfettered development of fully autonomous diagnostic machines akin to self-driving cars remains somewhat off in the misty future. For one, the lack of prospective trials in real-world situations means that stand-alone devices without an expert are unlikely to be used. Second, TBP population screening with AI is theoretically possible but highly risky. The reason is that AI has a lower specificity in unselected populations. The utility of AI for screening and surveillance of high-risk individuals post-expert clinician selection is yet to be established [137].

Finally, dermatologists tend to consider contextual information beyond morphology owing to their general knowledge. They also include human preferences in their decision-making process, such as the optimal trade-off between sensitivity and specificity. These preferences may differ between different types of patients [138].

CONCLUSION

The Internet of Things, cloud computing, artificial intelligence, machine learning, and deep learning are now considered emerging technologies that can help solve various practical problems. They are therefore used in smart cities, transportation, health, agriculture, and many other areas to deliver these solutions with positive impacts on various issues in this environment nowadays. IoT technologies also allow dermatologists to accurately and early identify skin cancer. However, IoT helps in the real-time monitoring of skin health, the strategy of an efficient treatment plan for skin cancer, and provides a productive outcome to the patients. While IoT offers great potential for monitoring skin cancer, several issues need to be considered, such as patient perspectives, image capturing and dataset availability, and ethical/regulatory implications of implementing IoT. Apart from skin cancer detection, the other future possibilities of IoT technology are processing and predicting many more types of cancers like blood, lung, breast, *etc*.

REFERENCES

[1] Hu W, Fang L, Ni R, Zhang H, Pan G. Changing trends in the disease burden of non-melanoma skin cancer globally from 1990 to 2019 and its predicted level in 25 years. BMC Cancer 2022; 22(1): 836. [http://dx.doi.org/10.1186/s12885-022-09940-3] [PMID: 35907848]

[2] Paolino G, Donati M, Didona D, Mercuri S, Cantisani C. Histology of non-melanoma skin cancers: an update. Biomedicines 2017; 5(4): 71. [http://dx.doi.org/10.3390/biomedicines5040071] [PMID: 29261131]

[3] Andreassi L. UV exposure as a risk factor for skin cancer. Expert Rev Dermatol 2011; 6(5): 445-54. [http://dx.doi.org/10.1586/edm.11.54]

[4] Paraiso KH, John JK, Smalley KS. Melanoma and other skin cancers. Biotargets Cancer Curr Clin Pract 2012; 439-68. [http://dx.doi.org/10.1007/978-1-61779-615-9_17]

[5] Kallini JR, Hamed N, Khachemoune A. Squamous cell carcinoma of the skin: epidemiology, classification, management, and novel trends. Int J Dermatol 2015; 54(2): 130-40.

[http://dx.doi.org/10.1111/ijd.12553] [PMID: 25428226]

[6] Green A, Whiteman D, Frost C, Battistutta D. Sun exposure, skin cancers and related skin conditions. J Epidemiol 1999; 9(6): 7-13.
[http://dx.doi.org/10.2188/jea.9.6sup_7]

[7] Cichorek M, Wachulska M, Stasiewicz A, Tymińska A. Skin melanocytes: biology and development. Adv Dermatol Alergol 2013; 30(1): 30-41.
[http://dx.doi.org/10.5114/pdia.2013.33376]

[8] Schadendorf D, Fisher DE, Garbe C, *et al.* Melanoma. Nat Rev Dis Primers 2015; 1(1): 15003.
[http://dx.doi.org/10.1038/nrdp.2015.3] [PMID: 27188223]

[9] Williams ML, Sagebiel RW. Melanoma risk factors and atypical moles. West J Med 1994; 160(4): 343-50.
[PMID: 8023484]

[10] Patel P, Hussain K. Merkel cell carcinoma. Clin Exp Dermatol 2021; 46(5): 814-9.
[http://dx.doi.org/10.1111/ced.14530] [PMID: 33252781]

[11] Becker JC, Stang A, DeCaprio JA, *et al.* Merkel cell carcinoma. Nat Rev Dis Primers 2017; 3(1): 17077.
[http://dx.doi.org/10.1038/nrdp.2017.77] [PMID: 29072302]

[12] Tow R, Hanoun S, Andresen B, *et al.* Recent advances in clinical research for skin cancer chemoprevention. Cancers (Basel) 2023; 15(15): 3819.
[http://dx.doi.org/10.3390/cancers15153819] [PMID: 37568635]

[13] Bashshur RL, Shannon GW, Tejasvi T, Kvedar JC, Gates M. The empirical foundations of teledermatology: a review of the research evidence. Telemed J E Health 2015; 21(12): 953-79.
[http://dx.doi.org/10.1089/tmj.2015.0146] [PMID: 26394022]

[14] Chouhan R, Patel R, Shakib K, Mitsimponas K. Surgical excision of non-melanoma skin cancer: no end in site?. Br J Oral Maxillofac Surg 2021; 59(10): 1264-9.
[http://dx.doi.org/10.1016/j.bjoms.2021.05.018] [PMID: 34275678]

[15] Diepgen TL, Fartasch M, Drexler H, Schmitt J. Occupational skin cancer induced by ultraviolet radiation and its prevention. Br J Dermatol 2012; 167(s2) (Suppl. 2): 76-84.
[http://dx.doi.org/10.1111/j.1365-2133.2012.11090.x] [PMID: 22881591]

[16] Abdul-Qawy AS, Pramod PJ, Magesh E, Srinivasulu T. The Internet of Things (IoT): An overview. Int J Eng Res Appl 2015; 5(12): 71-82.

[17] Krishnamurthi R, Kumar A, Gopinathan D, Nayyar A, Qureshi B. An overview of IoT sensor data processing, fusion, and analysis techniques. Sensors (Basel) 2020; 20(21): 6076.
[http://dx.doi.org/10.3390/s20216076] [PMID: 33114594]

[18] Ouaissa M, Ouaissa M, Khan IU, Boulouard Z, Rashid J, Eds. Low-power wide area network for large scale internet of things: Architectures, communication protocols and recent trends. CRC Press 2024.
[http://dx.doi.org/10.1201/9781003426974]

[19] Sarker IH. Machine learning for intelligent data analysis and automation in cybersecurity: current and prospects. Annals of Data Science 2023; 10(6): 1473-98.
[http://dx.doi.org/10.1007/s40745-022-00444-2]

[20] Gupta BB, Quamara M. An overview of Internet of Things (IoT): Architectural aspects, challenges, and protocols. Concurr Comput 2020; 32(21): 4946.
[http://dx.doi.org/10.1002/cpe.4946]

[21] Majumdar P, Mitra S, Bhattacharya D, Bhushan B. Enhancing sustainable 5G powered agriculture 4.0 : Summary of low power connectivity, internet of UAV things, AI solutions and research trends. Multimedia Tools Appl 2024; 1-45.
[http://dx.doi.org/10.1007/s11042-024-19728-1]

[22] Hui TKL, Sherratt RS, Sánchez DD. Major requirements for building Smart Homes in Smart Cities based on Internet of Things technologies. Future Gener Comput Syst 2017; 76: 358-69. [http://dx.doi.org/10.1016/j.future.2016.10.026]

[23] Allioui H, Mourdi Y. Exploring the full potentials of IoT for better financial growth and stability: A comprehensive survey. Sensors (Basel) 2023; 23(19): 8015. [http://dx.doi.org/10.3390/s23198015] [PMID: 37836845]

[24] Bertrand J, Steingrimsson E, Jouenne F, Paillerets B, Larue L. Melanoma risk and melanocyte biology. Acta Derm Venereol 2020; 100(11): adv00139. [http://dx.doi.org/10.2340/00015555-3494] [PMID: 32346747]

[25] Syrigos KN, Tzannou I, Katirtzoglou N, Georgiou E. Skin cancer in the elderly. in vivo 2005; 19(3): 643-52. [PMID: 15875788]

[26] Barnhill RL, Lugassy C, Taylor E, Zussman J. Cutaneous melanoma. Pathol Melanocytic Nevi Melanoma 2014; 331-487. [http://dx.doi.org/10.1007/978-3-642-38385-4_10]

[27] Keung EZ, Gershenwald JE. The eighth edition American Joint Committee on Cancer (AJCC) melanoma staging system: implications for melanoma treatment and care. Expert Rev Anticancer Ther 2018; 18(8): 775-84. [http://dx.doi.org/10.1080/14737140.2018.1489246] [PMID: 29923435]

[28] Ali AM, DiPersio JF, Schroeder MA. The role of biomarkers in the diagnosis and risk stratification of acute graft-*versus*-host disease: a systematic review. Biol Blood Marrow Transplant 2016; 22(9): 1552-64. [http://dx.doi.org/10.1016/j.bbmt.2016.04.022] [PMID: 27158050]

[29] Mandalà M, Massi D. Tissue prognostic biomarkers in primary cutaneous melanoma. Virchows Arch 2014; 464(3): 265-81. [http://dx.doi.org/10.1007/s00428-013-1526-x] [PMID: 24487785]

[30] Tombelli S, Mascini M. Biosensors for clinical biomarkers. Predict approaches drug discov dev biomarkers In Vitro In Vivo correl 2012; 11: 203-24. [http://dx.doi.org/10.1002/9781118230275.ch8]

[31] Wahab MR, Palaniyandi T, Viswanathan S, Baskar G, Surendran H, Gangadharan SG, Sugumaran A, Sivaji A, Kaliamoorthy S, Kumarasamy S. Biomarker-specific biosensors revolutionise breast cancer diagnosis. Clinica Chimica Acta. 2024;555:117792.

[32] Chatzilakou E, Hu Y, Jiang N, Yetisen AK. Biosensors for melanoma skin cancer diagnostics. Biosens Bioelectron 2024; 250: 116045. [http://dx.doi.org/10.1016/j.bios.2024.116045] [PMID: 38301546]

[33] Rodrigues D, Barbosa AI, Rebelo R, Kwon IK, Reis RL, Correlo VM. Skin-integrated wearable systems and implantable biosensors: a comprehensive review. Biosensors (Basel) 2020; 10(7): 79. [http://dx.doi.org/10.3390/bios10070079] [PMID: 32708103]

[34] Khan H, Shah MR, Barek J, Malik MI. Cancer biomarkers and their biosensors: A comprehensive review. Trends Analyt Chem 2023; 158: 116813. [http://dx.doi.org/10.1016/j.trac.2022.116813]

[35] Deacon DC, Smith EA, Judson-Torres RL. Molecular biomarkers for melanoma screening, diagnosis, and prognosis: current state and prospects. Front Med (Lausanne) 2021; 8: 642380. [http://dx.doi.org/10.3389/fmed.2021.642380] [PMID: 33937286]

[36] Nikolouzakis TK, Falzone L, Lasithiotakis K, *et al.* Current and future trends in molecular biomarkers for diagnostic, prognostic, and predictive purposes in non-melanoma skin cancer. J Clin Med 2020; 9(9): 2868. [http://dx.doi.org/10.3390/jcm9092868] [PMID: 32899768]

[37] Corrie SR, Coffey JW, Islam J, Markey KA, Kendall MAF. Blood, sweat, and tears: developing clinically relevant protein biosensors for integrated body fluid analysis. Analyst (Lond) 2015; 140(13): 4350-64.
[http://dx.doi.org/10.1039/C5AN00464K] [PMID: 25909342]

[38] Trager MH, Geskin LJ, Samie FH, Liu L. Biomarkers in melanoma and non-melanoma skin cancer prevention and risk stratification. Exp Dermatol 2022; 31(1): 4-12.
[http://dx.doi.org/10.1111/exd.14114] [PMID: 32415889]

[39] Du J, Miller AJ, Widlund HR, Horstmann MA, Ramaswamy S, Fisher DE. MITF transcriptionally regulates MLANA/MART1 and SILV/PMEL17/GP100 in melanocytes and melanoma. Am J Pathol 2003; 163(1): 333-43.
[http://dx.doi.org/10.1016/S0002-9440(10)63657-7] [PMID: 12819038]

[40] Pal M, Muinao T, Boruah HPD, Mahindroo N. Current advances in prognostic and diagnostic biomarkers for solid cancers: Detection techniques and future challenges. Biomed Pharmacother 2022; 146: 112488.
[http://dx.doi.org/10.1016/j.biopha.2021.112488] [PMID: 34894516]

[41] Griewank KG. Biomarkers in melanoma. Scand J Clin Lab Investig 2016; 76(245): S104-12.
[http://dx.doi.org/10.1080/00365513.2016.1210336]

[42] Qi J, Yang P, Min G, Amft O, Dong F, Xu L. Advanced internet of things for personalised healthcare systems: A survey. Pervasive Mobile Comput 2017; 41: 132-49.
[http://dx.doi.org/10.1016/j.pmcj.2017.06.018]

[43] Elhayatmy G, Dey N, Ashour AS. Internet of things based wireless body area network in healthcare. Internet Things Big Data Anal Toward Next-Gen Intell 2018; 3-20.
[http://dx.doi.org/10.1007/978-3-319-60435-0_1]

[44] Aceto G, Persico V, Pescapé A. Industry 4.0 and health: Internet of things, big data, and cloud computing for healthcare 4.0. J Ind Inf Integr 2020; 18: 100129.
[http://dx.doi.org/10.1016/j.jii.2020.100129]

[45] Ahmadi H, Arji G, Shahmoradi L, Safdari R, Nilashi M, Alizadeh M. The application of internet of things in healthcare: a systematic literature review and classification. Univers Access Inf Soc 2019; 18(4): 837-69.
[http://dx.doi.org/10.1007/s10209-018-0618-4]

[46] Comito C, Falcone D, Forrester A. Current trends and practices in smart health monitoring and clinical decision support. 2020 IEEE International Conference on Bioinformatics and Biomedicine (BIBM). 2577-84.
[http://dx.doi.org/10.1109/BIBM49941.2020.9313449]

[47] Pramanik PK, Upadhyaya BK, Pal S, Pal T. Internet of things, smart sensors, and pervasive systems: enabling connected and pervasive healthcare. In Healthcare Data Anal Manag. Academic Press. 2019; pp. 1-58.

[48] World Health Organization. Medical devices and eHealth solutions: Compendium of innovative health technologies for low-resource settings 2011-2012. World Health Organization 2013.

[49] Joyia GJ, Liaqat RM, Farooq A, Rehman S. Internet of medical things (IoMT): Applications, benefits and future challenges in the healthcare domain. J Commun 2017; 12(4): 240-7.

[50] Awasthi AK, Kumar S, Garov AK. IoT in the healthcare sector. In Mach Learn Deep Learn Big Data IoT Healthcare 2022; 107-23.
[http://dx.doi.org/10.1201/9781003227595-7]

[51] Krishnamoorthy S, Dua A, Gupta S. Role of emerging technologies in future IoT-driven Healthcare 4.0 technologies: a survey, current challenges and future directions. J Ambient Intell Humaniz Comput 2023; 14(1): 361-407.
[http://dx.doi.org/10.1007/s12652-021-03302-w]

[52] Kaukalias T, Chatzimisios P. Internet of Things (IoT) InEncyclopedia of information science and technology. 3rd ed. IGI Global 2015; pp. 7623-32.

[53] Adhikary T, Jana AD, Chakrabarty A, Jana SK. The internet of things (IOT) augmentation in healthcare: An application analytics. ICICCT 2019–System Reliability, Quality Control, Safety, Maintenance and Management: Applications to Electrical, Electronics and Computer Science and Engineering. 2020:576-83.

[54] Landaluce H, Arjona L, Perallos A, Falcone F, Angulo I, Muralter F. A review of IoT sensing applications and challenges using RFID and wireless sensor networks. Sensors (Basel) 2020; 20(9): 2495.
[http://dx.doi.org/10.3390/s20092495] [PMID: 32354063]

[55] Samann FEF, Abdulazeez AM, Askar S. Fog computing based on machine learning: A review. International Journal of Interactive Mobile Technologies (iJIM) 2021; 15(12): 21.
[http://dx.doi.org/10.3991/ijim.v15i12.21313]

[56] Bhuiyan MN, Rahman MM, Billah MM, Saha D. Internet of things (IoT): A review of its enabling technologies in healthcare applications, standards protocols, security, and market opportunities. IEEE Internet Things J 2021; 8(13): 10474-98.
[http://dx.doi.org/10.1109/JIOT.2021.3062630]

[57] Uckelmann D, Harrison M, Michahelles F. An architectural approach towards the future internet of things. Architecting Internet Things. Berlin, Heidelberg: Springer Berlin Heidelberg. 2011; pp. 1-24.
[http://dx.doi.org/10.1007/978-3-642-19157-2_1]

[58] Salam A, Hoang AD, Meghna A, *et al.* The future of emerging IoT paradigms: architectures and technologies. Preprints 2019; 2019120276.

[59] Salam A. Internet of Things for sustainable human health. Internet of Things for Sustainable Community Development: Wireless Communications, Sensing, and Systems. Cham: Springer International Publishing 2024; pp. 217-42.
[http://dx.doi.org/10.1007/978-3-031-62162-8_7]

[60] Jagadeeswari V, Subramaniyaswamy V, Logesh R, Vijayakumar V. A study on medical Internet of Things and Big Data in personalized healthcare system. Health Inf Sci Syst 2018; 6(1): 14.
[http://dx.doi.org/10.1007/s13755-018-0049-x] [PMID: 30279984]

[61] Chiuchisan I, Costin HN, Geman O. Adopting the Internet of Things technologies in health care systems. 2014 International Conference and Exposition on Electrical and Power Engineering (EPE). 532-5.
[http://dx.doi.org/10.1109/ICEPE.2014.6969965]

[62] Bebortta S, Senapati D. Precision healthcare in the era of IoT and big data: monitoring of self-care activities. Comput Intell Aided Syst Healthcare Domain 2023; 91-118.

[63] Parvez AS, Sarker B. Role of IoT and Cloud Computing in Digital Healthcare. Int J Adv Res Comput Commun Eng 2022; 11(4)

[64] Qureshi KN. New trends in the Internet of Things, applications, challenges, and solutions. TELKOMNIKA 2018; 16(3): 1114-9.
[http://dx.doi.org/10.12928/telkomnika.v16i3.8483]

[65] Tennina S, Santos M, Mesodiakaki A, *et al.* WSN4QoL: WSNs for remote patient monitoring in e-Health applications. 2016 IEEE International Conference on Communications (ICC). 1-6.
[http://dx.doi.org/10.1109/ICC.2016.7511597]

[66] Marks R, Motley RJ. Skin Cancer. Drugs 1995; 50(1): 48-61.
[http://dx.doi.org/10.2165/00003495-199550010-00005] [PMID: 7588089]

[67] King CE, Sarrafzadeh M. A survey of smartwatches in remote health monitoring. J Healthc Inform Res 2018; 2(1-2): 1-24.

[http://dx.doi.org/10.1007/s41666-017-0012-7] [PMID: 30035250]

[68] Appelboom G, Camacho E, Abraham ME, *et al.* Smart wearable body sensors for patient self-assessment and monitoring. Arch Public Health 2014; 72(1): 28. [http://dx.doi.org/10.1186/2049-3258-72-28] [PMID: 25232478]

[69] Black TA, George M, Rousseau MA, Rashid RM. Smart watches lack skin smarts: Current and future dermatologic applications in device metrics. Cureus 2024; 16(2): 55273. [http://dx.doi.org/10.7759/cureus.55273] [PMID: 38558692]

[70] Reichrath J, Leiter U, Eigentler T, Garbe C. Epidemiology of skin cancer. Sunlight Vitamin D Skin Cancer 2014; 120-40.

[71] Magno M, Salvatore GA, Mutter S, Farrukh W, Troester G, Benini L. Autonomous smartwatch with flexible sensors for accurate and continuous mapping of skin temperature. 2016 IEEE International Symposium on Circuits and Systems (ISCAS). 337-40. [http://dx.doi.org/10.1109/ISCAS.2016.7527239]

[72] Morganroth PA, Lim HW, Burnett CT. Ultraviolet radiation and the skin: an in-depth review. Am J Lifestyle Med 2013; 7(3): 168-81. [http://dx.doi.org/10.1177/1559827612460499]

[73] Nelson EE, Rousseau MA, Black TA, George MN, Rashid RM. Smartwatch technology in medicine: A call for future dermatologic research. JMIR Dermatol 2023; 6(1): 47252. [http://dx.doi.org/10.2196/47252] [PMID: 37843896]

[74] Gurova O, Merritt TR, Papachristos E, Vaajakari J. Sustainable solutions for wearable technologies: mapping the product development life cycle. Sustainability (Basel) 2020; 12(20): 8444. [http://dx.doi.org/10.3390/su12208444]

[75] Huang X, Chalmers AN. Review of wearable and portable sensors for monitoring personal solar UV exposure. Ann Biomed Eng 2021; 49(3): 964-78. [http://dx.doi.org/10.1007/s10439-020-02710-x] [PMID: 33432511]

[76] Nikitina-Helvey N. The effects of skin cancer prevention education and sunscreen availability on sunscreen use among outdoor high school athletes.

[77] Moloney FJ, Collins S, Murphy GM. Sunscreens. Am J Clin Dermatol 2002; 3(3): 185-91. [http://dx.doi.org/10.2165/00128071-200203030-00005] [PMID: 11978139]

[78] Wahlgren CF. Itch and atopic dermatitis: an overview. J Dermatol 1999; 26(11): 770-9. [http://dx.doi.org/10.1111/j.1346-8138.1999.tb02090.x] [PMID: 10635621]

[79] Lee J, Cho D, Kim J, *et al.* Itchtector: a wearable-based mobile system for managing itching conditions. Proceedings of the. 893-905. [http://dx.doi.org/10.1145/3025453.3025569]

[80] Patel RH, Foltz EA, Witkowski A, Ludzik J. Analysis of artificial intelligence-based approaches applied to non-invasive imaging for early detection of melanoma: a systematic review. Cancers. 2023;15(19):4694.

[81] Khadka B, Lee B, Kim KT. Drug delivery systems for personal healthcare by smart wearable patch system. Biomolecules 2023; 13(6): 929. [http://dx.doi.org/10.3390/biom13060929] [PMID: 37371509]

[82] Bunea AC, Dediu V, Laszlo EA, *et al.* E-skin: The dawn of a new era of on-body monitoring systems. Micromachines (Basel) 2021; 12(9): 1091. [http://dx.doi.org/10.3390/mi12091091] [PMID: 34577734]

[83] Lee H, Song C, Baik S, Kim D, Hyeon T, Kim DH. Device-assisted transdermal drug delivery. Adv Drug Deliv Rev 2018; 127: 35-45. [http://dx.doi.org/10.1016/j.addr.2017.08.009] [PMID: 28867296]

[84] Sarabia-Vallejos MA, Cerda-Iglesias FE, Pérez-Monje DA, *et al.* Smart polymer surfaces with

complex wrinkled patterns: Reversible, non-planar, gradient, and hierarchical structures. Polymers (Basel) 2023; 15(3): 612.
[http://dx.doi.org/10.3390/polym15030612] [PMID: 36771913]

[85] Yang X, Chen W, Fan Q, Chen J, Chen Y, Lai F, Liu H. Electronic skin for health monitoring systems: properties, functions, and applications. Advanced Materials. 2024 Aug;36(31):2402542.

[86] Wang B, Facchetti A. Mechanically flexible conductors for stretchable and wearable e-skin and e-textile devices. Adv Mater 2019; 31(28): 1901408.
[http://dx.doi.org/10.1002/adma.201901408] [PMID: 31106490]

[87] Trung TQ, Lee NE. Materials and devices for transparent stretchable electronics. J Mater Chem C Mater Opt Electron Devices 2017; 5(9): 2202-22.
[http://dx.doi.org/10.1039/C6TC05346G]

[88] Yagerman S, Marghoob A. Melanoma patient self-detection: a review of efficacy of the skin self-examination and patient-directed educational efforts. Expert Rev Anticancer Ther 2013; 13(12): 1423-31.
[http://dx.doi.org/10.1586/14737140.2013.856272] [PMID: 24236821]

[89] Vocaturo E, Zumpano E. Smart apps for risk assessment of skin cancer. 2020 IEEE/WIC/ACM International Joint Conference on Web Intelligence and Intelligent Agent Technology (WI-IAT). 699-704.
[http://dx.doi.org/10.1109/WIIAT50758.2020.00106]

[90] Vocaturo E, Zumpano E. Smart Apps for Risk Assessment of Skin Cancer. IEEE/WIC/ACM International Joint Conference on Web Intelligence and Intelligent Agent Technology. 699-704.
[http://dx.doi.org/10.1109/WIIAT50758.2020.00106]

[91] Kang AS, Lee DJ. Melanoma risk factors and prevention. Practical manual for dermatologic and surgical melanoma management 2021; pp. 15-27.

[92] Barnhill RL, Busam KJ. Spitz nevus and variants InPathology of melanocytic nevi and malignant melanoma. New York, NY: Springer, New York 2004; pp. 148-98.
[http://dx.doi.org/10.1007/978-0-387-21619-5_7]

[93] Young AT, Vora NB, Cortez J, *et al.* The role of technology in melanoma screening and diagnosis. Pigment Cell Melanoma Res 2021; 34(2): 288-300.
[http://dx.doi.org/10.1111/pcmr.12907] [PMID: 32558281]

[94] Elder DE. Skin cancer. Melanoma and other specific nonmelanoma skin cancers. Cancer 1995; 75(S1) (Suppl.): 245-56.
[http://dx.doi.org/10.1002/1097-0142(19950101)75] [PMID: 8000999]

[95] Deeks JJ, Dinnes J, Williams HC. Sensitivity and specificity of SkinVision are likely to have been overestimated. J Eur Acad Dermatol Venereol 2020; 34(10): 582-e583.
[http://dx.doi.org/10.1111/jdv.16382] [PMID: 32215960]

[96] Modaragama S. Decision intelligence: Transformational developments in skin cancer screening using mobile applications. SSRN 3687522.2023;

[97] Habgood E, McCormack C, Walter FM, Emery JD. Patients' experiences of using skin self-monitoring apps with people at higher risk of melanoma: Qualitative study. JMIR Dermatol 2021; 4(2): 22583.
[http://dx.doi.org/10.2196/22583] [PMID: 37632821]

[98] Santos F, Silva F, Georgieva P. Automated diagnosis of skin lesions. 2020 IEEE 10th Int Conf Intell Syst (IS). 545-50.
[http://dx.doi.org/10.1109/IS48319.2020.9200090]

[99] Snoswell CL, Whitty JA, Caffery LJ, *et al.* Consumer preference and willingness to pay for direct-to - consumer mobile teledermoscopy services in Australia. Dermatology 2022; 238(2): 358-67.
[http://dx.doi.org/10.1159/000517257] [PMID: 34515087]

[100] Ngoo A, Finnane A, McMeniman E, Soyer HP, Janda M. Fighting melanoma with smartphones: a snapshot of where we are a decade after app stores opened their doors. Int J Med Inform 2018; 118: 99-112.
[http://dx.doi.org/10.1016/j.ijmedinf.2018.08.004] [PMID: 30153928]

[101] Chuchu N, Takwoingi Y, Dinnes J, *et al.* Smartphone applications for triaging adults with skin lesions that are suspicious for melanoma. Cochrane Libr 2018; 2018(12)
[http://dx.doi.org/10.1002/14651858.CD013192] [PMID: 30521685]

[102] Magalhaes C, Mendes J, Vardasca R. The role of AI classifiers in skin cancer images. Skin Res Technol 2019; 25(5): 750-7.
[http://dx.doi.org/10.1111/srt.12713] [PMID: 31106913]

[103] Habuza T, Navaz AN, Hashim F, *et al.* AI applications in robotics, diagnostic image analysis and precision medicine: Current limitations, future trends, guidelines on CAD systems for medicine. Inform Med Unlocked 2021; 24: 100596.
[http://dx.doi.org/10.1016/j.imu.2021.100596]

[104] Abou Ali M, Dornaika F, Arganda-Carreras I, Ali H, Karaouni M. Naturalize revolution: Unprecedented AI-driven precision in skin cancer classification using deep learning. BioMedInformatics 2024; 4(1): 638-60.
[http://dx.doi.org/10.3390/biomedinformatics4010035]

[105] Goyal M, Knackstedt T, Yan S, Hassanpour S. Artificial intelligence-based image classification methods for diagnosis of skin cancer: Challenges and opportunities. Comput Biol Med 2020; 127: 104065.
[http://dx.doi.org/10.1016/j.compbiomed.2020.104065] [PMID: 33246265]

[106] Jutzi TB, Krieghoff-Henning EI, Holland-Letz T, *et al.* Artificial intelligence in skin cancer diagnostics: the patients' perspective. Front Med (Lausanne) 2020; 7: 233.
[http://dx.doi.org/10.3389/fmed.2020.00233] [PMID: 32671078]

[107] Brancaccio G, Balato A, Malvehy J, Puig S, Argenziano G, Kittler H. Artificial intelligence in skin cancer diagnosis: A reality check. J Invest Dermatol 2023.
[PMID: 37978982]

[108] Cerminara SE, Cheng P, Kostner L, *et al.* Diagnostic performance of augmented intelligence with 2D and 3D total body photography and convolutional neural networks in a high-risk population for melanoma under real-world conditions: A new era of skin cancer screening?. Eur J Cancer 2023; 190: 112954.
[http://dx.doi.org/10.1016/j.ejca.2023.112954] [PMID: 37453242]

[109] Jahn AS, Navarini AA, Cerminara SE, *et al.* Over-detection of melanoma-suspect lesions by a CE-certified smartphone app: performance in comparison to dermatologists, 2D and 3D convolutional neural networks in a prospective data set of 1204 pigmented skin lesions involving patients' perception. Cancers (Basel) 2022; 14(15): 3829.
[http://dx.doi.org/10.3390/cancers14153829] [PMID: 35954491]

[110] Maron RC, Utikal JS, Hekler A, *et al.* Artificial intelligence and its effect on dermatologists' accuracy in dermoscopic melanoma image classification: web-based survey study. J Med Internet Res 2020; 22(9): 18091.
[http://dx.doi.org/10.2196/18091] [PMID: 32915161]

[111] Bleicher B, Levine A, Markowitz O. Going digital with dermoscopy. Cutis 2018; 102(2): 102-5.
[PMID: 30235368]

[112] Gulia A, Giovanna Brunasso AM, Massone C. Dermoscopy: distinguishing malignant tumors from benign. Expert Rev Dermatol 2012; 7(5): 439-58.
[http://dx.doi.org/10.1586/edm.12.47]

[113] Ring C, Cox N, Lee JB. Dermatoscopy. Clin Dermatol 2021; 39(4): 635-42.

[http://dx.doi.org/10.1016/j.clindermatol.2021.03.009] [PMID: 34809768]

[114] Esteva A, Kuprel B, Novoa RA, *et al.* Dermatologist-level classification of skin cancer with deep neural networks. Nature 2017; 542(7639): 115-8. [http://dx.doi.org/10.1038/nature21056] [PMID: 28117445]

[115] Rademaker M, Oakley A. Digital monitoring by whole body photography and sequential digital dermoscopy detects thinner melanomas. J Prim Health Care 2010; 2(4): 268-72. [http://dx.doi.org/10.1071/HC10268] [PMID: 21125066]

[116] Chuchu N, Dinnes J, Takwoingi Y, *et al.* Teledermatology for diagnosing skin cancer in adults. Cochrane Libr 2018; 2018(12). [http://dx.doi.org/10.1002/14651858.CD013193] [PMID: 30521686]

[117] Fogel AL, Sarin KY. A survey of direct-to-consumer teledermatology services available to US patients: Explosive growth, opportunities and controversy. J Telemed Telecare 2017; 23(1): 19-25. [http://dx.doi.org/10.1177/1357633X15624044] [PMID: 26729755]

[118] Sun MD, Kentley J, Wilson BW, *et al.* Digital skin imaging applications, part I: Assessment of image acquisition technique features. Skin Res Technol 2022; 28(4): 623-32. [http://dx.doi.org/10.1111/srt.13163] [PMID: 35652379]

[119] Finnane A, Curiel-Lewandrowski C, Wimberley G, *et al.* Proposed technical guidelines for the acquisition of clinical images of skin-related conditions. JAMA Dermatol 2017; 153(5): 453-7. [http://dx.doi.org/10.1001/jamadermatol.2016.6214] [PMID: 28241182]

[120] Bliznuks D, Bolocko K, Sisojevs A, Ayub K. Towards the scalable cloud platform for non-invasive skin cancer diagnostics. Procedia Comput Sci 2017; 104: 468-76. [http://dx.doi.org/10.1016/j.procs.2017.01.161]

[121] Anuradha M, Jayasankar T, Prakash NB, *et al.* IoT enabled cancer prediction system to enhance the authentication and security using cloud computing. Microprocess Microsyst 2021; 80: 103301. [http://dx.doi.org/10.1016/j.micpro.2020.103301]

[122] Alzahrani S, Al-Bander B, Al-Nuaimy W. A comprehensive evaluation and benchmarking of convolutional neural networks for melanoma diagnosis. Cancers (Basel) 2021; 13(17): 4494. [http://dx.doi.org/10.3390/cancers13174494] [PMID: 34503300]

[123] Wei ML, Tada M, So A, Torres R. Artificial intelligence and skin cancer. Front Med (Lausanne) 2024; 11: 1331895. [http://dx.doi.org/10.3389/fmed.2024.1331895] [PMID: 38566925]

[124] Chanda T, Hauser K, Hobelsberger S, *et al.* Dermatologist-like explainable AI enhances trust and confidence in diagnosing melanoma. Nat Commun 2024; 15(1): 524. [http://dx.doi.org/10.1038/s41467-023-43095-4] [PMID: 38225244]

[125] Soenksen LR, Kassis T, Conover ST, *et al.* Using deep learning for dermatologist-level detection of suspicious pigmented skin lesions from wide-field images. Sci Transl Med 2021; 13(581): abb3652. [http://dx.doi.org/10.1126/scitranslmed.abb3652] [PMID: 33597262]

[126] Melarkode N, Srinivasan K, Qaisar SM, Plawiak P. AI-powered diagnosis of skin cancer: A contemporary review, open challenges and future research directions. Cancers (Basel) 2023; 15(4): 1183. [http://dx.doi.org/10.3390/cancers15041183] [PMID: 36831525]

[127] Kosan E, Krois J, Wingenfeld K, Deuter CE, Gaudin R, Schwendicke F. Patients' perspectives on artificial intelligence in dentistry: a controlled study. J Clin Med 2022; 11(8): 2143. [http://dx.doi.org/10.3390/jcm11082143] [PMID: 35456236]

[128] Tschandl P, Rinner C, Apalla Z, *et al.* Human–computer collaboration for skin cancer recognition. Nat Med 2020; 26(8): 1229-34. [http://dx.doi.org/10.1038/s41591-020-0942-0] [PMID: 32572267]

[129] Altamimi A, Alrowais F, Karamti H, Umer M, Cascone L, Ashraf I. An improved skin lesion detection solution using multi-step preprocessing features and NASNet transfer learning model. Image Vis Comput 2024; 144: 104969.
[http://dx.doi.org/10.1016/j.imavis.2024.104969]

[130] Semerci ZM, Toru HS, Çobankent Aytekin E, *et al.* The role of artificial intelligence in early diagnosis and molecular classification of head and neck skin cancers: A multidisciplinary approach. Diagnostics (Basel) 2024; 14(14): 1477.
[http://dx.doi.org/10.3390/diagnostics14141477] [PMID: 39061614]

[131] Painter MA II, Noy S, Holmes MD. Skin tone and asset inequality in Latin America. J Ethn Migr Stud 2020; 46(18): 3892-919.
[http://dx.doi.org/10.1080/1369183X.2019.1592881]

[132] Fliorent R, Fardman B, Podwojniak A, *et al.* Artificial intelligence in dermatology: advancements and challenges in skin of color. Int J Dermatol 2024; 63(4): 455-61.
[http://dx.doi.org/10.1111/ijd.17076] [PMID: 38444331]

[133] Okuboyejo DA, Olugbara OO. A review of prevalent methods for automatic skin lesion diagnosis. Open Dermatol J 2018; 12(1): 14-53.
[http://dx.doi.org/10.2174/1874372201812010014]

[134] Trager MH, Gordon ER, Breneman A, Weng C, Samie FH. Artificial intelligence for nonmelanoma skin cancer. Clin Dermatol 2024; 42(5): 466-76.
[http://dx.doi.org/10.1016/j.clindermatol.2024.06.016] [PMID: 38925444]

[135] Grzybowski A, Jin K, Wu H. Challenges of artificial intelligence in medicine and dermatology. Clin Dermatol 2024; 42(3): 210-5.
[http://dx.doi.org/10.1016/j.clindermatol.2023.12.013] [PMID: 38184124]

[136] Min A. Artificial intelligence and bias: Challenges, implications, and remedies. Journal of Social Research 2023; 2(11): 3808-17.
[http://dx.doi.org/10.55324/josr.v2i11.1477]

[137] Du-Harpur X, Watt FM, Luscombe NM, Lynch MD. What is AI? Applications of artificial intelligence to dermatology. Br J Dermatol 2020; 183(3): 423-30.
[http://dx.doi.org/10.1111/bjd.18880] [PMID: 31960407]

[138] Hogarty DT, Su JC, Phan K, *et al.* Artificial intelligence in dermatology—where we are and the way to the future: a review. Am J Clin Dermatol 2020; 21(1): 41-7.
[http://dx.doi.org/10.1007/s40257-019-00462-6] [PMID: 31278649]

CHAPTER 3

AI-powered Imaging for Early Skin Cancer Detection

Akhil Sharma[1], **Shaweta Sharma**[2], **Akanksha Sharma**[1], **Shivkanya Fuloria**[3] and **Sunita**[1,*]

[1] *R. J. College of Pharmacy, Raipur, Uttar Pradesh, India*

[2] *School of Medical and Allied Sciences, Galgotias University, Uttar Pradesh-201310, India*

[3] *Faculty of Pharmacy, AIMST University, Semeling Campus, Bedong, Kedah, Malaysia-08100*

Abstract: Artificial intelligence (AI) has made remarkable advances in recent years that have ushered in a new era of precision medicine, particularly when it comes to the early diagnosis of skin cancer. This chapter explores the potential role of artificial intelligence (AI), which is powered by imaging in dermatology, with a focus on early skin cancer diagnosis. This allows artificial intelligence to analyze complex dermatological photos with statistically greater accuracy, significantly streamlining the diagnostic process. It makes use of the latest algorithms and teaching approaches. AI-based technologies integrated with existing diagnostic methods, such as dermoscopy and molecular diagnostics, offer a comprehensive solution to the identification of skin tumors. This strategy improves the ability to detect neoplasms at their most early and treatable periods. Evidence of AI-driven solutions is applied successfully in clinical practice with case studies provided by Leicester ICS and Lancashire ICB. The examples depicted here demonstrate how AI may broaden diagnostic reach, reduce wait times, and provide more precise evaluations with flow-through benefits for patients. Lastly, the chapter explores several ethical and regulatory topics necessary for implementing artificial intelligence within health care. Special emphasis is placed on its importance in terms of data protection, security, reduction of bias, and patient approval. Future work in this field would include the development of real-time diagnostic and telemedicine applications, further optimization of AI algorithms, and better integration with other diagnostic modalities. Elimination of biases and improving generalizability of AI models across diverse populations remains a major area of ongoing challenge. Research and development of AI-powered imaging is maturing to the point where it could transform early-stage skin cancer detection and treatment. This promises a future where healthcare becomes more precise, efficient, and accessible.

Keywords: AI-powered imaging, Bias mitigation, Data privacy, Dermoscopy, Early diagnosis, Healthcare innovation, Machine learning, Molecular diagnostics, Precision medicine, Skin cancer detection, Telemedicine.

* **Corresponding author Sunita:** R.J. College of Pharmacy, Raipur, Uttar Pradesh, India;
E-mail: ssunitaathakur@gmail.com

Akhil Sharma, Shaweta Sharma, Shivkanya Fuloria & Sudhir Kumar (Eds.)

INTRODUCTION

Over the last few decades, the incidence of melanoma has increased worldwide, with global warming being one of the main contributors. Melanoma skin cancer [1] is the most common form of skin cancer and affects a large part of the fertile land of countries like the United States and Australia. As per the survey conducted by the World Health Organization (WHO), nearly thirteen million people are identified with melanoma, the deadliest type of skin cancer, annually. Therefore, the high mortality rate observed around the world and the growing cost of medical diagnosis have made early detection of melanoma skin cancer a necessary condition. Hence, it is suggested that action must be taken in order to perform early detection of melanoma as well as the diagnosis of this type of skin cancer [2].

Without any aid, a dermatologist's examination of the skin has often been shown to be poor at diagnosing melanoma. Many imaging modalities are currently examining the efficacy of this imaging to determine *in vivo* whether melanoma can be accurately diagnosed through imaging. These imaging techniques include extensive cutaneous photography, dermoscopy, confocal scanning laser microscopy (CSLM), ultrasound, magnetic resonance imaging (MRI), optical coherence tomography (OCT), and multispectral imaging [3].

For a complete analysis of a pigmented skin lesion, the first preprocessing step should be to extract the lesion area from the surrounding healthy skin. The transition ranges between the lesion and the surrounding skin area are smooth, which is a challenge for lesion detection in dermatoscopic images. It can be complicated — even for dermatologists who have had extensive training. Dermoscopy images have been shown to contain artifacts like uneven illumination, dermoscopic gel, black frames, ink marks, rulers, air bubbles, and intrinsic cutaneous features that will affect boundary recognition, blood vessels, hairs, and skin lines and texture [4, 5].

Segmentation is defined as dividing an image into segments that are similar on a specific property (*e.g.*, same luminance, same color, same texture of the image). A representation of an image is a simplified and/or modified version of an image that must be more interpretable and evaluable. This is the purpose of the segmentation process. However, the implementation of automatic segmentation algorithms is critically important in the development of an automated skin lesion diagnostic system. Due to the importance of segmentation as a necessary step prior to performing analysis on lesion images, it has become one of the more important areas of research, and numerous segmentation algorithms and techniques have been reported in the literature [6].

Feature extraction is like measuring certain characteristics, which are also referred to as features, that help differentiate one input pattern from another in order to reduce the size of the original dataset. Feature extraction is performed by measuring the pixels representing a segmented object. It helps in computing a few other features as well. However, the feature extraction stage is the most susceptible to a certain amount of error. Many features are extracted to use to input to a complex classifier. However, scant mention of the true meaning of those features or even objective ways to assess them is still scarce [7].

The classification phase of the diagnostic system is the one that completes the information on the steps to generate a diagnosis about the input image. The classification of dermoscopic images consists of two different methods. The first strategy considers only the second-order structure among the two classes (melanoma and not melanoma), and it gives a binary judgment of 0 or 1 for each data item. This gives you not only a class label for a data point but also a probability of belonging to a certain class. This result corresponds to the second attempt at modeling. Support vector machines embody the most famous implementation of the first approach. Methods coming under the second approach include logistic regression, artificial neural networks, nearest neighbors, and decision trees. However, the way in which these methods build an approximation from data is very different between the two [8].

SKIN CANCER

Skin cancer is the most common type of cancer in the world, and there are more cases of skin cancer in the United States of America than all other cancers combined. Skin cancer classification is based on two basic categories: melanoma and nonmelanoma skin cancer (abbreviated NMSC). Because of the absence of diagnostic criteria and underreporting of skin cancer, it is impossible to accurately know the rates at which the disease is manifesting. In contrast, a number of epidemiologic studies indicate that the incidence of non-melanoma skin cancer (NMSC) and melanoma has increased dramatically over the past several decades. Simultaneously, their detection and treatment represent an important public health issue both from the perspective of the patient's life quality and the costs associated with their management. Skin malignancies account for the most common lesions that arise in sun-exposed areas of the head and neck. In recognition and management of these disorders, there is a considerable burden of morbidity in the interim. The disease can be treated in surgical excision, cryotherapy, chemotherapy, immunotherapy, and radiation therapy, among others. There are also other treatments to consider, such as immunotherapy. Using sunscreen-beating skin cancer will protect them from any kind of neighboring risk [(9, 10)]. Squamous cell carcinoma (SCC), basal cell carcinoma (BCC), melanoma, Merkel cell carcinoma (MCC), cutaneous T-cell lymphoma (CTCL), and primary cutaneous B-cell lymphoma (PCBCL) are the diseases that are being managed, with a particular emphasis on the function of radiotherapy in the treatment of these disorders.

Types of Skin Cancer

The main types of skin cancer are represented in Fig. (**1**).

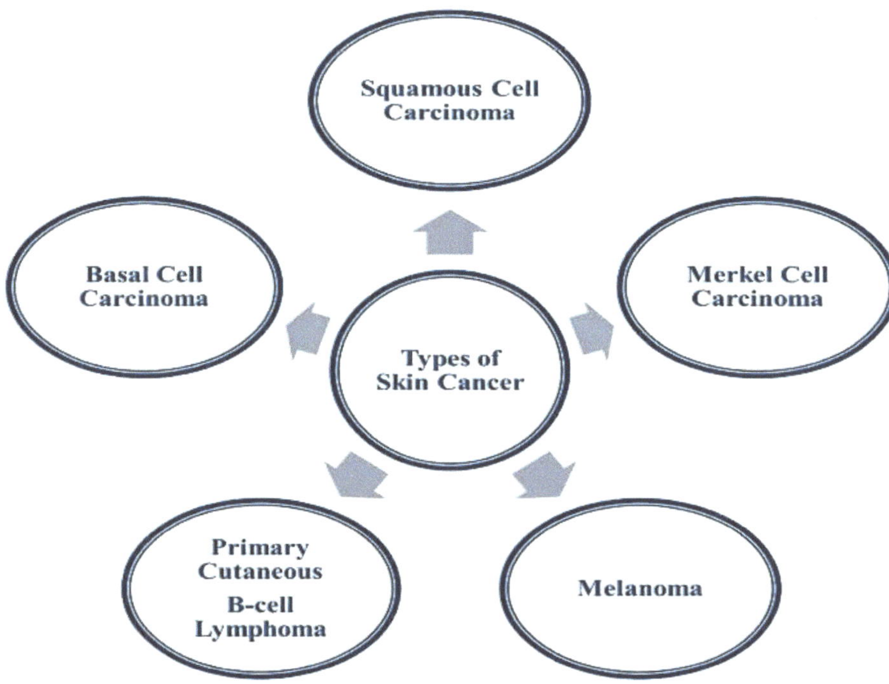

Fig. (1). Types of Skin Cancer.

Squamous Cell Carcinoma

About sixty percent of SCCs are linked to actinic keratoses premalignant macules that form following damage from UV light and are generally erythematous and scaly. About sixty percent of the cases included actinic keratoses. Features that warrant a biopsy include pain at the site of the lesion, bleeding, or growth in depth and diameter. All of these features are acquired during the progression of the lesion to a squamous cell carcinoma, and all are discovered in the course of a physical examination [11, 12]. A Marjolin tumor is another type of squamous cell carcinoma that can occur in chronically inflamed areas (ulcers or chronic wounds of the body) [13]. As described, an increased likelihood of post-surgical recurrence is considered to be associated with cancers that arise from sites of chronic inflammation. Even after all the tumors have been extracted, this is true. It comes as no surprise that advanced lesions that demonstrate poor differentiation express a greater risk of local recurrence and metastasis than more well-differentiated tumors such as squamous cell carcinoma (SCC). High-risk histologic tumor subtypes, including adenosquamous, metaplastic, adenoid, and desmoplastic tumors, are linked to worse outcomes. The desmoplastic subtype is known to exhibit exceptionally aggressive behavior when compared with the other types [14, 15].

Basal Cell Carcinoma

It is a low-grade disease as the incidence of metastasis in basal cell carcinoma is less than 0.01% compared to other neoplasms. UV is the major carcinogen driving several types of curable skin cancer, such as basal cell carcinoma (BCC), benign but disfiguring and painful and most of the BCCs occur on sun-exposed surfaces. BCCs are identified in the trunk in only 15% of all cases and in the head or neck in 70% to 80% of all cases [16].

Another factor that makes it more probable to return the tumor is its placement. Because basal cell carcinomas in site H (central face, eyebrows, eyelids, periorbital, nose, lips, chin mandible preauricular and postauricular skin temple ear genitalia hands or feet) have an increased -risk for surgical recurrence, they are classed as high-risk lesions regardless of their size. This is true regardless of the size of the lesions, which can be very large or small. Lesions greater than 10 mm in size are classified as high risk by the National Comprehensive Cancer Network. This also encompasses lesions seen in region M, which involves the cheeks, forehead, scalp, neck, and pretibial area. In comparison, 20-millimeter lesions [17] in region L [trunk, extremities] are considered high risk.

Other factors associated with higher recurrence rates include immunosuppression, poorly defined borders, recurrent tumors, previous radiotherapy, and PNI or LVI [18].

Melanoma

Melanomas are slow-growing epidermotropic tumors that spread radially, according to the first characterization. Melanomas can be dormant for years if the lesion has transitioned to a vertical growth phase and begun hitting the dermis; the chances of metastases occurring are significantly increased. Tumor thickness, ulceration, and mitotic index are markers that can be used to predict whether lymph node metastases will occur. Tumor thickness is among the most relevant markers [19].

Until today, invasive melanomas have been simplified into four basic pathologic categories. The subtype of melanoma can then be classified into superficial spreading, lentigo maligna, acral lentiginous, and nodular melanoma. More aggressive types of melanomas, such as nodular and acral lentiginous melanomas, are now recognized. As mutational markers within melanoma are defined, the disease and its classification will be more based on these features. This rise in these categories parallels the development of more targeted therapies. More importantly, BRAF mutations are present in 40% to 60% of nonresectable or metastatic melanomas. Not all BRAF mutations have been linked with more aggressive behavior; however, BRAF inhibitors (ex, vemurafenib, dabrafenib) have a strong anti-cancer response in patients with activating BRAF mutations [20 - 22].

Phase III trials have demonstrated greatly improved overall survival and progression-free survival in these people. It is notably effective in radiologic responses, achieving these in as many as 70% of patients with the BRAF V600 mutations. This combination of MEK inhibitors with BRAF inhibitors is common and has been shown to result in these goals. In addition, one should refrain from exposing patients on BRAF or MEK inhibitors to radiation due to the risk of causing significant toxicity, such as acute and lifelong severe dermatitis, as well as visceral toxicity. In these people, radiation is not recommended [23, 24].

Merkel Cell Carcinoma

Merkel cell carcinoma (MCC) is an uncommon type of neuroendocrine malignancy that has been associated with a high incidence of local recurrence and nodal metastasis in the literature. It was observed that immunosuppression is a major risk factor, and it was found 24 times more in transplant patients than in the immunocompetent group. Immunosuppression also presents as a risk factor. Again, this indicates that the disease scenario is a significant contributor to immunosuppression. The Merkel cell polyomavirus, which is normally prevalent in skin flora, is present in eighty percent of Merkel cell carcinomas. This is an interesting fact that must be kept in mind. Also, it is believed that the development of cancers induced by viruses follows a different pathway from that of non-viral tumors [25].

MCC is a common presentation of skin cancer where the skin has red or purple painless nodule. It has a shiny surface that helps in its rapid growth. Alternatively, you may see plaque-like lesions or nodules that are flesh tone. The MCC is often overlooked or misdiagnosed as a benign lesion due to its diffuse appearance. This is due to the characteristic appearance of the lesion [26].

Metastatic squamous cell carcinoma (MCC) is mostly localized within the skin. Nevertheless, 26% of patients also have lymph node metastases, and 8% present with distant metastatic disease. Regional lymph nodes are the most frequent location of metastases, followed by bones, brain, and lungs, with distant cutaneous sites being uncommon. Metastasis is most commonly found in lymph nodes [27, 28].

Primary Cutaneous B-cell Lymphoma

Primary cutaneous B cell lymphomas, or PCBCLs, are a heterogeneous group of non-Hodgkin lymphoma with involvement in the skin and no clinically credible evidence of extracutaneous disease at diagnosis. Primary cutaneous B-cell lymphoma (PCBCL) is a well-defined group of lymphoproliferative disorders that can be classified into 3 main subtypes: primary cutaneous marginal zone lymphoma (PCMZL), primary cutaneous follicular center lymphoma (PCFCL) and primarily cutaneous large B cell lymphoma, leg type (PCLBCL, leg type). Different from PCMZL and PCFCLPCLBCL, leg type is often BCL-2+, BCL-6+, MUM1+, MYC+, and FOXP1high, more aggressive than PCMZL and PCFCL and typically disseminate to extracutaneous sites, while for patients with PCLBCL, leg type, the 5-year OS rates are estimated to be between 41% and 60% using non-rituximab therapies and greater than 74% for those treated with rituximab [29 - 31].

TRADITIONAL IMAGING TECHNIQUES

Traditional imaging techniques for early skin cancer detection are shown in Fig. (**2**).

Skin Cancer Screening and Lesion Identification

There are no randomized controlled trials showing mortality benefits for routine skin cancer screening, especially not melanoma. Challenges for such trials include sample size, follow-up duration, and ethical considerations. Still, some studies have tried and done melanoma screening (*e.g.*, a community-based trial in Queensland, the Lawrence Livermore National Laboratory screening program, and a pilot study in Germany). Skin cancer screenings were included among nationwide services to be provided by Health Insurance Funds, as recently established by the German Federal Joint Committee (G-BA). The American Cancer Society encourages people to carefully check their skin for skin cancer. Still, the U.S. Preventive Services Task Force determined that there is not enough evidence to assess the balance of benefits *versus* harms from screening in the first place. Clinicians should be on the lookout for more malignant skin lesions encountered during a routine physical exam. Conversely, a high level of awareness, experience, and training is essential to detect NMSCs, but no similar detection rules exist for them. Morbidity may be minimized if such lesions are detected early [32, 33], resulting in improved long-term cosmetic outcomes as well as quality of life benefits [34].

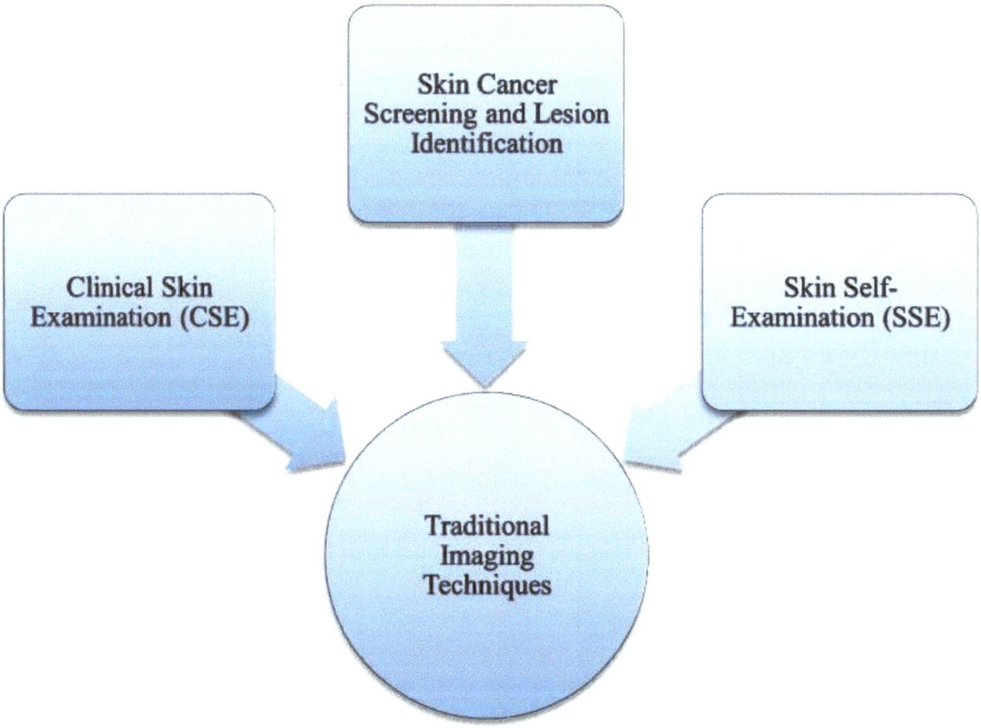

Fig. (2). Traditional imaging techniques.

Skin Self-Examination (SSE)

Skin cancer is frequently diagnosed incidentally or *via* deliberate self-examination (SSE), with rates of melanoma diagnosis by SSE being 40%-55%. In Australia, 44% of all melanoma and 73% of first melanoma recurrences are diagnosed by patients or their partners. Conclusion: SSE can reduce melanoma mortality by 63%. Its prevalence among the general population varies from 7% to 61%. It is associated with personal characteristics, including female gender, higher knowledge of skin cancer, fair skin, a personal history of skin cancer, a high perceived risk for skin cancer, and self-efficacy related to SSE. The sensitivity of SSE ranges from 25%–93%, and specificity 83%–97%. Improvements in SSE are partner-assisted SSE, mole maps, video, photographs, rulers, and magnifying lenses [35 - 38].

Clinical Skin Examination (CSE)

CSE is associated with less advanced melanoma thickness at diagnosis and earlier skin cancer diagnosis compared to SSE. This represents a randomized experiment done in Germany that demonstrated CSE to have a substantial positive impact on melanoma mortality. In a case-control study on Queensland population, a whole-body CSE within the last 3 years was associated with a nearly 14% reduced odds of diagnosis of thick melanoma. Using data from the Australian Melanoma Screening Trial, researchers found that CSE could be offered at a similar cost to other programs for early detection of melanoma in Australia, at least among adults aged 50 years or older [39 - 41].

Only thirty percent of people in Australia currently view a doctor for a skin check — as it stands, however. In addition, some sub-groups — for example, older men — are less likely to take up an invited screening even when the test could be more beneficial. Compared with the general population, those with a prior melanoma have a sixfold increase in risk of a second melanoma (but there is an approximately twofold increased risk associated with nonmelanoma skin cancer history). For those with hundreds of moles that are hard to track or in body locations that are difficult to inspect on their own, CSE might be an alternative or adjunct to SSE. In addition, melanoma survivors are not more likely to have an SSE than the general population and need regular clinical follow-up, usually done in 3–6-month intervals, depending on how long it has been since the primary diagnosis. However, the CSE adds less than 3 minutes to the entire time spent with a patient and is not routinely performed by most physicians, including dermatologists [42 - 45].

AI AND MACHINE LEARNING TECHNOLOGIES WITH THEIR FEATURES

Examples of Machine Learning in Practice

Image Recognition: Machine learning algorithms can analyze images and recognize objects, people, and other features in photos. An example of this can be applied to facial recognition, security cam, and self-driving cars [46, 47].

Speech Recognition: Machine learning algorithms can analyze speech and convert it to text or identify specific words or phrases. Speech recognition requires the use of Virtual Assistants, Dictation Software, and Call Center Automation Programs [48].

Fraud Detection: By analyzing large datasets of financial transactions, machine learning algorithms can identify patterns that may suggest fraudulent behavior [49].

Personalization: In fields such as e-commerce, entertainment, and social networks, machine learning algorithms so far analyze users' data based on their browsing history and purchase history in order to provide personalized recommendations also depending on given activity within social media [50, 51].

Health Care: Machine learning algorithms can analyze medical data that will then help in diagnosis, predict outcomes, and personalize treatment [52].

Deep Learning

Deep learning is a branch of machine learning where learners are trained in many-layered neural networks to identify patterns in numerical data. Some examples of tasks that often require deep learning models include image and audio recognition, natural language processing, and autonomous driving. These models are mostly used for complex tasks involving large datasets [53].

Deep learning is just building many layers of artificial neurons, each processing whatever data gets added (and passing it on to the next layer). These layers allow the model to learn representations of input data that are increasingly complex, enabling it to ultimately make predictions or decisions based on recognized patterns [54 - 56].

Examples of deep learning in practice

Image recognition:This includes facial identification, object detection, and medical imaging. Such models can identify objects, people, and other features in images with high accuracy.

Speech recognition: Deep learning models can transcribe speech to text with very high accuracy, allowing applications such as virtual assistants, dictation software, and call center automation.

Natural language processing: Deep learning models are also used in applications such as language translation, sentiment analysis, and chatbots, where human languages can be interpreted and synthesized by a computer.

Autonomous driving: Deep learning models are used to analyze data from the car's cameras and other sensors to determine what objects and obstacles exist on the road, react to them in real-time, and identify speed limit sign boards or traffic signs along with driving alone or around other autonomous vehicles.

Robotics: Deep learning approaches can enable robots to perform complex tasks such as grasping objects, localizing environments, and performing imitation learning [57, 58].

Natural Language Processing

NLP is used for face recognition, object detection, and medical imaging. These kinds of models can detect objects, individuals, and other elements in a photograph very accurately.

Deep learning for automatic speech recognition has allowed us to accurately convert speech to text, opening the door to virtual assistants, dictation-based software solutions, and call center automation, just to name a few [59].

Natural language processing in practice

Natural language processing (NLP) is an area of AI with a multitude of uses that vastly enhance our experience with text-based data.

Language translation: NLP systems can translate text between languages with high accuracy. Examples include software products such as Google Translate and Microsoft Translator to use these.

Sentiment analysis: These algorithms are capable of processing large volumes of text data, such as customer reviews and social media posts, to identify the sentiment or emotion being conveyed. Within brand monitoring and customer service, this feature is used to understand the public's feelings and to improve the user experience.

Chatbots: Natural Language Processing (NLP) techniques allow chatbots to understand and respond to natural language inputs from users. This is one of the most important features for virtual assistants and chatbots that are part of customer support, where there needs to be an efficient yet automated type of interaction.

Text summarizing: NLP algorithms analyzing huge amounts of text input can generate summaries that pick out the most important information. These summaries can be useful for cases of use, including news aggregation and document summarization.

Named entity recognition: NLP algorithms can automatically recognize and extract named entities from text data, such as persons, organizations, and locations (places). This approach is used in information retrieval and data analysis to help organize and make sense of a large set of datasets [60].

ARTIFICIAL INTELLIGENCE APPLICATIONS IN HEALTHCARE

Although traditional views would have predicted that artificial intelligence machines might replace the work of physicians and other healthcare staff members, it is generally anticipated that these tools are expected to ease and augment human work. AI is ready to ease various responsibilities for clinical staff, from administrative workflow and clinical documentation to patient outreach. Moreover, AI can also offer specialized assistance in the areas of image analysis, automation of medical devices, and patient monitoring processes. However, opinions differ on which particular applications of artificial intelligence hold the most promise from a medical perspective.Here are the areas predicted by Forbes to be the most important ones to work on back in 2018. Administration processes, image analysis, robotic surgery virtual assistance, and clinical decision support. In 2018, Accenture published a report, which, of course, included networked machines, dosage error reduction, and cybersecurity. Those same themes were echoed in a report. Based on research published by McKinsey in 2019, the vital categories comprise focused and specialized drugs, robotics-supported surgical treatment, electroceuticals, and related and intellectual devices [61, 62].

Technologies For Skin Cancer Detection

Skin cancer detection techniques include dermoscopy, RCM, OCT, and histopathology, which are shown in Fig. (**3**). Dermoscopy aids in early melanoma diagnosis, RCM provides high-resolution imaging, OCT captures micrometer-resolution images, and histopathology confirms cancer diagnosis through microscopic examination of biopsied tissue.

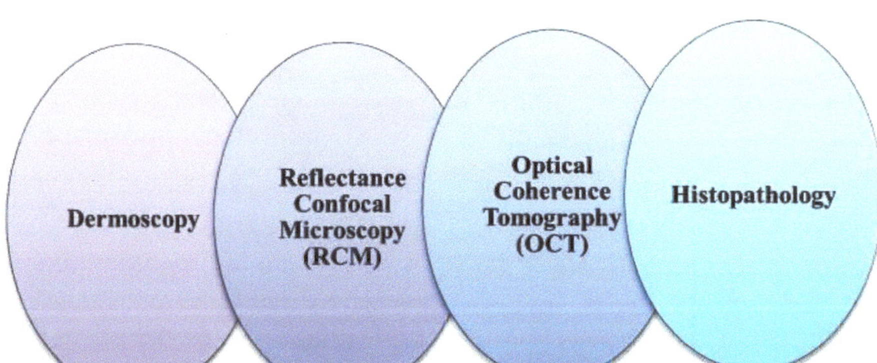

Fig. (3). Technologies for Skin Cancer Detection.

Dermoscopy

Dermoscopy, or dermatoscopy, is a non-invasive imaging procedure used to make the epidermis and papillary dermis more visible for diagnostic purposes. A handheld device, a dermatoscope, is used to further enlarge the skin surface and view it under polarized light. This allows dermatologists to analyze the morphological features of skin lesions in further detail and help differentiate between benign and malignant disorders [63, 64].

Dermoscopy is prescribed to identify skin cancer, particularly melanoma and non-melanoma skin cancers, early. It scans the lesion for features like asymmetry, border, color, diameter, and evolution to see if it can identify them as malignant or benign during diagnosis. The method has been proven to increase diagnostic accuracy compared with eye inspection alone, leading to a dramatic decrease in unnecessary biopsies and an improvement in treatment performance [65].

Limitations and Challenges

Various limitations and challenges of dermoscopy exist despite its advantages.

Operator Dependency: Dermoscopy is highly operator-dependent. However, the poor performance of this result, in particular, is not itself surprising, given the presence of likely high variability at the interpretation level due to dermatologists often seeing only images instead of a profile and potential misdiagnoses. It has been studied that diagnostic outcomes have a high dependency on inter-observer variability.

Learning Curve: Dermoscopy is a difficult technique to learn, and visual skills take time to develop. However, the program that introduces you to cardiac MR interpretation in practice can be a hindrance to new practitioners who are bewildered and do not know how to interpret and render images for clinical use.

Limited to Surface Features: Dermoscopy is restricted to surface features, which means that it does not supply information related to the depth of the dermoscope. While appropriate for various clinical assessments, it does not evaluate deeper dermal structures where malignancies may be clinically important to diagnose in the presence of subcutaneous malignancies.

Technological Constraints: Dermoscopy is used widely, but certain settings, especially low-resource levels, tend to lack access to advanced dermatoscopes and training. This limitation can hinder its utilization and advantage in the early detection of skin cancer.

False Positives and Negatives: Dermoscopy enhances diagnostic accuracy; however, it is not foolproof. Despite these advances, the potential for false positives (benign lesions misclassified as malignant) and false negatives (overlooked malignant lesions) still exists, requiring histological validation [66, 67].

Reflectance Confocal Microscopy (RCM)

Reflectance confocal microscopy is currently the most advanced noninvasive *in vivo* imaging technique for the investigation of cutaneous structures at a depth between the stratum corneum and superficial reticular dermis. This device provides real-time, skin-parallel images with microscopic resolution on the order of magnitude, which is the case with traditional histology tools. It permits imaging of the epidermis through the papillary dermis in real-time. In comparison with conventional histology, resolution is nearly the same. Aside from decreasing the number of unnecessary skin biopsies, it has the advantage that the physician can perform a "virtual biopsy" of the skin to obtain diagnostic information [68].

In Minsky's hands, the world first saw the confocal microscope sometime around the middle of the 1950s. Eventually, RCM as an imaging modality for skin was described by Dr. Rajadhyaksha and his colleagues in 1995. Since then, there has been considerable interest in the application of this method for diagnosing human skin cancers, including melanoma and some inflammatory skin diseases [69].

RCM employs a diode laser to illuminate the skin and detects the reflected light to glean information from cellular structures. Using this technique, an image can be acquired from the epidermis and upper dermal layers, which are typically between 200 and 300 μm deep. This approach is founded on the light backscattering property of structures with differential refractive indices (melanin and keratin), allowing for high-resolution *in vivo* imaging of cell morphology [70].

Applications for Clinical Use

RCM is very helpful for the following:

Diagnosis of Skin Cancers: It helps in the diagnosis of malignant lesions, including melanoma and non-melanoma skin cancers.

In monitoring treatment, RCM can be used to assess therapeutic response in different skin diseases.

Evaluation of Inflammatory Skin Diseases: It will help identify any disorders like psoriasis and dermatitis by understanding cellular changes that accompany these diseases [71].

Limitations and Challenges

Despite its advantages, RCM has several limitations:

Depth of Imaging: Maximum imaging depth is 200–300 μm, and thus, deeper skin lesions or processes may be missed with this technique.

Training Requirements: Operators need to be trained in RCM for image interpretation. This could restrict its global deployment, specifically in low-resource settings.

Field of View: RCM usually has a smaller field of view compared to other imaging systems. Thus, multiple scans may be needed to evaluate larger lesions.

Cost and Accessibility: RCM devices are expensive to purchase, making it difficult for smaller medical practices or institutions that do not often encounter patients who require healthy matic clinical examination services.

Image Quality Issues: The speed of imaging and noise will impact the quality of images acquired, making interpretation difficult [68, 71].

Optical Coherence Tomography (OCT)

Optical Coherence Tomography (OCT) is a non-invasive imaging modality that provides high-resolution cross-sectional images of biological tissues. It has been widely used in the field of ophthalmology to visualize the retina. It makes use of light waves and hence provides the possibility to visualize tissue structures at micrometer resolution [72].

OCT uses low-coherence interferometry to create images, yielding axials in the 5–15 μm range nearly all of the time. This ability enables the detailed mapping of layers in the retina, making it useful for identifying and monitoring a range of eye conditions, such as:

Glaucoma: Evaluation of the thickness of retinal nerve fiber layer.

Age-related Macular Degeneration (AMD): Tracking retinal structure and thickness changes.

Diabetic Eye Disease: Assessment of diabetic retinopathy and macular edema.

Optic Nerve Disorders: Detecting changes to the optic nerve fibers (*e.g.*, due to optic neuritis or non-glaucomatous optic neuropathies) [73].

Limitations and Challenges

Media Opacities: In conditions like thick cataracts or vitreous hemorrhage, where the light cannot pass through properly, the image quality and properties of OCT may also be limited.

Patient Cooperation: The quality of scans may be compromised if patients do not comply because even slight movement can capture an image of poor quality. While recent machines reduce the acquisition time to the minimal possible time to render minimum motion artifact, the patient's compliance holds the utmost importance for obtaining optimal results.

Operator Dependency: The operator may not always be optimal, leading to errors in image acquisition and interpretation. The first generation of OCT systems required that the position be very precise, and artifacts in serial images over time could lead to their misinterpretation. Newer systems with eye-tracking solutions have reduced some of these problems.

Cost and Accessibility: As OCT devices are expensive, they may not be widely available in some lower-resource healthcare settings, which can limit access to patients.

Depth Limitations: The limited depth of penetration reduces its utility for evaluating deeper structures within the eye or other tissues [74, 75].

Histopathology

Histopathology is a subdivision of pathology that deals with the microscopic examination of tissue to study the manifestations of disease. This method is widely used in medicine to identify disease by examining the morphology of tissue and cells for any abnormal organization [76].

Histopathology involves in

Tissue Collection: These samples are collected through biopsies, surgical resections, or autopsies.

Tissue Processing: After collection, the samples are fixed (usually in formalin), embedded in paraffin, cut into thin slices, and stained for visualization under the microscope.

Microscopic Examination: When pathologists examine the stained sections, they look for characteristics of diseases like infections, cancer cells, autoimmune diseases, and various pathological changes [77].

Clinical Applications

Cancer Diagnosis: A major use of the test is to assess tissues for atypical cells, growth patterns, and degree of differentiation, all of which are important for cancer staging and treatment planning.

Infectious Diseases: Infectious Diseases are capable of diagnosing infections by identifying pathogens and inflammatory responses in human tissue samples.

Autoimmune Diseases: Histopathology helps discover the tissue-specific changes associated with autoimmune diseases.

Research and Education: It aids in the understanding of disease mechanisms and therapeutic responses for medical research [78].

Limitations and Challenges

Sample Quality: Histopathological diagnoses are reliant on tissue quality. Samples that have not been preserved or processed appropriately can be incorrectly interpreted.

Interpretation Variability: Depending on the situation, different pathologists might reach a conclusion of nature using the same sample.

Time-Consuming Process: The processing and interpretation of tissue samples can take several days to weeks, leading to delays in diagnosis and treatment.

Depth of Information: Histopathology is limited in the molecular and genetic descriptive power, it can provide within a specimen, which is becoming more significant in personalized medicine.

Technological Limitations: Conventional histopathology is based on 2D imaging, which cannot necessarily characterize the complex three-dimensional tissue anatomy. New techniques such as digital pathology and immunohistochemistry are starting to overcome some of these challenges but need higher resources and training [79].

AI INTEGRATION WITH IMAGING TECHNIQUES

AI algorithms have been used with growing frequency to detect skin cancer, and major methods are already proving to be highly effective. CNN, SVM, and ensemble methods are the three types of algorithms.

Convolutional Neural Networks (CNNs)

These CNNs are examples of deep learning algorithms that have successfully solved image classification problems, such as skin cancer diagnosis. This is achieved by the automated feature extraction of images, making it possible to detect complex patterns correlated with different forms of skin lesions. Several studies have demonstrated the ability of CNNs to classify skin lesions from dermoscopic images with an accuracy similar to a panel of expert dermatologists. For example, CNNs have reportedly surpassed human experts in multiclass skin cancer image classification. It shows the effectiveness of CNNs in malignant *vs.* benign lesion classification [80].

Convolutional neural networks (CNNs) can offer unique advantages in the diagnosis of skin cancer because of their ability to process large datasets and learn from multiple image modalities, such as clinical, dermoscopic, and histologic images. The rising incidence of skin cancer, together with the need for timely and accurate detection, renders this functionality crucial [81].

Support Vector Machines (SVMs)

SVMs used to be another kind of machine learning algorithm that was applied to skin cancer detection. They work by finding a hyperplane in a higher dimensional space that best separates the different species of data points. Abstract Support Vector Machines (SVMs) are applied to classify skin lesions based on photographs from which various features are from the enzyme-linked immunosorbent assay characterization of IgG antibody response in type 1 autoimmune state. While support vector machines (SVMs) have indeed been shown to be effective, they usually need specific hand-crafted feature construction. Furthermore, they will not always work well in cases where we have large amounts of complex visual data compared with CNNs.

To improve classification accuracy, feature extraction methods are often used together with support vector machines (SVM). These techniques have been employed in various research activities, providing a consistent approach to the classification of skin lesions. This is especially helpful in conditions where computational resources are heavy as compared to deep-learning approaches like CNN [82].

Ensemble Methods

Ensemble learning methods are well known because they combine more than one learning algorithm into a predictive model, which generally exhibits better performance than any of the individual components. For instance, for skin cancer detection, ensemble methods can be used to combine the predictions of different classifiers like CNNs and SVMs to improve the accuracy and robustness of the detection process. While this approach enhances the overall diagnostic performance, it also relieves the disadvantages related to solo models [83].

Many studies have shown that ensemble methods can improve the sensitivity of skin cancer detection system and act as a tool for reducing false positives. They utilize the advantages of diverse algorithms, making them particularly well-suited to clinical settings where diagnostic accuracy is crucial [84].

Training AI Models

Dataset Collection and Annotation

Collecting and annotating datasets is one of the earlier challenges in training artificial intelligence models. Pulling a good amount of relevant data for this process for the respective task that the model should perform is needed. For example, if the model is built for image classification, then thousands of well-labeled images are necessary. The annotation process is also important as without it, none of the data can be tagged with the correct output. This provides the model with the ground truth that is required to train upon anything. This can be a tedious process that often requires human labor to ensure accuracy and relevance [85, 86].

Preprocessing and Augmentation

Once the dataset is collected, preprocessing transforms the raw data into a format that can be fed into the training. Functions such as normalizing values, handling missing data, and transforming the data into numerical shapes (if not done before) are all part of this category. Data augmentation techniques are used to expand the dataset artificially and fortify the model. These methods are rotating the picture, flipping it, and adding noise. These steps are important for improving the data quality, reducing overfitting, and providing a high ability to generalize from the training data set to unseen data [87, 88].

Model Training and Validation

The two most essential pieces of building an artificial intelligence model are training and validation. During training, the model adjusts its parameters to minimize whatever error it is making when predicting the input data. This method needs the data to be split independently between the training and validation sets in order to check performance and prevent overfitting. Model performance on validation set: The model performance, which is the accuracy along with other metrics like precision and recall, is evaluated when validating the model. Other approaches to improve the performance of modeling include cross-validation and hyperparameter tuning. The final goal is to produce a model that easily generalizes new unseen data, hence making it possible for deployment in real-world scenarios [89, 90].

Performance Metrics

Accuracy

Accuracy is one of the simplest and most common performance evaluation metrics in classification tasks. The accuracy is the ratio of correct predictions (both True Positive and True Negative) over a total number of instances in the dataset. The formula for finding accuracy is

$$Accuracy = \frac{True\ Positives + True\ Negatives}{Total\ Instances}$$

Although accuracy is an explicative metric of the performance of any given model, it poses great limitations, particularly in class imbalance scenarios. Illustrating with a simple example, consider a dataset where 95% of instances belong to one class. A model achieving 95% accuracy is trivial - simply predicting the majority class always. It may even lead to overconfidence in the performance of a particular model. So, accuracy is a good metrics to check, but it should not be the only factor to measure a model's performance, especially in the case of imbalanced datasets [91, 92].

Sensitivity and Specificity

Sensitivity (also called recall or true positive rate) tells us the proportion of real positives that the model correctly identifies. It is calculated as follows:

$$Sensitivity = \frac{True\ Positives}{True\ Positives + False\ Negatives}$$

Specificity (also called recall or true negative rate) tells us the proportion of real negatives that the model correctly identifies. It is calculated as follows:

$$Specificity = \frac{True\ Negatives}{True\ Negatives + False\ Positives}$$

Combined, sensitivity and specificity provide a more complete picture of model performance in cases where the cost of erroneous positives and the cost of false negatives are not equal. For example, in case of medical diagnostics, having high sensitivity is important to identify a disease, and having high specificity is necessary for healthy people to not be worried unnecessarily or subject to unnecessary tests. In several applications, it is essential to strike the right balance between these two metrics as they result in a much better model selection and deployment decision [93, 94].

ROC Curves

One of the most widely used graphical measures of binary classifier performance is the Receiver Operating Characteristic (ROC) curve, which assesses classifier performance over a range of different thresholds. It plots the True Positive Rate (sensitivity) *versus* the False Positive Rate (1 - specificity) for different threshold values. The Receiver Operating Characteristic (ROC) curve displays this trade-off between sensitivity and specificity so that practitioners can see the effect of changing a decision threshold on detection performance [93].

In the ROC space, a random classifier is represented by a diagonal line, which acts as a baseline for comparison purposes. An ROC curve that bows to the top left corner of the plot indicates high sensitivity (true positive rate) and low false positive rates, so a good model will have its ROC bowing towards the top left corner. The ROC curve allows a stakeholder to pick an optimal threshold for their specific function, whether it be minimizing false negatives, minimizing false positives, or somewhere in between [95, 96].

AUC

Area Under the Curve (AUC) measures the overall performance of the model represented by the ROC curve. The single value indicates how capable the model is in distinguishing between the positive and negative classes. An AUC can range between 0 and 1; an AUC of 0.5 means the model is doing no better than a random guess, while an AUC of 1 indicates that it is a perfect classifier. One thing worth emphasizing is the AUC value itself, as it is threshold-independent, and this implies its usefulness since it gives an idea of the entire classifier performance for all classification thresholds. Thus, it is a more reliable metric for model comparison in scenarios with an imbalanced class distribution. In general, any dataset with an AUC score over 0.7 is considered acceptable; above 0.8 is good, and above 0.9 is excellent. However, it is also the most difficult evaluation metric because the AUC that has a specific understanding means nothing without context and meaning in relation to the use cases associated with every AUC [97, 98].

Various categories of AI with imaging techniques for skin cancer detection are represented in Table **1** with their details.

Table 1. Representation of AI integration with imaging techniques for skin cancer detection.

Category	Details	Reference
AI Algorithms		
Convolutional Neural Networks (CNNs)	Convolutional Neural Networks (CNNs)	[99 - 101]
Support Vector Machines (SVMs)	Used for classification tasks. Effective in high-dimensional spaces and commonly used in early skin cancer detection.	
Ensemble Methods	Combines multiple models (*e.g.*, Random Forest, Gradient Boosting) to improve prediction accuracy and robustness.	
Training AI Models		
Dataset Collection and Annotation	Collecting diverse and representative datasets with proper annotation by dermatologists.	[102, 103]
Preprocessing and Augmentation	Enhancing dataset quality through normalization, resizing, noise reduction, and augmentation techniques like rotation, flipping, *etc*.	
Model Training and Validation	Training models with training datasets and validating with separate validation datasets to avoid overfitting and ensure generalizability.	
Performance Metrics		
Accuracy	Measures the overall correctness of the model predictions. Calculated as (True Positives + True Negatives) / Total Predictions.	[104, 105]
Sensitivity (Recall)	Measures the model's ability to correctly identify positive cases (True Positives / (True Positives + False Negatives).	
Specificity	Measures the model's ability to correctly identify negative cases (True Negatives / (True Negatives + False Positives).	
Receiver Operating Characteristic (ROC) Curves	Graphical plot illustrating the diagnostic ability of a binary classifier system. It shows the trade-off between sensitivity and specificity.	
Area Under the Curve (AUC)	Represents the degree of separability and the performance of the classifier. A higher AUC indicates better performance.	

ETHICAL AND REGULATORY CONSIDERATIONS

In domains such as healthcare, finance, or personal data management, where AI models are introduced for development and deployment, ethical issues arise. Data privacy and security are important to build trust and remain compliant with the law. They safeguard sensitive data by employing measures like encryption, access controls, and data anonymization to prevent unauthorized access and misuse while also ensuring regulatory compliance with GDPR, HIPAA, *etc*. Using more diverse datasets, taking bias detection tools, and performing regular audits to avoid any discrimination must be taken into account when addressing the issue of AI bias. Transparency in the usage of model training and engagement of a variety of stakeholders during development are common ethical practices. Section-specific and global regulatory frameworks need to be managed, creating and preserving documentation trails that you could defend in court if required, alongside other layers of risk mitigation, such as talking to a lawyer. Any info used by AI in healthcare will need to include an informed consent framework that gives patients clear communication on how their data is used, opt-in mechanisms to allow patients to enroll if they want, and the ability for them to withdraw such consent. Explainable AI models and feedback mechanisms promote transparency within organizations, which leads to trust in the technology and continuous improvement [106, 107].

FUTURE DIRECTIONS AND CHALLENGES

There is a lot of potential to make progress on AI for sensitive domains, but learning to overcome challenges will be required. This takes artificial intelligence algorithm advancements to improve accuracy, efficiency, and the capability of managing complex datasets. It also said that these would leverage more advanced approaches (*e.g.*, deep learning and reinforcement learning) to evolve the capabilities of these diagnostics. The synergy of AI with other diagnostic technologies, like molecular diagnostics, is expected to offer a more holistic and multi-modal picture that will eventually help improve the accuracy and reliability of patient outcomes. This effort to create real-time diagnostic and telemedicine software will enable rapid evaluations remotely, allowing for more accessible and responsive medical treatment, especially in areas that are underserved today. Addressing biases in AI models is, therefore, an essential theme that demands continuous work on enhancing dataset diversity and effective bias identification/mitigation mechanisms to treat everyone equitably. And it is also necessary to improve model generalizability. This guarantees that AI systems can reliably operate across a whole spectrum of populations and settings, thereby enhancing their validity, effectiveness, and acceptability in real-world contexts [108, 109].

CONCLUSION

The integration of imaging technology, powered by artificial intelligence, into dermatology, represents a great stride in the early detection and treatment of skin cancer. In this chapter, we explored the role high-end artificial intelligence algorithms and machine learning methods play in how accurate and efficient dermatological cancer diagnostics are. Case studies from some of the leading healthcare institutions have shown that the use of AI-powered technology can increase the capability for diagnosis, reduce patient wait times, and ultimately improve clinical outcomes. AI-powered digital imaging provides a holistic solution as it can perfectly work in tandem with existing diagnostic devices like dermoscopy and molecular diagnostics. This combination enables skin cancer to be diagnosed in its early stages, allowing for a greater chance of successful treatment. However, embedding artificial intelligence in clinical practice is fraught with challenges surrounding patient data confidentiality, bias mitigation 4, regulatory compliance, and provision of informed consent. These issues must be resolved to make sure that the use of AI in healthcare is ethical and effective.

AI has great potential for future applications in dermatology. Continued advances in algorithm refinement, the integration of analytical tools, and real-time/telemedicine developments will further revolutionize the identification and treatment of skin cancer. Addressing these areas will enhance the trustworthiness and fairness of AI-driven solutions by facilitating the generalizability of AI models across diverse populations and reducing bias. Imaging methods driven by artificial intelligence are a paradigm of innovation in combating skin cancer. If it does, that will be a turning point in medical history that could change the processes of early detection and treatment. It promises a future in which healthcare can be accurate, efficient, and accessible to all. As research and technology progress, the use of artificial intelligence (AI) in dermatology will ultimately lead to better patient outcomes and a significant decrease in the global prevalence rate of skin malignancies.

REFERENCES

[1] Arnold M, Singh D, Laversanne M, *et al.* Global Burden of Cutaneous Melanoma in 2020 and Projections to 2040. JAMA Dermatol 2022; 158(5): 495-503. [http://dx.doi.org/10.1001/jamadermatol.2022.0160] [PMID: 35353115]

[2] Arnold Melina. Dermatology, including those for text and data mining. AI Training, And Similar Technologies 2024.

[3] Sial M, Shakeel S, Asim M, Khalil A, Irfan MA, Jan A. Skin scan: cutting-edge AI-powered skin cancer classification app for early diagnosis and prevention. 2024.

[4] Parker ER. The influence of climate change on skin cancer incidence – a review of the evidence. Int J Womens Dermatol. Elsevier Inc. 2021; 7: pp. 17-27.

[5] Watson TPG, Tong M, Bailie J, Ekanayake K, Bailie RS. Relationship between climate change and skin cancer and implications for prevention and management: a scoping review. Public Health. Elsevier B.V. 2024; 227: pp. 243-9.

[6] Heidelberg Berlin. Malignant melanoma 2005.

[7] Garnavi R, Aldeen M, Celebi ME, Varigos G, Finch S. Border detection in dermoscopy images using hybrid thresholding on optimized color channels. Comput Med Imaging Graph 2011; 35(2): 105-15.

[http://dx.doi.org/10.1016/j.compmedimag.2010.08.001] [PMID: 20832992]

[8] Sreelatha T, Subramanyam MV, Giri Prasad MN. Survey work on Early Detection methods of Melanoma Skin Cancer. Research Journal of Pharmacy and Technology. Research Journal of Pharmacy and Technology 2019; 12: pp. 2589-96.

[9] Rogers H W, *et al.* Associations of Internal Medicine Residency Milestone Ratings and Certification Examination Scores With Patient Outcomes 2024.

[10] Glazer AM, Winkelmann RR, Farberg AS, Rigel DS. Analysis of trends in US melanoma incidence and mortality. JAMA Dermatol. American Medical Association 2017; 153: pp. 225-6. [http://dx.doi.org/10.1001/jamadermatol.2016.4512]

[11] Jennings L. Chrysalyne; Schmults D. Management of High-Risk Cutaneous Squamous Cell Carcinoma. Vol. 3. J Clin Aesthet Dermatol 2010.

[12] South C, Selwood TS. Malignant transformation of solar keratoses to squamous cell carcinoma. Anti-Cancer Council of Victoria 1988.

[13] Marques E, Teris , Chen M. Actinic keratosis continuing education activity. 2023. Available from: https://www.ncbi.nlm.nih.gov/books/NBK557401/

[14] Eigentler TK, Leiter U, Häfner HM, Garbe C, Röcken M, Breuninger H. Survival of Patients with Cutaneous Squamous Cell Carcinoma: Results of a Prospective Cohort Study. J Invest Dermatol 2017; 137(11): 2309-15. [http://dx.doi.org/10.1016/j.jid.2017.06.025] [PMID: 28736229]

[15] Pekarek DPM B, Buck DPM S, Osher DPM L. A Comprehensive Review on Marjolin's Ulcers: Diagnosis and Treatment 2011.

[16] Awad R, Andrade JCB, Mousa H, Mahmoud F. Invasive Basal Cell Carcinoma of the Skin Treated Successfully with Vismodegib: A Case Report. Perm J 2018; 22(3): 17-181. [http://dx.doi.org/10.7812/TPP/17-181] [PMID: 30005721]

[17] Wang YJ, Tang TY, Wang JY, Huang YK, Wu YH. Genital basal cell carcinoma, a different pathogenesis from sun-exposed basal cell carcinoma? A case-control study of 30 cases. J Cutan Pathol 2018; 45(9): 688-95. [http://dx.doi.org/10.1111/cup.13304] [PMID: 29920730]

[18] Schmults CD, Blitzblau R, Aasi SZ, *et al.* Basal Cell Skin Cancer, Version 2.2024, NCCN Clinical Practice Guidelines in Oncology. J Natl Compr Canc Netw 2023; 21(11): 1181-203. [http://dx.doi.org/10.6004/jnccn.2023.0056] [PMID: 37935106]

[19] Breslow AMD. Thickness. Cross-Sectional Areas and Depth of Invasion in the Prognosis of Cutaneous Melanoma 2024.

[20] Scolyer RA, Long GV, Thompson JF. Evolving concepts in melanoma classification and their relevance to multidisciplinary melanoma patient care. Mol Oncol. John Wiley and Sons Ltd 2011; 5: pp. 124-36. [http://dx.doi.org/10.1016/j.molonc.2011.03.002]

[21] Swetter SM, Kashani-Sabet M, Johannet P, Reddy SA, Phillips TL. Leibel and Phillips Textbook of Radiation Oncology (Third Edition). Melanoma Get rights and content First-page preview Share 2010; p. 67.

[22] Greenwald HS, Friedman EB, Osman I. Superficial spreading and nodular melanoma are distinct biological entities. Melanoma Res 2012; 22(1): 1-8. [http://dx.doi.org/10.1097/CMR.0b013e32834e6aa0] [PMID: 22108608]

[23] Lasithiotakis KG, Leiter U, Gorkievicz R, *et al.* The incidence and mortality of cutaneous melanoma in southern Germany. Cancer 2006; 107(6): 1331-9. [http://dx.doi.org/10.1002/cncr.22126] [PMID: 16909413]

[24] Long GV, Menzies AM, Nagrial AM, *et al.* Prognostic and clinicopathologic associations of

oncogenic BRAF in metastatic melanoma. J Clin Oncol 2011; 29(10): 1239-46. [http://dx.doi.org/10.1200/JCO.2010.32.4327] [PMID: 21343559]

[25] Asgari MM, Sokil MM, Warton EM, Iyer J, Paulson KG, Nghiem P. Effect of host, tumor, diagnostic, and treatment variables on outcomes in a large cohort with Merkel cell carcinoma. JAMA Dermatol 2014; 150(7): 716-23. [http://dx.doi.org/10.1001/jamadermatol.2013.8116] [PMID: 24807619]

[26] Leroux-Kozal V, Lévêque N, Brodard V, *et al.* Merkel cell carcinoma: histopathologic and prognostic features according to the immunohistochemical expression of Merkel cell polyomavirus large T antigen correlated with viral load. Hum Pathol 2015; 46(3): 443-53. [http://dx.doi.org/10.1016/j.humpath.2014.12.001] [PMID: 25623078]

[27] Heath M, Jaimes N, Lemos B, *et al.* Clinical characteristics of Merkel cell carcinoma at diagnosis in 195 patients: the AEIOU features. J Am Acad Dermatol 2008; 58(3): 375-81. [http://dx.doi.org/10.1016/j.jaad.2007.11.020] [PMID: 18280333]

[28] Haymerle G, Fochtmann A, Kunstfeld R, Pammer J, Erovic BM. Management of Merkel cell carcinoma of unknown primary origin: the Vienna Medical School experience. Eur Arch Otorhinolaryngol 2015; 272(2): 425-9. [http://dx.doi.org/10.1007/s00405-014-2974-x] [PMID: 24633244]

[29] Grange F, *et al.* How Can Operating Rooms Be Greener? Primary Cutaneous Diffuse Large B-Cell Lymphoma, Leg Type: Clinicopathologic Features and Prognostic Analysis in 60 Cases. 2014. Available from: https://jamanetwork.com/journals/jamadermatology/article-abstract/654378

[30] Grange F, *et al.* Primary Cutaneous Diffuse Large B-Cell Lymphoma, Leg Type. 2007. Available from: https://jamanetwork.com/journals/jamadermatology/article-abstract/1839265

[31] Kim YH, Willemze R, Pimpinelli N, Whittaker S, Olsen EA, Ranki A, *et al.* TNM classification system for primary cutaneous lymphomas other than mycosis fungoides and Sézary syndrome: A proposal of the International Society for Cutaneous Lymphomas (ISCL) and the Cutaneous Lymphoma Task Force of the European Organization of Research and Treatment of Cancer (EORTC). Blood. American Society of Hematology 2007; 110: pp. 479-84.

[32] Shakya S. Screening for Melanoma for At-Risk Population: A Practice Guide. 2019. Available from: https://digscholarship.unco.edu/capstoneshttps://digscholarship.unco.edu/capstones/61

[33] Brozek W, Clemens P, Ulmer H, *et al.* Evaluation of a Population-Based Targeted Screening Approach for Skin Cancer with Long-Time Follow-Up in Austria including Potential Effects on Melanoma Mortality. Cancers (Basel) 2024; 16(7): 1283. [http://dx.doi.org/10.3390/cancers16071283] [PMID: 38610961]

[34] Curiel-Lewandrowski C, Chen SC, Swetter SM. Screening and prevention measures for melanoma: is there a survival advantage?. Curr Oncol Rep 2012; 14(5): 458-67. [http://dx.doi.org/10.1007/s11912-012-0256-6] [PMID: 22907282]

[35] Coroiu A, Moran C, Bergeron C, *et al.* Short and long-term barriers and facilitators of skin self-examination among individuals diagnosed with melanoma. BMC Cancer 2020; 20(1): 123. [http://dx.doi.org/10.1186/s12885-019-6476-5] [PMID: 32059700]

[36] Manne S, Heckman CJ, Frederick S, *et al.* A Digital Intervention to Improve Skin Self-Examination Among Survivors of Melanoma: Protocol for a Type-1 Hybrid Effectiveness-Implementation Randomized Trial. JMIR Res Protoc 2024; 13(1): 52689. [http://dx.doi.org/10.2196/52689] [PMID: 38345836]

[37] Robinson JK, Gaber R, Hultgren B, *et al.* Skin self-examination education for early detection of melanoma: a randomized controlled trial of Internet, workbook, and in-person interventions. J Med Internet Res 2014; 16(1): 7. [http://dx.doi.org/10.2196/jmir.2883] [PMID: 24418949]

[38] Bhurosy T, Heckman CJ, Riley M. Prevalence and correlates of skin self-examination behaviors

among melanoma survivors: A systematic review. Transl Behav Med. Oxford University Press 2020; 10: pp. 1120-33.

[39] Pham JP, Allen N, Star P, *et al.* Full-body skin examination in screening for cutaneous malignancy: a focus on concealed sites and the practices of Australian dermatologists. Int J Dermatol 2024; 63(4): 467-73. [http://dx.doi.org/10.1111/ijd.16942] [PMID: 38036942]

[40] Pham JP, Allen N, Star P, *et al.* Full-body skin examination in screening for cutaneous malignancy: A focus on concealed sites and the practices of international dermatologists. JEADV Clin Pract 2024; 3(4): 1132-9. [http://dx.doi.org/10.1002/jvc2.437]

[41] Policy P. Gestational Age From Blind Ultrasound Sweeps Read the study Get the latest from JAMA Dermatology, including those for text and data mining, AI training, and similar technologies Skin Examination Behavior: The Role of Melanoma History, Skin Type, Psychosocial Factors, and Region of Residence in Determi 2020. Available from: https://jamanetwork.com/journals/jamadermatology/article-abstract/1216970

[42] Youl PH, Baade PD, Parekh S, English D, Elwood M, Aitken JF. Association between melanoma thickness, clinical skin examination and socioeconomic status: Results of a large population-based study. Int J Cancer 2011; 128(9): 2158-65. [http://dx.doi.org/10.1002/ijc.25540] [PMID: 20607832]

[43] Janda M, *et al.* Clinical Skin Examination Outcomes After a Video-Based Behavioral Intervention: Analysis From a Randomized Clinical Trial | Can 2024. Available from: https://jamanetwork.com/journals/jamadermatology/article-abstract/1832204

[44] Stratton DB, Loescher LJ. Educational interventions for primary care providers to improve clinical skin examination for skin cancer. J Am Assoc Nurse Pract. Lippincott Williams and Wilkins 2020; 32: pp. 369-79. [http://dx.doi.org/10.1097/JXX.0000000000000235]

[45] Zalaudek I, *et al.* Time Required for a Complete Skin Examination With and Without Dermoscopy: A Prospective, Randomized Multicenter Study 2008. Available from: https://jamanetwork.com/journals/jamadermatology/article-abstract/419639

[46] Haleem A, Javaid M, Asim Qadri M, Pratap Singh R, Suman R. Artificial intelligence (AI) applications for marketing: A literature-based study. International Journal of Intelligent Networks. KeAi Communications Co. 2022; 3: pp. 119-32.

[47] Sennott SC, Akagi L, Lee M, Rhodes A. AAC and Artificial Intelligence (AI). Top Lang Disord 2019; 39(4): 389-403. [http://dx.doi.org/10.1097/TLD.0000000000000197] [PMID: 34012187]

[48] Chojnowska M. The Basics of Artificial Intelligence: Understanding the Key Concepts and Terminology 2023. Available from: https://sunscrapers.com/blog/the-basics-of-artificial-intellig-nce-understanding-the-key-concepts-and-terminology/#artificial-intelligence---definition

[49] Habehh H, Gohel S. Machine Learning in Healthcare. Curr Genomics 2021; 22(4): 291-300. [http://dx.doi.org/10.2174/1389202922666210705124359] [PMID: 35273459]

[50] Manakitsa N, Maraslidis GS, Moysis L, Fragulis GF. A review of machine learning and deep learning for object detection, semantic segmentation, and human action recognition in machine and robotic vision. Technologies. Multidisciplinary Digital Publishing Institute (MDPI) 2024; 12.

[51] Anusuya MA, Katti SK. Speech recognition by machine: a review. Int J Comput Sci Inf Secur 2009; 6 Available from: http://sites.google.com/site/ijcsis/

[52] Byrapu Reddy SR, Kanagala P, Ravichandran P, Pulimamidi DR, Sivarambabu PV, Polireddi NSA. Effective fraud detection in e-commerce: Leveraging machine learning and big data analytics. Meas Sensors 2024; 33: 101138.

[http://dx.doi.org/10.1016/j.measen.2024.101138]

[53] Xu K, Zhou H, Zheng H, Zhu M, Xin Q. Intelligent Classification and Personalized Recommendation of E-commerce Products Based on Machine Learning 2024.
[http://dx.doi.org/10.54254/2755-2721/64/20241365]

[54] Javaid M, Haleem A, Pratap Singh R, Suman R, Rab S. Significance of machine learning in healthcare: Features, pillars and applications. International Journal of Intelligent Networks 2022; 3: 58-73.
[http://dx.doi.org/10.1016/j.ijin.2022.05.002]

[55] Taye MM. Understanding of Machine Learning with Deep Learning: Architectures, Workflow, Applications and Future Directions. Computers. MDPI 2023; 12.

[56] Misra S, Li H. Chapter 7 Deep neural network architectures to approximate the fluid-filled pore size distributions of subsurface geological formations 2020. Available from: https://www.sciencedirect.com/science/article/abs/pii/B9780128177365000077
[http://dx.doi.org/10.1016/B978-0-12-817736-5.00007-7]

[57] Soori M, Arezoo B, Dastres R. Artificial intelligence, machine learning and deep learning in advanced robotics, a review. Cognitive Robotics. KeAi Communications Co. 2023; 3: pp. 54-70.

[58] Davenport T, Kalakota R. The potential for artificial intelligence in healthcare. Future Healthc J 2019; 6(2): 94-8.
[http://dx.doi.org/10.7861/futurehosp.6-2-94]

[59] Nadkarni PM, Ohno-Machado L, Chapman WW. Natural language processing: an introduction. J Am Med Inform Assoc 2011; 18(5): 544-51.
[http://dx.doi.org/10.1136/amiajnl-2011-000464] [PMID: 21846786]

[60] Chowdhury GG. Natural language processing. Annu Rev Inf Sci Technol 2003; 37 Available from: http://eprints.cdlr.strath.ac.uk/2611/

[61] Bohr A, Memarzadeh K. The rise of artificial intelligence in healthcare applications. Artificial Intelligence in Healthcare. Elsevier 2020; pp. 25-60.
[http://dx.doi.org/10.1016/B978-0-12-818438-7.00002-2]

[62] Yousef Shaheen M. Applications of Artificial Intelligence (AI) in healthcare 2021. Available from: https://www.scienceopen.com/

[63] Soglia S, Pérez-Anker J, Lobos Guede N, Giavedoni P, Puig S, Malvehy J. Diagnostics Using Non-Invasive Technologies in Dermatological Oncology. Cancers. MDPI 2022; 14.

[64] Dobre eg, Surcel M, Constantin C, Ilie MA, Caruntu A, Caruntu C, *et al.* Skin Cancer Pathobiology at a Glance: A Focus on Imaging Techniques and Their Potential for Improved Diagnosis and Surveillance in Clinical Cohorts. International Journal of Molecular Sciences. MDPI 2023; 24.

[65] Narayanamurthy V, Padmapriya P, Noorasafrin A, Pooja B, Hema K, Firus Khan AY, *et al.* Skin cancer detection using non-invasive techniques. RSC Adv. Royal Society of Chemistry 2018; 8: pp. 28095-130.
[http://dx.doi.org/10.1039/C8RA04164D]

[66] Foltz EA, Witkowski A, Becker AL, Latour E, Lim JY, Hamilton A, *et al.* Artificial intelligence applied to non-invasive imaging modalities in identification of nonmelanoma skin cancer: A systematic review. Cancers. Multidisciplinary Digital Publishing Institute (MDPI) 2024; 16.
[http://dx.doi.org/10.3390/cancers16030629]

[67] Mahmoud NM, Soliman AM. Early automated detection system for skin cancer diagnosis using artificial intelligent techniques. Sci Rep 2024; 14(1): 9749.
[http://dx.doi.org/10.1038/s41598-024-59783-0] [PMID: 38679633]

[68] Waddell A, Star P, Guitera P. Advances in the use of reflectance confocal microscopy in melanoma. Melanoma Manag. Newlands Press Ltd 2018; 5.

[http://dx.doi.org/10.2217/mmt-2018-0001]

[69] Rossi A, Hammond S, Rao Babar. An introduction to reflectance confocal microscopy 2019. Available from: https://practicaldermatology.com/topics/skin-cancer-photoprotection/an-introductio--to-reflectance-confocal-microscopy/23150/

[70] Hofmann-Wellenhof R, Wurm EMT, Ahlgrimm-Siess V, *et al.* Reflectance confocal microscopy--state-of-art and research overview. Semin Cutan Med Surg 2009; 28(3): 172-9. [http://dx.doi.org/10.1016/j.sder.2009.06.004] [PMID: 19782941]

[71] Levine A, Markowitz O. Introduction to reflectance confocal microscopy and its use in clinical practice. JAAD Case Rep 2018; 4(10): 1014-23. [http://dx.doi.org/10.1016/j.jdcr.2018.09.019] [PMID: 30456275]

[72] Schmitt JM. Optical coherence tomography (OCT): a review. IEEE J Sel Top Quantum Electron 1999; 5(4): 1205-15. [http://dx.doi.org/10.1109/2944.796348]

[73] James G. ISP Focus Issue: Optical Coherence Tomography (OCT) in Ophthalmology 2009.

[74] Turbert D, By R, Gregori NZ. What Is Optical Coherence Tomography? ¿Qué es una tomografía de coherencia óptica? 2023. Available from: https://www.aao.org/eye-health/treatments/what-is-opti-al-coherence-tomography

[75] Peter M. A Note on Optical Coherence Tomography 2021.

[76] Paparella MM. Mondini's deafness: a review of histopathology. Ann Otol Rhinol Laryngol 1980; 89(2): 1-10.

[77] Titford M. A short history of histopathology technique. J Histotechnol. National Society for Histotechnology 2006; 29: pp. 99-110. [http://dx.doi.org/10.1179/his.2006.29.2.99]

[78] Meng X, Zou T. Clinical applications of graph neural networks in computational histopathology: a review. Comput Biol Med 2023. Available from: https://doi.org/./j.compbiomed

[79] Bosman FT, Nieuwenhuijzen Kruseman AC. Clinical Labeled Antibody Method Immunoperoxidase Methods in Diagnostic Histopathology. 1979; 27.

[80] Foltz EA, Witkowski A, Becker AL, Latour E, Lim JY, Hamilton A, *et al.* Artificial intelligence applied to non-invasive imaging modalities in identification of nonmelanoma skin cancer: A systematic review. Cancers. Multidisciplinary Digital Publishing Institute (MDPI) 2024; 16. [http://dx.doi.org/10.3390/cancers16030629]

[81] Goyal M, Knackstedt T, Yan S, Hassanpour S. Artificial intelligence-based image classification methods for diagnosis of skin cancer: Challenges and opportunities. Comput Biol Med. Elsevier Ltd 2020; 127.

[82] Liopyris K, Gregoriou S, Dias J, Stratigos AJ. Artificial Intelligence in Dermatology: Challenges and Perspectives. Dermatol Ther (Heidelb) 2022; 12(12): 2637-51. [http://dx.doi.org/10.1007/s13555-022-00833-8] [PMID: 36306100]

[83] Hosseinzadeh M, Hussain D, Mahmood FMZ, Alenizi FA, Varzeghani AN, Asghari P, *et al.* A model for skin cancer using a combination of ensemble learning and deep learning. PLoS One 2024; 19(5)

[84] Venkatesh KP, Raza M, Kvedar J. AI-based skin cancer detection: the balance between access and overutilization. NPJ Digit Med. Nature Research 2023; 6.

[85] Daniş FS, Naskali AT, Cemgil AT, Ersoy C. An Indoor Localization Dataset and Data Collection Framework with High Precision Position Annotation. 2022. Available from: http://arxiv.org/abs/2209.02270

[86] Cleland I, Donnelly MP, Nugent CD, Hallberg J, Espinilla M, Garcia-Constantino M. Collection of a diverse, realistic and annotated dataset for wearable activity recognition. 2018 IEEE International

Conference on Pervasive Computing and Communications Workshops, PerCom Workshops 2018. 555-60.

[87] Fan C, Chen M, Wang X, Wang J, Huang B. A Review of Data Preprocessing Techniques Toward Efficient and Reliable Knowledge Discovery From Building Operational Data. Frontiers in Energy Research. Frontiers Media S.A. 2021; 9.

[88] Maharana K, Mondal S, Nemade B. A review: Data pre-processing and data augmentation techniques. Glob Transit Proc 2022; 3(1): 91-9. [http://dx.doi.org/10.1016/j.gltp.2022.04.020]

[89] Sarker IH. Deep learning: A comprehensive overview on techniques, taxonomy, applications and research directions. SN Comput Sci. Springer 2021; 2.

[90] Ho SY, Phua K, Wong L, Bin Goh WW. Extensions of the external validation for checking learned model interpretability and generalizability. Patterns. Cell Press 2020; 1. [http://dx.doi.org/10.1016/j.patter.2020.100129]

[91] Orozco-Arias S, Piña JS, Tabares-Soto R, Castillo-Ossa LF, Guyot R, Isaza G. Measuring performance metrics of machine learning algorithms for detecting and classifying transposable elements. Processes (Basel) 2020; 8(6): 638. [http://dx.doi.org/10.3390/pr8060638]

[92] Erickson BJ, Kitamura F. Magician's corner: 9. performance metrics for machine learning models. Radiol Artif Intell. Radiological Society of North America Inc 2021; 3.

[93] Monaghan TF, Rahman SN, Agudelo CW, Wein AJ, Lazar JM, Everaert K, *et al.* Foundational statistical principles in medical research: Sensitivity, specificity, positive predictive value, and negative predictive value. Medicina, Lithuania: MDPI AG 2021; 57.

[94] Shreffler J, Huecker MR. Diagnostic Testing Accuracy: Sensitivity, Specificity, Predictive Values and Likelihood Ratios 2023. Available from: https://www.ncbi.nlm.nih.gov/books/NBK557491/

[95] Richardson E, Trevizani R, Greenbaum JA, Carter H, Nielsen M, Peters B. The receiver operating characteristic curve accurately assesses imbalanced datasets. Patterns (N Y) 2024; 5(6): 100994. [http://dx.doi.org/10.1016/j.patter.2024.100994] [PMID: 39005487]

[96] Hajian-Tilaki K. Receiver Operating Characteristic (ROC) Curve Analysis for Medical Diagnostic Test Evaluation. Caspian J Intern Med 2013; 4(2): 627-35. [PMID: 24009950]

[97] Hand DJ. Measuring classifier performance: a coherent alternative to the area under the ROC curve. Mach Learn 2009; 77(1): 103-23. [http://dx.doi.org/10.1007/s10994-009-5119-5]

[98] Turner JR. Area Under the Curve (AUC). Encyclopedia of Behavioral Medicine. Springer International Publishing 2020; pp. 146-6. [http://dx.doi.org/10.1007/978-3-030-39903-0_986]

[99] Chapman & Hall Ensemble Methods Foundations and Algorithms. 2012.

[100] Kattenborn T, Leitloff J, Schiefer F, Hinz S. Review on Convolutional Neural Networks (CNN) in vegetation remote sensing. ISPRS Journal of Photogrammetry and Remote Sensing. Elsevier B.V. 2021; 173: pp. 24-49.

[101] Ingo Steinward AC. Ingo Steinward AC 2018.

[102] Kattenborn T, Schiefer F, Frey J, Feilhauer H, Mahecha MD, Dormann CF. Spatially autocorrelated training and validation samples inflate performance assessment of convolutional neural networks. ISPRS Open J Photogramm Remote Sens 2022; 5 [http://dx.doi.org/10.1016/j.ophoto.2022.100018]

[103] Duong HT, Nguyen-Thi TA. A review: preprocessing techniques and data augmentation for sentiment analysis. Comput Soc Netw 2021; 8(1): 1.

[http://dx.doi.org/10.1186/s40649-020-00080-x]

[104] Kleijnen JPC, Smits MT. Performance metrics in supply chain management. J Oper Res Soc 2003; 54(5): 507-14.
[http://dx.doi.org/10.1057/palgrave.jors.2601539]

[105] Banker RD, Chang H, Janakiraman SN, Konstans C. A balanced scorecard analysis of performance metrics. Eur J Oper Res. 2004; pp. 423-36.
[http://dx.doi.org/10.1016/S0377-2217(03)00179-6]

[106] Mennella C, Maniscalco U, De Pietro G, Esposito M. Ethical and regulatory challenges of AI technologies in healthcare: A narrative review. Heliyon. Elsevier Ltd 2024; 10.

[107] Naik N, Hameed BMZ, Shetty DK, *et al.* Legal and Ethical Consideration in Artificial Intelligence in Healthcare: Who Takes Responsibility?. Front Surg 2022; 9: 862322.
[http://dx.doi.org/10.3389/fsurg.2022.862322] [PMID: 35360424]

[108] Sundar R, Choudhury ZH, Chiranjivi M, Parasa G, Ravuri P, Sivaram M, *et al.* Future directions of artificial intelligence integration: Managing strategies and opportunities. J Intell Fuzzy Syst 2024; 46(3): 7109-22.
[http://dx.doi.org/10.3233/JIFS-238830]

[109] Fink O, Wang Q, Svensén M, Dersin P, Lee WJ, Ducoffe M. Potential, challenges and future directions for deep learning in prognostics and health management applications. Eng Appl Artif Intell 2020; 92: 103678.
[http://dx.doi.org/10.1016/j.engappai.2020.103678]

CHAPTER 4

Role of IoT in Remote Dermatology Monitoring

Sunita[1], **Akhil Sharma**[1], **Shaweta Sharma**[2], **Neeraj Kumar Fuloria**[3] and **Ashish Verma**[4,*]

[1] *R. J. College of Pharmacy, Raipur, Uttar Pradesh , India*

[2] *School of Medical and Allied Sciences, Galgotias University, Uttar Pradesh-201310, India*

[3] *Department of Pharmaceutical Chemistry, Faculty of Pharmacy, AIMST University, Semeling Campus, Bedong-08100, Malaysia*

[4] *Mangalmay Pharmacy College, Greater Noida, Uttar Pradesh-201306, India*

Abstract: Skin diseases are among the most prevalent issues in contemporary times that must be examined. The diagnostic process is still based on the opinions and expertise of medical professionals. A wrong diagnosis, diagnostic lag, or an inability to diagnose can have serious or fatal outcomes. The Internet of Things implies connectivity, heterogeneity, and a huge number of devices joining daily as technology advances and puts away insightful gadgets' floods massively. This has led to a need for context-aware platforms anywhere and everywhere. Nonetheless, this divergence of knowledge needs to be integrated and unified to prepare the ground for achieving the goals above and firmly establishing the IoT paradigm. This chapter highlighted the employment of IoT devices for remote monitoring of skin conditions using wearable devices, smart sensors, and mobile applications. It also highlights IoT Technologies (such as AI and machine learning, cloud computing, big data analytics, and telemedicine platforms) for remote monitoring of dermatology. It concluded by discussing the application of IoT in remote dermatology.

Keywords: Cloud computing, Dermatology, IoT, Remote monitoring, Smart sensors.

INTRODUCTION

The Healthcare sector is considered the backbone of any nation for growth and development. In rural areas, because of the dirtiness, inadequate basic amenities, and overpopulation, skin issues are highlighted. Season and temperature are the geographical factors that influence skin disease prevalence [1]. Skin is one of the

* **Corresponding author Ashish Verma:** Mangalmay Pharmacy College, Greater Noida, Uttar Pradesh-201306, India; E-mail: ashishsing264@gmail.com

Akhil Sharma, Shaweta Sharma, Shivkanya Fuloria & Sudhir Kumar (Eds.)

last frontiers in healthcare, and diagnosing and treating skin conditions remains a nascent yet needy area. They are often neglected and considered non-fatal diseases. Neglected skin disease leads to discomfort, side effects, chronic disfigurement, and often malignant skin [2]. With the pace of technological advancement, medical and healthcare industries are growing at an accelerating pace. The healthcare industry is now focused on providing large-scale, high-quality diagnostic services, which will provide access to healthcare for a larger population. One of the most suggested technologies for real-time, remote health tracking is IoT-based health monitoring [3].

Today, the Internet of Things (IoT) is increasingly applied in a great number of applications, and its significance is growing in our common locks. IoT technology is also evolving in the healthcare monitoring system to offer efficient emergency services to patients [4]. It is also an E-health application in various aspects, such as early detection of medical problems, emergency alarms, and computer-assisted rehabilitation processes. The subject is connected to the sensor to monitor health, and these smartphones have become an indispensable part of people's daily lives. An end-to-end surveillance system has been developed, which focuses on real-time data acquisition from wards 1 and diagnostic devices, mining these data for effective and automated healthcare [5]. The IoT healthcare system provides very good monitoring and tracking systems that are important in managing people's resources. Cloud computing is used to manage healthcare data, and it offers resource-sharing functionalities such as flexibility, scalable data storage, early data service integration, parallel processing, and security issues [6].

Hence, wearable sensors can be implanted in patients with a very short battery life in the IoT-based healthcare system. Patients also have to charge these and mobile devices often, which may fatigue them over time and require nurse engagement, hampering the use experience. Cloud data centers also consume a lot of energy, indirectly promoting the cost of cloud computing. However, the health monitoring system needs high cloud availability with low latency and power consumption. Another problem of healthcare monitoring is the security that the attacker or hackers can easily corrupt the data. So, a privacy-preserving IoT-based healthcare system has to be formulated, and it needs to be accepted by the patient side for better transferring of data. A smaller number of research works are proposed to enhance the data transmission security in IoT systems. Research studies about IoT-based healthcare systems examine the aspects of precision, computation time, and present challenges during implementation [7].

The connected objects in real-time technology across the internet make IoT one of the growing techs. The convergence from an object to a smart object (the two-way interaction) is why it is popular in various industries. It has a lifetime effect on health tracking, controlling, and clinical delivery of patients' bodily statistics. The sensors are connected to the patients, and the data is attached to the controlling devices and then sent to the health monitoring unit [8]. In some cases, to manage a part of data with security on cloud storage. The IoT is a developing field, and one of the essential aspects is security because transmitting data from the sensor to the cloud center is a potential threat to integrity and confidentiality. In addition, since data obtained from low-resource devices are complex to encrypt [9].

Cloud is a distributed environment, so it is the best option for storing medical data where doctors can access it and *vice versa*, providing more flexibility in remotely caring for patients. The complexity of the architecture of sending and receiving data turns into a handshake between IoT and Cloud for real-time processing. A new hybrid approach framework for managing real-time IoT data and scientific-based irrelevant IoT data is proposed to simplify the complexity of IoT as well [10].

Components of IoT System

Things with Networked Sensors and Actuators (TNSA), Raw Information and Processed Data Stores (RI-PD-S), and Analytical and Computing Engines (ACE) are the three primary components of the Internet of Things. Table **1** describes the component functions of the IoT system.

Table 1. The function of IoT components.

S. No.	Components	Function
1	Things with Networked Sensors and Actuators (TNSA)	Gathers data from items or substances concentrated by a particular application area [11].
2	Raw Information and Processed Data Stores (RI-PD-S)	It retains the information gathered in various formats, including text, data, pictures, videos, models, *etc* [12].
3	Analytical and Computing Engines (ACE)	It facilitates communication between humans and machines and permits feedback based on human needs. It also permits analysis based on the computing model selected according to the specifications [13].

The building blocks of IoT commence with the Things with Networked Sensors and Actuators, which sense the exact information on user requests. It can sense the data over a period defined by the user. After that, the sensed data is stored as Raw Data and processed in the data storage element in the Internet of Things so TNSA can communicate with RI-PD-S. The report states are delivered, allowing the interaction to occur and remain in different shapes (text, data, photos, and videos). The Analytical and Computing Engine (ACE) is the third component of

IoT and is responsible for the logical analysis of stored data and decision-making, depending on several models. It allows the ACE to communicate with the RI- PD-S unit. A series of iterative steps is then followed to reach the end targets of the user, and all this is implemented through logical reasoning. The third of these components enables server and cloud analytics, human-machine interaction, and machine learning. Human-machine interactive learning sessions of Things with Networked Sensors and Actuators (TNSA) form a coordinating controller to bring feedback from TNSA based on H-ML or control commands/requests to the Things with Networked Sensors and Actuators Component [14].

DERMATOLOGY

Dermatology is the medical specialty that cares for conditions affecting the skin, hair, and nails in pediatric and adult patients [15]. The skin has many functions besides enclosing and encapsulating all the deeper structures. The superficial epidermis is an upper layer of self-renewing keratinocyte-dominated tissue that becomes red and scaly during superficial inflammatory responses due to irritation or infection [16]. Directly underneath is the dermis, which has skin appendages, blood vessels, and connective tissues. These appendages - which consist of the eccrine and apocrine sweat glands, nails, and the pilosebaceous unit (the site of inflammation in rosacea, acne vulgaris, and alopecia)- derive from epidermal buds that penetrate the dermis during early development. The subcutaneous tissue is found over the muscular fascia below the dermis in most body regions. It comprises larger trunks of veins and nerves that pass through, along with adipocytes [17].

Every dermatological condition can be viewed as an alteration of these three cell and structural components. A healthy skin barrier is essential to normal physiology and development, as loss of function leads to nearly all of the more than 3000 dermatologic disorders through excessive inflammation or autoinflammation, abnormal neurologic signals, or metabolic disturbances in normal functionality [18]. The exact reasons may be difficult to determine, as many dermatological conditions have unknown etiology. This can lead to dermatoses being seen in atypical forms; some diseases may have similar clinical presentations [19].

Common Dermatological Condition

Skin illnesses are associated with abnormalities in the layers or components of human skin. It has impacted individuals of all ages, genders, ethnicities, and social or economic status. Dry skin, acne problems, and hyperpigmentation are the three main types of skin disorders that almost all people around the globe deal with to a certain extent. Sometimes, it manifests itself in itching and irritated skin.

Most skin diseases were shown to be caused by particular defects in structural proteins, enzymes, or lipid metabolism. Moreover, alterations of the barrier function deficiency associated with proteins or lipids may increase transepidermal water loss due to stratum corneum barrier dysfunction. This adverse situation causes skin integrity over time to decline [20].

Dry Skin

Dry skin is often associated with low sebum or natural oils. Variables that cause people to develop dry skin include low humidity, low ambient temperature, and chemical/microbial exposure. Another study showed that the overuse of abrasive cleansers, soaps, and astringents, along with sun exposure, may speed up the development of dry skin syndrome. These are a few crucial elements to consider when choosing an efficient skin disease management strategy catered to each patient's unique requirements [21].

Dry skin can affect both adults and children, which, if untreated, can lead to an irregularity followed by skin diseases eventually. Any skin condition beyond the normal dry state is considered extremely dry [22]. Follicular barrier function impairment, seen in atopic dermatitis (AD), psoriasis (PS), ichthyosis (IC), and contact dermatitis, is often correlated with dry skin. The terms dermatitis and eczema are often used interchangeably to describe a polymorphic inflammatory pattern triggered by dryness (xerosis) in the acute stage and atopic dermatitis, psoriasis, ichthyosis, xerosis and contact dermatitis in the chronic phase [23]. At Germany Home Care, a study found that more than 50% of participants experienced dry skin. Similarly, another study on US patients with adult atopic dermatitis reported that 60.1% of participants were adversely affected by mild disease while 28.9% and 11%, respectively, had a moderate and then severe form [24].

Dry skin is often confused with dehydrated skin. In general, dehydrated skin means a lack of water; dry skin is related to skin that lacks natural oils or sebum [25]. Dehydration results from a fluid imbalance where the amount of circulating blood supply is inadequate, either due to excessive loss or ingestion of fluid [26]. In another research, scientists found that dehydration affects your skin's ability to sweat and secrete saliva. In dry skin, the sebaceous glands deficiently produce natural oils, leading to white flakes, redness, scales on the skin, and irritation. Dehydration conditions can result in sunken eyes, dullness, itching, and a greater appearance of wrinkles [27].

While dry skin is very different, they also share many similarities. In some cases, these dry skin conditions have been attributed to a lack of water and a natural oily moisturizing lipid barrier. Patients with dehydrated skin can also change their diet and lifestyle to increase hydration, such as increasing water intake. Such patients need to hydrate their skin through appropriate treatments (*e.g.*, frequent application of moisturizers). For patients with dehydrated and dry skin, treatments for the dehydration subtypes mentioned above can be used in combination [28].

Acne Skin

Acne is a chronic inflammatory disease of the pilosebaceous follicle, characterized by large sebaceous glands and relatively short hair that rarely erupts from the follicle. Acne has four stages of development: (i) release of inflammatory mediators into the skin, (ii) keratinization alteration process with comedones; and (iii) hormone-mediated sebum production by sebaceous gland under androgen control, and (iv) Propionibacterium acnes additionally colonize hair follicles on the human face (usually the forehead, cheek, nose, and chin), neck, chest, and back [29].

While a certain amount of sebum is essential for healthy skin, overproduction can compromise suitability. The Sebaceous gland, connected to hair follicles, secretes a type of oily material known as sebum [30]. Propionibacterium acnes reside in each sebaceous follicle and come to the skin surface as sebum, bringing with it bacteria and debris. In the next stage of acne, you can develop inflammatory pustules, papules, and nodules. Examples of inflammatory skin include pus, swelling, and redness. Skin sebum regulation is thus vital to effectively managing acne. Some studies state that oxidized lipids stimulate keratinocyte proliferation in aphakia, and vitamin D can cause more effective sebum production as a treatment [31].

Acne lesions, such as nodules, blemishes, pimples, blackheads, or whiteheads, can differ in type. Blackheads are the pores where keratin and sebum accumulate, which darkens in color. Whiteheads form when sebaceous glands become blocked and swell under the tissue. Nodules are solid tumors that usually invade the deeper layers of skin and damage the surrounding tissue. It triggers horrible acne and will probably cause scarring. On the other hand, bumps do not contain pus but are still firm and contain inflamed acne pimples that appear swollen. Plus, it combines white blood cells, pathogenic bacteria, and dead tissues around hair follicles [32].

Hyperpigmented Skin

Pigment-related skin diseases can be defined as pigmentation loss or decline of the skin color. Pigmented skin is linked to inflammation, sun protection, and other mechanisms. Pigmentation is associated with the inability to synthesize or transport melanin appropriately within the melanosomes [33]. Mast cells,

Langerhans cells, and lymphocytes all play a role along with keratinocytes. Pigmented skin is generally classified into three types: hypopigmentation, hyperpigmentation, and depigmentation. Hypopigmentation refers to a reduced level of melanin, and depigmentation indicates a complete loss of pigment [34].

Epidermal Melanosis

The hyperpigmented skin shows only excessive amounts of melanin but a normal density of melanocytes. Two clinical examples of updated conditions include urticaria pigmentosa and cafe-au-lait spots. During Woods' light examination, the boundaries of these spots are clearly defined and dark brown. A drawing of average skin is included for reference. Treatment for this hyperpigmentation works best locally [35].

Dermal Melanosis

The hyperpigmentation found in this type is due to dermal melanin among collagen bundles or within melanophages or clear cells. Melanin is natural on the epidermis. Examples of clinical cases include lichen planus, incontinentia pigment, permanent medicine eruption, and various types of post-inflammatory hyperpigmentation. In the wood light, lesions appear brown-grey with blurred margins. A visual of skin that is considered average is provided for comparison. The insensitivity to melanin resulting from macrophage phagocytosis of melanosomes makes local therapy- such as bleaching creams containing hydroquinone- less effective [36].

Post-inflammatory Hyperpigmentation

It is one of the most common and persistent in dark-skinned patients. In dark individuals, residual hyperpigmentation is often attributable to skin diseases such as inflammatory dermatoses, trauma, and medical interventions, including laser therapy. Sometimes, spots are aggravated and worsened by chemicals, sunlight exposure, or some medicines [37]. Dyschromia is diffuse and conforms to the configuration of the original dermatoses; however, its severity does not always correspond with the degree of prior inflammation. Most of it is dark epidermal pigmentation and will fade in a few months. Dermal pigmentation is usually a dark grey-brown and permanent over the years. Post-inflammatory hyperpigmentation is difficult to treat [38]. The therapeutic goal is to treat the etiology. The most important clinical improvement of the lesions correlates directly with topical therapy other than depigmentation medicines. This is particularly important when these therapies suggest normal sunblock [39].

Melasma

It is another frequent occurrence that might impact the emotional and confidence levels of individuals and their quality of life. A common form of hyperpigmentation is melasma, which presents as blotchy dark patches on sun-exposed skin. Women using birth control pills may create the commonest kind of melasma on their face during gestation. The characteristic findings are well-defined bilateral hyperpigmented areas, which usually appear on the forehead (frontalis) and cheeks (malar) and cause changes in color around the upper lip (pseudo melasma), on the nose, and or chin [40].

Although the exact etiology of melasma remains unknown, its pathophysiology is multifactorial. Genetic predisposition and UV or visible light exposure are primary causes of melasma. Other causes of melasma include oral contraceptive use, pregnancy, and estrogen-progesterone treatment, anticonvulsants, thyroid disorders, medicines and cosmetics. An increasing number of cases of melasma in females are attributed to oral contraceptive pills (8.5%), whitening creams and perfume-containing moisturizing creams (10%), and pregnancy-related hormonal effects (32%) [41].

IMPORTANCE OF DERMATOLOGY

Patients can examine their skin, identify changes, and most probably seek help regarding the types of initial changes they had. Roughly 20–25% of primary care patients see their family doctor for skin-related issues; nearly all have at least one abnormal skin finding [42].

Skin problems are common. Almost every teen has acne. Depending on the demographic, atopy may occur in up to 20–30% of people. Psoriasis impacts one to two percent of the global populace, and people with it live significantly worse lives than those who live differently [43].

By retirement age, nearly all patients in a Western country have measurable sun-induced aging changes, including clinically detectable pre-malignant changes. Basal cell carcinoma is the most common variety of all human malignancies, comprising 30 to 50 percent of all cancers. However, it is not included in most statistics on cancer due to the low death rate [44].

Dermatology has become increasingly popular as a specialty because of the frequency of skin symptoms and signs and the focus on skincare. It is a very popular career choice for those who want to work in medicine. Most senior dermatologists promptly admit they would be lucky to get into a dermatology residency program in the modern era. A dermatologist might pursue a variety of career routes, from basic skin diagnosis and treatment to surgical procedures targeted at malignancies or aesthetics. Subspecialties include immunohematology, photo dermatology, dermatology in children, and dermatology pathology. Among the other study areas are hair and nail disorders [45].

Dermatology research builds on a solid background in immunology and genetics. Dermatopathology laboratories have produced a considerable amount of basic research over time on a wide array of topics, ranging from electron microscopy, cytokines, and autoimmune diseases to Langerhans cell function and the entire range of dermatopathology [46].

Multiple cutaneous manifestations are characteristic of several syndromes; dermatologists have been instrumental in identifying many disease-causing genes by carefully collating large family pedigrees [47].

Skin physiology provides valuable new insight into how our skin works. Still, it has also become an integral part of the assessment for drug and cosmetic companies proposing to treat such conditions as dry skin or dull hair. Dermatologists have been instrumental in identifying the genes responsible for the associated diseases by carefully piecing together extended family pedigrees, as the syndromes can exhibit unique cutaneous manifestations [48].

Skin physiology not only crucially illustrates the mechanisms of our skin's functioning but is also a valuable tool for quantifying the claims made by pharmaceutical and cosmetic companies to treat conditions such as dry skin and dull hair [49].

NEED FOR REMOTE MONITORING

The healthcare system in India consists of three levels. PHCs form the first-tier institutions, district hospitals are the second-tier institutions, and tertiary care centers (TCCs) are the third-tier institutions. The only diagnostic services for rural people, the PHCs, were started as a solution to their healthcare needs. Therefore, the diagnostic facilities available at the district hospitals are much better than those at the PHCs, whereas the diagnostic facilities available at the TCCs are state-of-the-art. Research indicates dermatologist services are necessary since skin problems greatly affect the rural population [50].

Still, the PHCs do not have enough dermatologists or other physicians to treat each patient, nor the diagnostic tools to identify skin-related diseases. However, the unavailability of medical specialists and health facilities with diagnostic facilities causes delays in providing the required interventions and treatment for patients presenting to PHCs. The delay in starting intervention can be treated and avoided by increasing the quality of care at PHCs through remote access to dermatologists and diagnostic facilities *via* Teledermatology. This can be provided to the patient in the remote center with the help of technology [51].

The PHC and TCC are connected by remote monitoring, with an expert system offering diagnostic advice. Images of skin lesions and patient information are obtained at the PHC and sent to the TCC *via* the Internet. The TCC processes the patient's text and visual data and archives their personal information [52]. The TCC's expert system determines the case as a potential diagnosis. The proposed diagnosis is relayed to the PHC [53].

Alternatively, even later, the PHC can still obtain the diagnostic recommendations from the TCC. This diagnostic data would assist the PHC health worker in starting preventive treatment and prevent the patient's condition from worsening until a doctor arrives. Web services based on the Simple Object Access Protocol (SOAP) and a mobile device are used to implement remote monitoring [54].

REMOTE HEALTHCARE

Two of the ways to deliver remote health care are telemedicine and remote monitoring. Telemedicine stands for its method when a patient has their visit with doctors who are miles away from their area due to conditions of isolation. Meanwhile, clinicians use remotely available health monitoring equipment to monitor the patient continuously by any appropriate means. This is called remote health monitoring. Though at first glance, telemedicine and remote monitoring are increasingly converging with the advent of IoT-embedded systems, ubiquitous systems, healthcare data analytics, and other viable applications of these technologies in the medical sector. Remote health monitoring has increasingly become viable and cost-effective due to developments in extremely high bandwidth, narrow-bandwidth power-efficient wireless technologies, and the increased availability and functionality of nanosensors and the Internet of Things [55].

Current medical treatment models do not meet the challenges of the constantly growing demand for low-cost health services in hospitals and other medical care settings [56]. The discovery of new medical models that have proposed advanced biosensors, efficient patient records management, and digital and high-tech medical tools have largely been linked to information and communication technology (ICT) [57]. The rapid development of seamless information exchange has further facilitated bridging the distance and infrastructure gap between unserved or under-served regions and hospitals equipped with appropriate infrastructures. This model is called e-health or remote healthcare. In simple terms, remote healthcare involves managing a patient *via* phone or video rather than seeing the health professional in person. Remote healthcare aims to provide medical care to individuals in their homes or other locations apart from standard healthcare facilities [58].

Remote healthcare, which enables compliance with treatment regimens without the need for frequent relocation of the patient or healthcare providers, is heavily reliant on capturing, administering, and transferring non-genetic biometric identification information of a patient, their medication, and any associated personal and medical data. Remote healthcare revolves around the exchange of information. Interactions of the pathway with the stakeholder, especially self-management, lifestyle promotion, and disease detection, should be well-structured. Information exchanges should also ensure proper coordination and transition across the different stages to allow for process continuance [59]. The advantages of remote healthcare are outlined in Fig. (**1**).

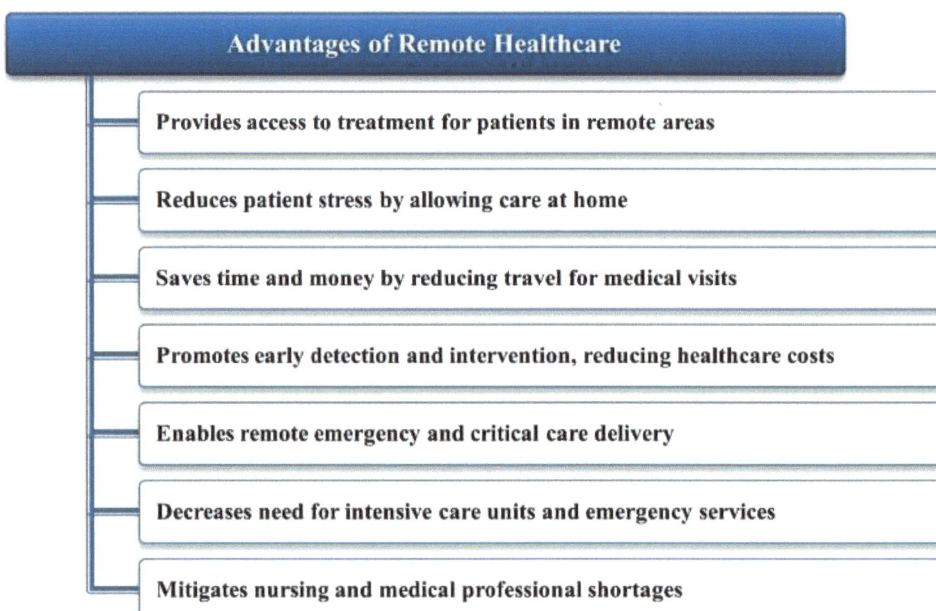

Fig. (1). Advantages of remote healthcare.

IOT DEVICES IN REMOTE DERMATOLOGY MONITORING

Currently, skin disorders are the most prevalent health problem globally under national health services and also cause a significant individual burden. Most dermatologic disorders negatively impact a patient's quality of life, and some can be fatal or lead to long-lasting disabilities. Every day, the global population is aging, while environmental dynamics and health-risk factors (such as changing climate) are increasing the demand for more human, financial, scientific, and technical resources to sustain and strengthen dermatology practice [60].

Therefore, integrating new business models and technology into dermatology practices now and in the future is imperative as they can provide efficient and cost-effective relief. IoT technologies like smart wearable medical devices, smart sensors, and mobile applications can solve some of the greatest challenges in health care. Such technologies enable more precise, real-time, lower-cost, comprehensive monitoring and diagnostics [61]. IoT devices used in remote dermatology monitoring are depicted in Fig. (**2**).

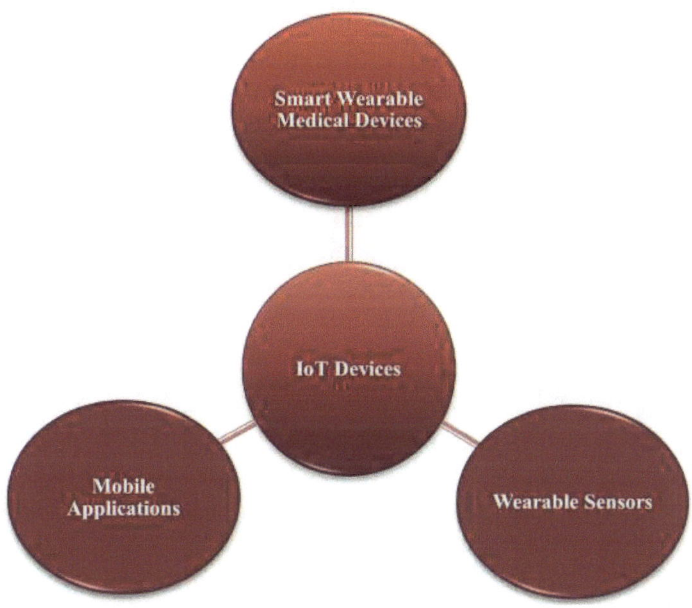

Fig. (2). IoT devices used in remote dermatology monitoring.

Smart Wearable Medical Devices

Wearable devices are a type of electronic device that can be physically paired with human skin, worn on the body as an accessory, and embedded in the material used to make clothing (as in flexible electronics). Wearable Devices include wristbands, hearing aids, electronic/optical tattoos, head-mounted displays (HMD), subcutaneous sensors, electronic footwear, or smart cloth (electronic textiles). These also include accessories, outside of the skin, or in a close environment which monetarize, generate electronic signaling and gives physical and biochemical information about the drugs [62].

Smart wearable devices (a combination of sensors and microcontrollers) harness the IoT potential in healthcare by inducing proactive preventive care, a better diagnosis, and a more relevant assessment of the treatment results. Developed for both monitoring and diagnostic functions, these wearable medical devices can be set at different parts of the human body (*e.g.*, electrodes for electrocardiography, electromyography, devices for monitoring of blood pressure, temperature, glucose, lactate, pH, Na, K, blood oxygenation, skin hydration or evolution of wounds) [63].

Implications of Smart Wearable Medical Devices in Dermatology

Dermatology is an incredibly visual field, focused primarily on the visual observation of the skin and its current state of health. Compared to other organs, the skin seems more applicable for real-time monitoring and provides an interface to other organs that can be measured with wearable smart medical devices [64].

Through continuous monitoring and real-time data access, many hospital stays and routine exams will be prevented, thus enabling dermatologists to make better decisions and diagnoses. They can have quicker and more individualized access to patients through access to specific health parameters obtained *via* smart wearable devices such as skin mechanics, wound healing, temperature, blood oxygen level, and hydration levels. Medical experts can be notified almost immediately whenever an abnormal event occurs by getting timely information on their smartphones; rural monitoring and treatment are a possibility for the underserved populations, *i.e.*, those who live in rural or ultraportable areas; smart wearable medical devices are non-invasive and improve attitudes and behaviors of patients toward skin disease treatment; results of such a specific application (treatment of skin diseases, wounds, or the postoperative healing process) may facilitate improving medicines, dressing patches or devices [65]. Some examples of smart wearable medical devices are discussed below:

Smart Bandage

Researchers from Tufts University in Massachusetts have developed a smart bandage containing sensors and a processor. The bandage automatically delivers doses of medication and constantly observes the wound. The smart bandage has embedded sensors and a unique processor that detects how well the wound is healing. Smart bandages have integrated specific sensors that record the wound's pH and thermal values, enabling the detection of acute warning signs of inflammation or infection. Consequently, the antibiotics required will be used as topical [66].

A smart bandage consists of several components, including (i) pH and temperature sensors, (ii) a flexible microheater, (iii) heat-responsive drug carriers integrated into a hydrogel patch, and (iv) wireless electronics capable of reading sensor data and then activating and controlling the thermal actuation system if necessary [67].

Smart Patches

U.S. researchers at Ohio State University developed a nanochip that can reprogram cells to assist in internal healing. The new method, called tissue nanotransfection, involves using a specially designed patch with coin-sized nanochip on the diseased tissue. Cell reprogramming begins as soon as the patch has been on for one second, and the skin will heal itself when removed. A strong localized electric field is generated along the device as soon as it is attached to the skin. It allows the nanochip to go against one of these codes into the skin cells, which gives them the power to differentiate in any cell and repair damaged blood vessels [68].

Wearable Sensors

Sensitive Sensor for Measuring Exposure to UV Radiation

UV light is beneficial for human health and is important in vitamin D synthesis, but too much exposure to UV has many adverse effects, including skin cancer and photosensitization. In general, excessive exposure to UVA and UVB has acute effects that are temporary and reversible. These can lead to sunburn, erythema, and darkening. Long-term exposure to UV rays, particularly below erythemal UV doses, leads to accelerated skin aging through collagen and elastin thickening and degradation of keratinocytes and blood vessels [69].

Researchers have created a breathable, extensible, ultra-thin wearable UV sensor that accurately quantifies UV radiation exposure and solar protection. A soft, flexible interface that mimics the skin and a UV sensor. These dyes inside the sensor change color when exposed to UV light. Then, this color change is quantified (with a smartphone and a quantization technique). Its operation has been demonstrated in different environmental conditions, such as ocean swimming, beach sunbathing, showering, sunscreen, and cosmetic products [70].

Scan - Wearable Device for Diagnosing Skin Cancer

The portable scan device will soon make skin cancer diagnosis possible. The gadget was the creation of four teenage engineers at McMaster University in Ontario, Canada. This device is compact and convenient for single-handed use and mobility. In addition, the device is made of cheap and easily available materials, so it will be affordable when it launches. The tool can detect early melanoma by using temperature sensors that record the temperature on the skin's surface. Skin damaged by melanoma will heat up much faster than neighboring skin when cooled down by a cold source. That's exactly what the idea of scan is based on. sKan uses thermistors to take repeated measurements of heat emissions from the cancer cells. Then, it uses known genes about heat shock response (HSR) to create a heat map that can estimate the recovery rate of cells from HSR, implying melanoma [71].

Mobile Application

Recently, social media resources and smartphone applications (mobile apps) have been increasingly used to improve the care of patients with skin lesions. According to the editor of JAMA Dermatology in 2005: "We are starting to transition from clinicopathologic diagnosis into a world of clinical-imaging diagnosis," at least when it comes to dermatology. Now, dermatologists usually diagnose patients with clinical imaging, which needs much fewer skin samples, followed by pathological studies. This change in clinical practice requires an explanation, which can be attributed to the increasing usage of dermoscopy and the incorporation of social media platforms and smartphone applications into daily clinical use [72].

There are so many dermatology apps; some are designed for patients, while others are for doctors. VisualDx and YouDermoscopy are two mobile apps designed specifically for dermatologists; they may be useful in everyday clinical practice [73].

VisualDx is a cost-effective application with a dual purpose. One way to use it is by searching for specific diseases. It provides a summary of the key aspects of the disease with images, a summary of clinical features, diagnostic tools, differential diagnosis, laboratory tests, management, and therapy. Nevertheless, it can also generate a differential diagnosis from clinical signs entered by the dermatologist (*e.g.*, patient age, dermatosis type, site of lesions, other symptoms, history of disease, and others) [74]. YouDermoscopy, an app originally developed as a dermatologist training tool, is available worldwide. Users must diagnose the lesions correctly based on dermoscopy images. The program features multiple levels, each with its own group of photos that must be identified in under 10 seconds. A prime example of how mobile applications can facilitate education and training in dermatology, this application encourages users who score poorly on any given level to attempt that level again [75].

Recently, many more smartphone applications have been developed to encourage worldwide knowledge dissemination amongst dermatologists and other health professionals. Enrolled users of the Pierre Fabre Dermo-cosmetic Club Dermaweb website can download the free mobile teledermatology app Skindiag. App users can send in a mobile image and inquiry for diagnostic and therapeutic assistance, and two hospital specialists will respond, depending on the continent, within 48 hours. Skindiag allows dermatologists to archive cases according to categories for educational purposes and discuss topical cases with other colleagues [76].

In addition to dermatologists and other medical professionals, many apps are designed for patients. For example, one such software (SkinVision) is meant to help patients determine whether a mole on their skin could be cancerous, by inputting aphotograph of a user's skin lesion to assess cancer risk. Despite being the most frequently chosen app by users searching for "melanoma," data suggests automated diagnostic tools of this type probably won't work. MelaFind is the market's first automatic melanoma diagnosis device. Nevertheless, given the best of funds, two decades of research produced a system that detected 98.4% of melanomas but possessed less than 10% specificity. Hence, it is unlikely that automatic diagnosis would be feasible for melanoma, and these smartphone apps may need to be utilized cautiously [77].

The advent of social media platforms like WhatsApp and dermatology specialty apps is very useful in the remote management of skin-related issues. This technology allows patients to take photos in some areas, and dermatologists can analyze them remotely. Thus, social media platforms can alleviate the demand for in-office evaluations of patients with obviously non-malignant illnesses. Moreover, they can also alleviate patients' anxiety by providing professional consultations as soon as possible. They can even recommend topical therapies and record patient progress clinic-free. For instance, patients with naevi and illnesses that need a dermoscopy for a precise diagnosis should be given priority for regular clinical consultations [78].

KEY TECHNOLOGY OF IOT IN REMOTE DERMATOLOGY MONITORING

The term "Internet of Things" (IoT) describes a picture of the Internet in which everything and everyone is strongly connected at all times and from any location. It shows how digital and physical objects can be connected to enable and support new services and applications [79]. Fig. (**3**) illustrates the important IoT technologies in dermatology.

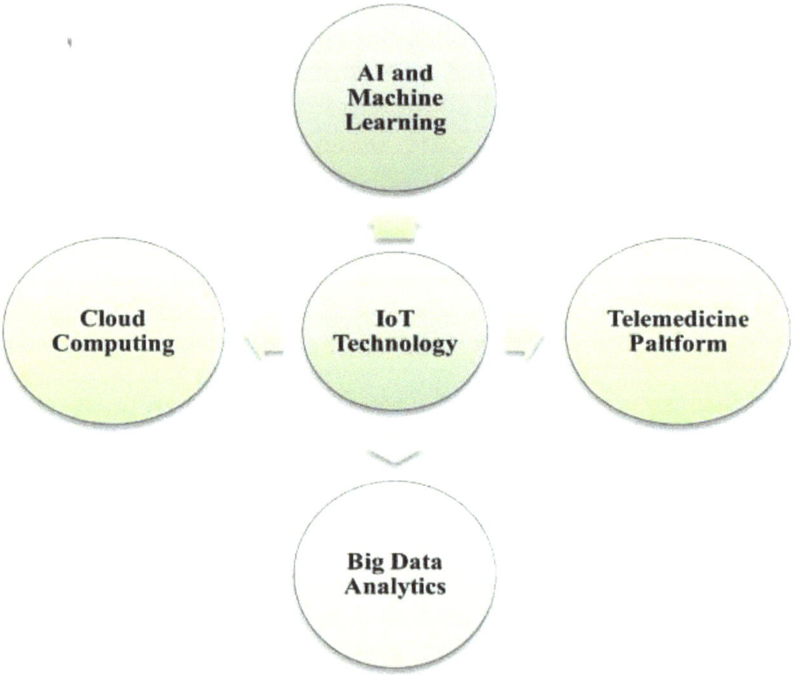

Fig. (3). Key technology of IoT used in remote dermatology monitoring.

AI and Machine Learning (ML) for Remote Dermatology Monitoring

The Association for the Advancement of Artificial Intelligence defines artificial intelligence (AI) as "the scientific understanding of the mechanisms underlying thought and intelligent behavior and their embodiment in machines." In other words, AI is a subfield of computer science that deals with complex data manipulation and requires developing programs that attempt to mimic human thinking processes [80].

Terms such as convolutional neural networks (CNN), machine learning, and artificial intelligence (AI) have become popular when discussing the future of dermatology. Despite being in the early days of development, AI is anticipated to have a significant role in everyday dermatology practice. Medicine is producing data at an increasing rate that will become increasingly difficult to structure, manage, and analyze. Some AI and machine learning applications are genome analysis, patient treatment, diagnosis, and preventive medicine [81].

These include radiography, oncology, neurology, cardiology, and ophthalmology applications in medicine. Although the role of AI is continually evolving, it will not likely replace dermatologists in the field but aid clinicians as a part of their practice. The impact could reduce treatment costs by 50%, but only if effectively deployed. AI is increasingly important in dermatology, but its application remains highly limited. It is, therefore, essential that stakeholders (including physicians, patients, employers, insurers, pharmaceutical companies, and the government) understand the terminology, uses, limitations, and potential applications of artificial intelligence (AI) in dermatology as systems are built and deployed continually [82].

Artificial intelligence (AI) has appeared in dermatology literature as early as 1987, with microcomputer-based systems of dermato pathologic diagnostics. A few years later, computer technology was developed to aid dermatologists in diagnosis, prognosis, and literature searches. In the 2000s, artificial neural networks and pattern recognition were studied to diagnose conditions such as vitiligo, atopic dermatitis, nonmelanoma skin cancer, and melanomas [83].

Due to abundant data available in clinical records, patient demographics, imaging examination results, and questionnaire data, dermatology is on the verge of having personalized medicine revolutionized [84]. Translational research in dermatitis is already quite broad-based, with information obtained from the genome, epigenome, transcriptome, proteomics, and microbiome. These areas of research are often grouped under the acronym "OMICS." Recent advancements in the speed of processors and the cost of storage have allowed for the development of ML algorithms that mimic human intelligence. These algorithms have various applications in dermatology. To be able to evaluate the effectiveness of these emerging technologies, dermatologists need a basic understanding of artificial intelligence and machine learning [85].

Machine learning techniques can be divided into three categories: reinforcement learning, unsupervised learning, and supervised learning [86]. The inputs (called Features) and outputs (called Labels) for supervised learning must be given in a dataset. For example, a photograph of a pigmented lesion is an example of a "feature" in an algorithm where pixels/values are input determining whether or not the pigmented lesion is benign or malignant and categorical data indicating what type of lesion is used as "labels." The system uses what it has learned about benign pigmented lesions and melanoma from labeled photos. It applies that knowledge to a new set of skin images which the computer has not seen before. Supervised learning is the most common type of dermatology training [87].

Machine Learning Algorithms

A variety of machine learning methods are commonly used in dermatology. Examples of the most commonly used statistical learning methods include logistic regression, k-nearest neighbor (k-NN), support vector machines (SVM), random forests (RF), and natural language processing (NLP). Most machine learning

(ML) algorithms are specific types of statistical learning. The k-NN method can be used for both regression and data classification simultaneously (the output depends on whether it is a mean regressed based on neighbors' labels or a class assigned based on the most common label of neighbors). SVMs classify data by finding a hyperplane that separates two classes. RFs construct a network of random decision trees to find the most common among all the randomly generated results. NLP analyses large text corpora to discover patterns [88].

Dermatology and Machine Learning

There is so much exciting potential for machinc learning in dermatology. Image categorization has drawn the greatest interest from the perspective of access to skin examination and optimal usage of dermatologists' workflow with potential improvement in skin cancer screening *via* convolutional neural network (CNN) [89]. CNN has already succeeded in many other fields, such as radiology, pathology, and ophthalmology. In 2018, a convolutional neural network (CNN) in the IDx-DR diagnostic system independent screening for diabetic retinopathy was approved by the US Food and Drug Administration (FDA) following validation in large prospective clinical studies including over 900 patients [10]. They compared this diagnostic approach against an independent, superior gold standard of imaging techniques and achieved a sensitivity of 87.2% and specificity of 90.7% [90].

CNN has limitations and has yet to be validated in prospective clinical trials for melanoma or non-melanoma skin malignancy screening. Besides distinguishing benign from malignant lesions, machine learning (ML) has been applied in dermatopathology, teledermatology, differential diagnosis, mobile apps, and personalized medicine. For regulators to ensure and optimize these technologies for patients, they need an understanding of what kind of deep learning techniques are already being implemented and how they are evolving [91].

Application of AI and Machine Learning in Dermatology

The ability of an experienced board-certified dermatologist to directly diagnose skin diseases is largely based on experience. An experienced board-certified dermatologist has visually examined thousands of skin conditions over many years and diagnosed them by resemblance to previous cases [92]. Similarly, AI tries to visually evaluate the skin state in these hundreds of photos concerning trends and identify diseases by comparing them to earlier photographs. Whether AI can diagnose clinical dermatologic skin illness as accurately as a board-certified dermatologist is an important subject to address [93].

A recent study tested a CNN in two use cases: (1) comparing keratinocyte carcinomas and benign seborrheic keratoses and (2) malignant melanomas *versus* nevi against 21 board-certified dermatologists. The study's validity was further strengthened by only using imaging data that had been biopsy-proven. The only barrier for CNN [94] was the fine-grained difference of skin lesions [94].

Analyzing two-dimensional photographs of three-dimensional skin problems is a significant constraint of AI in clinical skin disease diagnosis. Because of the wide variations in zoom, angle, and lighting, there are grounds for concern over the quality and uniformity of images sent into the neural network. Skin curvature frequently causes uneven lighting, which degrades the performance of neural network segmentation techniques [95].

In a pigmented skin lesion study, the AI system was 86% accurate, with 94% sensitivity and 68% specificity for distinguishing benign and malignant lesions. A consumer-grade digital camera [96] was utilized. Investigators devised a new methodology to address the uneven illumination commonly observed in clinical photographs. Specifically, an image has two types of spatial frequency components: low frequencies represent uneven illumination, and high frequencies represent a pigmented skin lesion. In designing their neural network classification method, the researchers removed clinical photographs' low spatial frequency component. This compensated for unevenly illuminated lights and improved diagnostic classification accuracies of the neural network [97].

Telemedicine Platform for Remote Dermatology Monitoring

Telemedicine (sometimes called e-health) uses telecommunications technologies to exchange medical information for diagnosis, consultation, treatment, and education. By definition, the exchange happens across a distance. Also called "medicine at a distance," telemedicine provides individuals with knowledge that would otherwise be unavailable in a particular region. A telemedicine consultation usually involves a doctor helping to diagnose or treat a patient using the transmission of sound or an image. Data can be exchanged between patients, doctors, and experts [98].

Telemedicine has a subcategory called teledermatology. Dermatology is a visual field, so utilizing the many telemedicine application opportunities makes sense. In "classic" clinical teledermatology, dermatologists assess patient data with still or video images depicting skin conditions [99].

Many publications within the past few years have addressed the benefits of various communications methods employed in teledermatology. The store-and - forward (SAF) method has been useful in teledermatology. Several published comparative studies have described the level of agreement between telephone and in-person diagnoses. Existing data and literature show that store-and-forward techniques using conventional digital cameras and findings from direct physical examination agree in 54–95% of circumstances. In addition to clinical teledermatology, other major sub-disciplines include teledermatopathology and teledermatoscopy, in which the suspicious part of the skin is evaluated on a monitor screen rather than through a microscope [100].

Telemedicine is now a way to offer healthcare rather than an alternative approach. However, this change has not been entirely achieved. Teledermatology is one of the most prevalent telemedicine applications and one of the more mature subspecialties in this domain. Primary care physicians who do not currently employ teledermatology will likely have that opportunity soon if they haven't already encountered it. Although teledermatology is an emerging model of care, it alters the method in which care is received, thus influencing the experiences of patients, dermatologists, and referring physicians [101].

Teledermatology Modalities

Teledermatology is performed using a store and forward technique or real-time interactive technology.

In teledermatology, the store-and-forward method has been the most widely adopted modality. It usually consists of high-quality digital images paired with standardized clinical and clinical data. These are more standardized history questions and may include how long the lesion has been, whether it has changed in size, and if it is itchy. A traditional imaging convention or process is utilized to acquire the image collection. The consult requests are sent electronically from the location of the referring clinician and patient to that of the consulting dermatologist, such as through an electronic health record or any other electronic mechanism using means compliant with applicable security and privacy regulations. Store and forward teledermatology is unique because the patient, the referring clinician, and even the dermatologist may be separated by time and distance [102]. For example, a practitioner may submit a consult request on day 1 from one geographic site, and the dermatopathologist at the second geographic site will review the consult request report. In-store and forward sessions, though, with the constraints of the teledermatology consultation, there is usually no connection between the dermatologist and the patient. Results and recommendations from the dermatologist are sent to the referring clinician, who then communicates those results to the patient, ensuring that any recommended follow-up is undertaken [103].

The real-time interactive type of teledermatology [11] is conducted using videoconferencing technology. The videoconference includes the dermatologist, the patient, and usually a representative from the referral site, facilitator, technician, or referring clinician [104]. The difference in functionality between this modality and store and forward is that functionally, in-store and forward, the patient is separated from their dermatologist spatially and temporally. Thus, when using real-time interactive technology, having both sites open simultaneously is a logistical challenge. If the consultations occur across time zones, scheduling could get more complicated. This technology enables virtual conversations between the patient and dermatologist, like during an in-person clinic appointment [105].

Big Data Analytics in Remote Dermatology Monitoring

Any collection of datasets whose size and complexity surpass conventional data processing programs' capability is called “big data.” Big data archives containing clinical, biological, and epidemiological data present never-before-seen research opportunities to direct scientific progress. Big data has several benefits, such as the potential for precision medicine, the convenience and affordability of data collection, the capacity to tackle problems both proactively and retrospectively, and the usefulness of hypothesis creation and testing [106].

Even though big data analyses can be “traditional hypothesis testing” and amenable to various forms of statistical testing, they are often hypothesis-generating as big data serves better for research on rare diseases or exposure . Instead of testing an existing hypothesis, they can support new hypotheses that can be examined using a more conventional approach. Searching for patterns is a common pursuit of big data analysis. In classical predictive modeling, based on a finite number of covariates, big data predictive modeling often introduces high dimensionality, with thousands to millions of factors not selected beforehand. This makes big data analysis more exploratory than traditional data analysis. Because many potential patterns are tested, there is diversity in these data investigations that can be accounted for through specialized statistical techniques utilizing p-value adjustments or false discovery rates; such approaches have been developed for subsets of these large datasets [107].

Big data is a new way of looking at complex data, not only extremely massive data or many data sources. It offers a new framework for generating hypotheses and a challenge to advance analytics. Though it comes with its advantages, there are plenty of disadvantages, too, and conventional data analytics is still very much a thing. Big data will enable dermatologists to manage a variety of skin diseases better, improve risk prediction models, allow for more targeted screening of high-risk individuals (*e.g.*, targeted screening for malignant melanoma), and also assist in clinical decision support (*e.g.*, whether or not to biopsy a pigmented lesion) [108].

Different disease phenotypes are examined within diverse disorders that may benefit from specialized therapy, such as psoriasis or eczema, and also the genetics of skin diseases (*e.g.*, genome-wide association studies). For rare events, however, big data may be a powerful tool for monitoring and evaluating the safety of medical products. The potential of big data for dermatology represents an unprecedented opportunity for academics to capitalize on existing data sources and novel, efficient, and powerful study methods moving forward [109]. The advantages and limitations of big data are depicted in Table 2.

Table 2. Advantages and limitations of big data.

Advantages	Limitations
Large-scale sample size [111].	Storage: Storing datasets can take a lot of resources [112].
Combining many data points from various sources might use smaller datasets or various sources to gather advantages [113].	Precision and coherence of techniques: numerous methods are still in their infancy and may continue to evolve with time [114].
Data acquisition and collection can be low-cost: in many situations, the data have already been gathered through normal clinical care (electronic health records) or participant self-surveillance (personal monitoring devices or internet searches) [115].	Before the data can be analyzed, formatting and data cleansing may require considerable computer science [116].
There are frequent options for both prospective and retrospective methods [117].	Quality control is a challenging task that frequently requires tiny representative samples. Privacy and security issues are frequently more intricate than standard databases [118].

Cloud Computing in Remote Dermatology Monitoring

Cloud computing is a set of on-demand, dynamically scalable, and often virtualized resources, such as networks, storage, applications, and even medical organizations, readily available to users with minimal management effort over the Internet. Suppose distributed computing could be generalized. Cloud computing is utilized to access numerous registering resources [119]. These resources are accessible on-demand to provide clients with foundations, apps, figuring force, and services. Depending on the user's needs, it helps retrieve information, various apps, and data from anywhere [120].

In addition, cloud computing is all about a simple reformative change in existing and distributed systems for geographically dispersed 'self-managing resources dynamically at run time depending on their demands, supply, and quality of service requirements' provisioning, assurance, and execution. These days, advanced cloud computing is growing exponentially in the IT sector. It ensures that a vast array of the internet is beyond the safe limit. An emerging opportunity for clinical research is big tech and pharma in the industrial sector . All social orders are now acquired through their cell innovation in this cutting-edge world. So, the next major point is that this real-time data should be stored and saved, which means distributed computing plays a key role in storing applications like Facebook, Twitter, Amazon, and WhatsApp. It is an increasingly popular approach for elegantly and discreetly managing externalized IT assets [121].

In many parts of the world, people are miles away from their nearest hospital. In an emergency, reaching the healthcare service centers takes some time. Likewise, it is difficult for physicians to schedule patients who have chronic conditions. Remote patient care through IoT can solve long-travel issues [122]. Remote devices and sensors can allow healthcare providers to help outpatients with advice, therapy, and biometric counting. For example, patients can update the data instantly and pair any wearable device with the cloud. IoT gadgets let them talk directly to you *via* the internet. This may help the medical professional to have an idea of care plans. These tools generate a calendar of the daily physical condition information for those who face skin problems. Therefore, charts and graphs based on the merged data are readily available to healthcare professionals. Patients can be monitored for their condition through real-time audio and video transmissions without exchanging [123].

Utilizing cloud computing in remote dermatology monitoring in healthcare transforms care delivery in five ways, *i.e.*, reliability, seasonableness, efficacy, security and safety are paramount, and adaptability.

Reliability: This may lead to greater effectiveness. By eliminating in-person visits and reducing the face-to-face time between doctors and patients, practices may transition to a more automated scheduling system thanks to remote care's easy, almost instantaneous communication capabilities.

Seasonableness: One of the biggest benefits of IoT healthcare is the opportunity for early intervention. Especially in more severe and urgent medical circumstances, constant monitoring can buy valuable, lifesaving minutes.

Efficacy: Another key advantage of the Internet of medical things in healthcare is enhancing quality and early detection. Bringing all devices and alarms into the same state-of-the-art GPS network allows for early management of patient symptoms that have been highlighted. It also allows workers to respond quickly and more accurately in an emergency, especially among patients [124].

Security and safety are paramount: Digital surveillance for patients gives a secure computer network access, allowing health-related information regarding the patient's condition to be retrievable. Physical surveillance acts as an imminent safety measure for falls when added with sophisticated network security protection tools. Some smaller hospitals have used RPM integration to protect their proprietary data internally [125].

***Adaptability*:** This could boost customer satisfaction rates. Patients want more access to health care using their everyday consumer electronics. Offering people that option and then delivering engaging and easy-to-navigate content and interaction would yield higher satisfaction rates. Fitbit and other mHealth technologies have grown with this trend [126].

Cloud computing's efficiency and low cost contribute to the quality of patient services, where medical services can be delivered easily. Meanwhile, cloud computing can help access and share data among different systems, mutually recognize test results, strongly support remote consultation, expand diversified and high-quality medical resources, and ease visitation difficulties [127].

APPLICATION OF IOT IN REMOTE DERMATOLOGY MONITORING

The Internet of Things (IoT) is a paradigm shift that enables remote management and operation of any connected tangible object in any smart application space, such as smart homes, smart cities, and smart healthcare. Much medical care depends on diagnosing and monitoring the patient's state regarding illnesses; advanced access to these parameters *via* sensor networks connected to the human body will be a tremendous assistance. Moreover, the data are readily available anywhere and anytime [128].

The Internet of Things (IoT) also helps doctors schedule appointments more effectively and monitor patients remotely. Patients should also improve their home-based care to reduce the risk of unnecessary or inappropriate medical interventions at hospitals or clinics. So, if overall healthcare spending decreases, patient safety and the quality of care may also tighten. The scope of IoT in the healthcare sector is immense [129].

It won't be too long that we can access a home-use health monitoring system that expedites hospital procedures. A dense deployment of IoT sensors will be required to monitor the body and environment continuously. This undertaking will aid in tracking chronic disease management and the progression of rehabilitation. In the long run, the Internet of Things (IoT) can also make strong data connections from multiple locations for virtual consultations for distant medical remedies [130].

There is also a shift from patient access to healthcare, as wireless IoT-driven solutions bring healthcare to the patient itself. The IoT-based sensors can gather data securely, analyze it using a small algorithm, and then share it with healthcare providers, giving relevant suggestions [131].

The Internet of Things (IoT) leverages sensor values and telecommunications, which solves the problem of efficient and practical real-time monitoring of senior health status. Research has shown that integrating smart technology with the Internet of Things could provide upgraded and improved services. Various emergency systems have been developed whereby sensors using communication technology that is intelligent and wireless but far from each other can communicate with one another. This technology has been used in many other medical applications, and one of the most popular ones is senior citizens' health monitoring. Taking crucial vital signs gives information on general health and unhealthy conditions [132].

The Internet of Wearable Things (IoWT) aims to enhance the quality of human life. It features devices that a human can wear and are embedded with sensors to track an individual's activity, health, and other elements. This IoWT data is fed into medical infrastructure so that even when physicians are going about their regular lives, they can see their patients' data from afar. A new integrative framework for the IoWT is under development based on the architecture of the IoT. The IoWT will be a disruptive technology that can create an ecosystem of automated telehealth treatments in healthcare systems [133].

Wireless transceiver technologies such as Bluetooth, infrared, near–field communication (NFC), RFID, Wi-Fi, and Zigbee can support wearable devices that communicate with smartphones and other devices. Technology also advances healthcare through remote diagnosis and monitoring. Currently, the Internet of Things in healthcare is a key concern. Disease recognition and management are among the most important facets of health care. It will be helpful to this in the body sensor network. In addition, the data could be accessed anywhere in the world [134].

CONCLUSION

Skin is a crucial barrier protecting the human body from harmful environmental factors. Monitoring skin health is the biggest, never-before-studied thing ever. Emerging and remotely used technologies have been applied for remote dermatological monitoring to improve diagnosis, treatment, and patient care; IoT use in those areas is promising. IoT technology uses online sensors that collect real-time data, allowing for continuous monitoring and instantaneous responses when necessary, thus requiring in-person consultations with physicians less frequently. This adds convenience to healthcare and provides easy access to people living in remote or underserved regions. Also, IoT-driven technologies have made it easier for dermatologists to access objectively tracked disease progression and treatment outcomes, further aiding them in improving their clinical decision-making skills. However, for the potential of IoT in dermatology to be realized, challenges such as interoperability between devices, privacy, and data security need to be addressed. ICON encourages industry professionals to follow insights from technological advancements, such as IoT development in dermatology, that will continue to change the specialty and improve patient outcomes.

REFERENCES

[1] Sharma A, Gupta S. Skin disease in tropics: Impacted by heat, humidity, and healthcare neglect. Critical Thinking in Contemporary Dermatology: Cognitive Essays. Singapore: Springer Nature Singapore. 2024; pp. 229-50.

[2] Riazul Islam SM, Daehan Kwak , Humaun Kabir M, Hossain M, Kyung-Sup Kwak . The internet of things for health care: a comprehensive survey. IEEE Access 2015; 3: 678-708. [http://dx.doi.org/10.1109/ACCESS.2015.2437951]

[3] Juyal S, Sharma S, Shankar Shukla A. Smart skin health monitoring using AI-enabled cloud-based IoT. Mater Today Proc 2021; 46: 10539-45. [http://dx.doi.org/10.1016/j.matpr.2021.01.074]

[4] Khan SF. A healthcare monitoring system on the Internet of Things (IoT) uses RFID. 6th International Conference on Industrial Technology and Management (ICITM). 198-204.

[5] Kumar S, Srivastava R, Pathak S, Kumar B. Cloud-based computer-assisted diagnostic solutions for e-health. Intelligent Data Security Solutions for e-Health Applications 2020; 219-35. [http://dx.doi.org/10.1016/B978-0-12-819511-6.00012-1]

[6] Elhoseny M, Abdelaziz A, Salama AS, Riad AM, Muhammad K, Sangaiah AK. A hybrid model of Internet of Things and cloud computing to manage big data in health services applications. Future Gener Comput Syst 2018; 86: 1383-94. [http://dx.doi.org/10.1016/j.future.2018.03.005]

[7] Selvaraj S, Sundaravaradhan S. Challenges and opportunities in IoT healthcare systems: a systematic review. SN Appl Sci 2020; 2(1): 139. [http://dx.doi.org/10.1007/s42452-019-1925-y]

[8] Borgia E. The Internet of Things vision: Key features, applications and open issues. Comput Commun 2014; 54: 1-31. [http://dx.doi.org/10.1016/j.comcom.2014.09.008]

[9] Ray S, Mishra KN, Dutta S. Big data security issues from the IoT and cloud computing perspective: A review. Recent Advances in Computer Science and Communications 2020; 12(1): 1-22.

[10] Sultan N. Making use of cloud computing for healthcare provision: Opportunities and challenges. Int J Inf Manage 2014; 34(2): 177-84. [http://dx.doi.org/10.1016/j.ijinfomgt.2013.12.011]

[11] Chauhan RA. Utilization of possible security and privacy issues considering the component interaction in high-speed communication networks. Int J Manag Technol Eng 2023; 13.

[12] Pandian SA, Murugan R, Kumar NS, Sahil SM. IoT and its Evolution in Healthcare. I-Manager's Journal on IoT and Smart Automation 2024; 2(1): 38.

[13] Prabhu CS. Overview-fog computing and internet-of-things (IOT). EAI Endorsed Trans Cloud Syst 2017; 3(10)

[14] Kumar NM, Mallick PK. The Internet of Things: Insights into the building blocks, component interactions, and architecture layers. Procedia Comput Sci 2018; 132: 109-17. [http://dx.doi.org/10.1016/j.procs.2018.05.170]

[15] Wilmer EN, Gustafson CJ, Ahn CS, Davis SA, Feldman SR, Huang WW. Most common dermatologic conditions encountered by dermatologists and nondermatologists. Cutis 2014; 94(6): 285-92. [PMID: 25566569]

[16] Gilaberte Y, Prieto-Torres L, Pastushenko I, Juarranz Á. Anatomy and function of the skin. Nanoscience in Dermatology. Academic Press 2016; pp. 1-14. [http://dx.doi.org/10.1016/B978-0-12-802926-8.00001-X]

[17] Kumar MA. The skin. Techniques in small animal wound management 2024; 1.

[18] Richmond JM, Harris JE. Immunology and skin in health and disease. Cold Spring Harb Perspect Med 2014; 4(12): a015339. [http://dx.doi.org/10.1101/cshperspect.a015339] [PMID: 25452424]

[19] Proksch E, Brandner JM, Jensen JM. The skin: an indispensable barrier. Exp Dermatol 2008; 17(12): 1063-72. [http://dx.doi.org/10.1111/j.1600-0625.2008.00786.x] [PMID: 19043850]

[20] Kasolang S, Adlina WA, Rahman NA, Nik NR. Common skin disorders: a review. J Tribol 2020; 25: 59-82.

[21] Lodén M. Role of topical emollients and moisturizers in the treatment of dry skin barrier disorders. Am J Clin Dermatol 2003; 4(11): 771-88. [http://dx.doi.org/10.2165/00128071-200304110-00005] [PMID: 14572299]

[22] Lodén M. Moisturizers: treatment of dry skin syndrome and barrier defects. Cosmeceuticals and Active Cosmetics 2015; 3: 235.

[23] Proksch E, Fölster-Holst R, Bräutigam M, Sepehrmanesh M, Pfeiffer S, Jensen JM. Role of the epidermal barrier in atopic dermatitis. J Dtsch Dermatol Ges 2009; 7(10): 899-910. [http://dx.doi.org/10.1111/j.1610-0387.2009.07157.x] [PMID: 19682176]

[24] Lichterfeld-Kottner A, Lahmann N, Blume-Peytavi U, Mueller-Werdan U, Kottner J. Dry skin in home care: A representative prevalence study. J Tissue Viability 2018; 27(4): 226-31. [http://dx.doi.org/10.1016/j.jtv.2018.07.001] [PMID: 30487067]

[25] Black D, Diridollou S, Lagarde JM, Gall Y. Skin care products for normal, dry, greasy skin. Textbook of Cosmetic Dermatology 1998; 2(1): 125-50.

[26] Hooper L, Bunn D, Jimoh FO, Fairweather-Tait SJ. Water-loss dehydration and aging. Mech Ageing Dev 2014; 136: 50-8. [http://dx.doi.org/10.1016/j.mad.2013.11.009]

[27] Benelam B, Wyness L. Hydration and health: a review. Nutr Bull 2010; 35(1): 3-25. [http://dx.doi.org/10.1111/j.1467-3010.2009.01795.x]

[28] Verdier-Sévrain S, Bonté F. Skin hydration: a review on its molecular mechanisms. J Cosmet Dermatol 2007; 6(2): 75-82. [http://dx.doi.org/10.1111/j.1473-2165.2007.00300.x] [PMID: 17524122]

[29] Reddy D, Jain V. An overview of medicinal plants for the treatment of acne. Journal of Critical Reviews 2019; 6(6): 7-14. [http://dx.doi.org/10.22159/jcr.2019v6i6.35696]

[30] Celleno L, Tamburi F. Structure and function of the skin. Nutritional Cosmetics. William Andrew Publishing. 2009; pp. 3-45.

[http://dx.doi.org/10.1016/B978-0-8155-2029-0.50008-9]

[31] Ravisankar P, Koushik OS, Himaja V, Ramesh J, Pragna P. Acne-causes and amazing remedial measures for acne. J Pharm Res 2015; 5: 209-301.

[32] Kameswararao K, Sujani C, Koteswararao NVN, Rajarao A, Satyanarayanamma PNS. A brief review on acne vulgaris. Research Journal of Pharmacology and Pharmacodynamics 2019; 11(3): 109-19. [http://dx.doi.org/10.5958/2321-5836.2019.00020.X]

[33] Lee AY. Skin pigmentation abnormalities and their possible relationship with skin aging. Int J Mol Sci 2021; 22(7): 3727. [http://dx.doi.org/10.3390/ijms22073727] [PMID: 33918445]

[34] Thawabteh AM, Jibreen A, Karaman D, Thawabteh A, Karaman R. Skin pigmentation types, causes and treatment—a review. Molecules 2023; 28(12): 4839. [http://dx.doi.org/10.3390/molecules28124839] [PMID: 37375394]

[35] Mannone F, De Giorgi V, Cattaneo A, Massi D, De Magnis A, Carli P. Dermoscopic features of mucosal melanosis. Dermatol Surg 2004; 30(8): 1118-23. [PMID: 15274702]

[36] Stanford DG, Georgouras KE. Dermal melanocytosis: A clinical spectrum. Australas J Dermatol 1996; 37(1): 19-25. [http://dx.doi.org/10.1111/j.1440-0960.1996.tb00989.x] [PMID: 8936066]

[37] Maghfour J, Olayinka J, Hamzavi IH, Mohammad TF. A Focused review on the pathophysiology of post-inflammatory hyperpigmentation. Pigment Cell Melanoma Res 2022; 35(3): 320-7. [http://dx.doi.org/10.1111/pcmr.13038] [PMID: 35306737]

[38] Bose SK, Ortonne JP. Pigmentation: dyschromia. Textbook of Cosmetic Dermatology. London, UK: Martin-Dunitz Ltd 1998; pp. 391-415.

[39] AlGhamdi KM, Kumar A. Depigmentation therapies for normal skin in vitiligo universalis. J Eur Acad Dermatol Venereol 2011; 25(7): 749-57. [http://dx.doi.org/10.1111/j.1468-3083.2010.03876.x] [PMID: 21054565]

[40] Rendon M, Berneburg M, Arellano I, Picardo M. Treatment of melasma. J Am Acad Dermatol 2006; 54(5) (Suppl. 2): S272-81. [http://dx.doi.org/10.1016/j.jaad.2005.12.039] [PMID: 16631968]

[41] Artzi O, Horovitz T, Bar-Ilan E, *et al.* The pathogenesis of melasma and implications for treatment. J Cosmet Dermatol 2021; 20(11): 3432-45. [http://dx.doi.org/10.1111/jocd.14382] [PMID: 34411403]

[42] Jafferany M. Psychodermatology. Prim Care Companion J Clin Psychiatry 2007; 9(3): 203-13. [http://dx.doi.org/10.4088/PCC.v09n0306] [PMID: 17632653]

[43] Kawshar T, Rajesh J. Sociodemographic factors and their association to prevalence of skin diseases among adolescents. Nasza Dermatol Online 2013; 4(3): 281-6. [http://dx.doi.org/10.7241/ourd.20133.68]

[44] Blume-Peytavi U, Bagot M, Tennstedt D, *et al.* Dermatology today and tomorrow: from symptom control to targeted therapy. J Eur Acad Dermatol Venereol 2019; 33(S1) (Suppl. 1): 3-36. [http://dx.doi.org/10.1111/jdv.15335] [PMID: 30561009]

[45] Weller RB, Hunter HJ, Mann MW. Clinical dermatology. John Wiley & Sons 2014.

[46] Tavakolpour S, Daneshpazhooh M, Mahmoudi H. Skin cancer: genetics, immunology, treatments, and psychological care. Cancer Genetics and Psychotherapy. 2017; pp. 851-934. [http://dx.doi.org/10.1007/978-3-319-64550-6_18]

[47] Sybert VP. Genetic skin disorders. Oxford University Press 2017. [http://dx.doi.org/10.1093/med/9780190276478.001.0001]

[48] Kotnala A, Verma K, Sharma A, *et al.* Indian Medicinal Plants for skin care and cosmeceuticals: A review. Journal of Biomedical and Therapeutic Sciences 2019; 6(2): 24-60.

[49] Surber C, Dragicevic N, Kottner J. Skin care products for healthy and diseased skin. pH of the Skin. Curr Probl Dermatol 2018; 54: 183-200.
[http://dx.doi.org/10.1159/000489532] [PMID: 30130786]

[50] Sudhakara UP, Hebbar H, Arunkumar G, Sampathila N. A technology framework for remote patient care in dermatology for early diagnosis. Inform Med Unlocked 2019; 15: 100171.
[http://dx.doi.org/10.1016/j.imu.2019.100171]

[51] Mahé A, Faye O, N'Diaye HT, *et al.* Definition of an algorithm for the management of common skin diseases at primary health care level in sub-Saharan Africa. Trans R Soc Trop Med Hyg 2005; 99(1): 39-47.
[http://dx.doi.org/10.1016/j.trstmh.2004.03.008] [PMID: 15550260]

[52] Indraratna P, Biswas U, Liu H, *et al.* Process evaluation of a randomized controlled trial for TeleClinical care, a smartphone-app-based model of care. Front Med (Lausanne) 2022; 8: 780882.
[http://dx.doi.org/10.3389/fmed.2021.780882] [PMID: 35211483]

[53] Sudhakara Upadya P, Hebbara H, Govindakarnavarb A, Sampathilac N. Informatics in Medicine Unlocked .

[54] Duarte ER, Kaiser DE, Menegon DB, Schneider SM, Ferla AA, Ferreira GE. Dermatological assistance in the primary health care: A Brazilian nursing approach. Dermatology in Public Health Environments: A Comprehensive Textbook 2023; 1975-94.
[http://dx.doi.org/10.1007/978-3-031-13505-7_81]

[55] Field MJ, Grigsby J. Telemedicine and remote patient monitoring. JAMA 2002; 288(4): 423-5.
[http://dx.doi.org/10.1001/jama.288.4.423] [PMID: 12132953]

[56] Kuo AMH. Opportunities and challenges of cloud computing to improve health care services. J Med Internet Res 2011; 13(3): 67.
[http://dx.doi.org/10.2196/jmir.1867] [PMID: 21937354]

[57] Metkar SK, Girigoswami K. Diagnostic biosensors in medicine – A review. Biocatal Agric Biotechnol 2019; 17: 271-83.
[http://dx.doi.org/10.1016/j.bcab.2018.11.029]

[58] Banbury A, Roots A, Nancarrow S. Rapid review of applications of e-health and remote monitoring for rural residents. Aust J Rural Health 2014; 22(5): 211-22.
[http://dx.doi.org/10.1111/ajr.12127] [PMID: 25303412]

[59] Blount M, Batra VM, Capella AN, *et al.* Remote health-care monitoring using Personal Care Connect. IBM Syst J 2007; 46(1): 95-113.
[http://dx.doi.org/10.1147/sj.461.0095]

[60] Basra MKA, Shahrukh M. Burden of skin diseases. Expert Rev Pharmacoecon Outcomes Res 2009; 9(3): 271-83.
[http://dx.doi.org/10.1586/erp.09.23] [PMID: 19527100]

[61] Farahani B, Firouzi F, Chang V, Badaroglu M, Constant N, Mankodiya K. Towards fog-driven IoT eHealth: Promises and challenges of IoT in medicine and healthcare. Future Gener Comput Syst 2018; 78: 659-76.
[http://dx.doi.org/10.1016/j.future.2017.04.036]

[62] Ianculescu MA, Alexandru AD, Coardo D, Coman OA. Smart wearable medical devices are the next step in providing affordable support for dermatology practice. Dermatovenerologie-J Romanian Soc Dermat 2018; 63: 295-306.

[63] Pramanik PK, Upadhyaya BK, Pal S, Pal T. Internet of things, smart sensors, and pervasive systems: Enabling connected and pervasive healthcare. Healthcare Data Analytics and Management. Academic

Press. 2019; pp. 1-58.

[64] Igarashi T, Nishino K, Nayar SK. The appearance of human skin: A survey. Found Trends Comput Graph Vis 2007; 3(1): 1-95. [http://dx.doi.org/10.1561/9781601980878]

[65] Welzel J, Winkler JK, Hänßle HA, *et al.* Digital dermatology. Digital Medicine. Jenny Stanford Publishing. 2023; pp. 563-81. [http://dx.doi.org/10.1201/9781003386070-32]

[66] Punjiya M, Mostafalu P, Sonkusale S. Smart bandages for chronic wound monitoring and on-demand drug delivery. 60th International Midwest Symposium on Circuits and Systems (MWSCAS). (): 495-8. [http://dx.doi.org/10.1109/MWSCAS.2017.8052968]

[67] Mostafalu P, Tamayol A, Rahimi R, *et al.* Smart bandage for monitoring and treatment of chronic wounds. Small 2018; 14(33): 1703509. [http://dx.doi.org/10.1002/smll.201703509] [PMID: 29978547]

[68] Hwang I, Kim HN, Seong M, *et al.* Multifunctional smart skin adhesive patches for advanced health care. Adv Healthc Mater 2018; 7(15): 1800275. [http://dx.doi.org/10.1002/adhm.201800275] [PMID: 29757494]

[69] Huang X, Chalmers AN. Review of wearable and portable sensors for monitoring personal solar UV exposure. Ann Biomed Eng 2021; 49(3): 964-78. [http://dx.doi.org/10.1007/s10439-020-02710-x] [PMID: 33432511]

[70] Pathan S, Prabhu KG, Siddalingaswamy PC. Techniques and algorithms for computer aided diagnosis of pigmented skin lesions—A review. Biomed Signal Process Control 2018; 39: 237-62. [http://dx.doi.org/10.1016/j.bspc.2017.07.010]

[71] Shafi N, Costantine J, Kanj R, *et al.* A portable non-invasive electromagnetic lesion-optimized sensing device for the diagnosis of skin cancer (SkanMD). IEEE Trans Biomed Circuits Syst 2023; 17(3): 558-73. [http://dx.doi.org/10.1109/TBCAS.2023.3260581] [PMID: 37030747]

[72] Moreno-Ramírez D, Argenziano G. Teledermatology and mobile applications in the management of patients with skin lesions. Acta Derm Venereol 2017. (Suppl. 218). [http://dx.doi.org/10.2340/00015555-2718] [PMID: 28676881]

[73] Glines KR, Haidari W, Ramani L, Akkurt ZM, Feldman SR. Digital future of dermatology. Dermatol Online J 2020; 26(10): 13030/qt75p7q57j. [http://dx.doi.org/10.5070/D32610050455] [PMID: 33147661]

[74] Tleyjeh IM, Nada H, Baddour LM. VisualDx: decision-support software for the diagnosis and management of dermatologic disorders. Clin Infect Dis 2006; 43(9): 1177-84. [http://dx.doi.org/10.1086/508283] [PMID: 17029139]

[75] Pellacani G, Argenziano G. New insights from non-invasive imaging: from prospection of skin photodamages to training with mobile application. J Eur Acad Dermatol Venereol 2022; 36(S6) (Suppl. 6): 38-50. [http://dx.doi.org/10.1111/jdv.18197] [PMID: 35738810]

[76] Brzozowska JM, Gotlib J. The importance of remote counseling in cosmetology and cosmetic dermatology. Pol Merkuriusz Lek 2023; 51(1): 74-87. [http://dx.doi.org/10.36740/Merkur202301111] [PMID: 36960904]

[77] Deeks JJ, Dinnes J, Williams HC. Sensitivity and specificity of SkinVision are likely to have been overestimated. J Eur Acad Dermatol Venereol 2020; 34(10): 582-e583. [http://dx.doi.org/10.1111/jdv.16382] [PMID: 32215960]

[78] Alhayaza G, Chisti M, Binamer Y. The impact of social media on dermatologists and in captivating their patients: a cross-sectional study. J Dermatolog Treat 2022; 33(4): 2217-24. [http://dx.doi.org/10.1080/09546634.2021.1940809] [PMID: 34114511]

[79] Vermesan O, Friess P, Eds. Internet of Things: converging technologies for smart environments and integrated ecosystems. River Publishers 2013.

[80] Castro D, New J. The promise of artificial intelligence. Center for Data Innovation 2016; 115(10): 32-5.

[81] Du-Harpur X, Watt FM, Luscombe NM, Lynch MD. What is AI? Applications of artificial intelligence to dermatology. Br J Dermatol 2020; 183(3): 423-30. [http://dx.doi.org/10.1111/bjd.18880] [PMID: 31960407]

[82] Li Z, Koban KC, Schenck TL, Giunta RE, Li Q, Sun Y. Artificial intelligence in dermatology image analysis: current developments and future trends. J Clin Med 2022; 11(22): 6826. [http://dx.doi.org/10.3390/jcm11226826] [PMID: 36431301]

[83] Gomolin A, Netchiporouk E, Gniadecki R, Litvinov IV. Artificial intelligence applications in dermatology: where do we stand?. Front Med (Lausanne) 2020; 7: 100. [http://dx.doi.org/10.3389/fmed.2020.00100] [PMID: 32296706]

[84] Litman T. Personalized medicine—concepts, technologies, and applications in inflammatory skin diseases. Acta Pathol Microbiol Scand Suppl 2019; 127(5): 386-424. [http://dx.doi.org/10.1111/apm.12934] [PMID: 31124204]

[85] Mazhar T, Haq I, Ditta A, *et al.* The role of machine learning and deep learning approaches for detecting skin cancer. Healthcare. MDPI. 2023; 11: p. (3)415.

[86] Li Y. Deep reinforcement learning: An overview. arXiv preprint arXiv:170107274 2017.

[87] Lindholm V, Raita-Hakola AM, Annala L, *et al.* Differentiating malignant from benign pigmented or non-pigmented skin tumors—A pilot study on 3D hyperspectral imaging of complex skin surfaces and convolutional neural networks. J Clin Med 2022; 11(7): 1914. [http://dx.doi.org/10.3390/jcm11071914] [PMID: 35407522]

[88] Mahesh B. Machine learning algorithms-a review. Int J Sci Res 2020; 9(1): 381-6. [http://dx.doi.org/10.21275/ART20203995]

[89] Sampson DM, Sampson DD. AI-driven innovations in signal/image processing and data analysis for optical coherence tomography in clinical applications. Biophotonics and Biosensing. Elsevier. 2024; pp. 417-80.

[90] Chan S, Reddy V, Myers B, Thibodeaux Q, Brownstone N, Liao W. Machine learning in dermatology: current applications, opportunities, and limitations. Dermatol Ther (Heidelb) 2020; 10(3): 365-86. [http://dx.doi.org/10.1007/s13555-020-00372-0] [PMID: 32253623]

[91] Aljohani K, Turki T. Automatic classification of melanoma skin cancer with deep convolutional neural networks. AI 2022; 3(2): 512-25. [http://dx.doi.org/10.3390/ai3020029]

[92] A dermatologist with board certification has frequently studied thousands of patients' skin issues visually for years, looking for trends and then diagnosing them based on similarities to earlier cases. 2022.

[93] Olveres J, González G, Torres F, *et al.* What is new in computer vision and artificial intelligence in medical image analysis applications. Quant Imaging Med Surg 2021; 11(8): 3830-53. [http://dx.doi.org/10.21037/qims-20-1151] [PMID: 34341753]

[94] Albahar MA. Skin lesion classification using a convolutional neural network with a novel regularizer. IEEE Access 2019; 7: 38306-13. [http://dx.doi.org/10.1109/ACCESS.2019.2906241]

[95] Mehrabi JN, Baugh eg, Fast A, *et al.* A clinical perspective on the automated analysis of reflectance confocal microscopy in dermatology. Lasers Surg Med 2021; 53(8): 1011-9. [http://dx.doi.org/10.1002/lsm.23376] [PMID: 33476062]

[96] Phillips M, Greenhalgh J, Marsden H, Palamaras I. Detection of malignant melanoma using artificial intelligence: an observational study of diagnostic accuracy. Dermatol Pract Concept 2019; 10(1): 2020011.
[http://dx.doi.org/10.5826/dpc.1001a11] [PMID: 31921498]

[97] Abdou MA. Literature review: efficient deep neural networks techniques for medical image analysis. Neural Comput Appl 2022; 34(8): 5791-812.
[http://dx.doi.org/10.1007/s00521-022-06960-9]

[98] Scalvini S, Vitacca M, Paletta L, Giordano A, Balbi B. Telemedicine: a new frontier for effective healthcare services. Monaldi Arch Chest Dis 2004; 61(4): 226-33.
[http://dx.doi.org/10.4081/monaldi.2004.686] [PMID: 15909613]

[99] Wurm EM, Soyer HP, Smith AC. Introduction to teledermatology. Telemedicine in Dermatology 2012; pp. 1-6.

[100] Baba M, Seçkin D, Kapdağli S. A comparison of teledermatology using store-and-forward methodology alone, and in combination with Web camera videoconferencing. J Telemed Telecare 2005; 11(7): 354-60.
[http://dx.doi.org/10.1177/1357633X0501100706] [PMID: 16238837]

[101] van Sinderen F, Kuziemsky C, W Jaspers M, W Peute L. An exploration of dutch dermatologists' experience and satisfaction with teledermatology: Sociotechnical and complex adaptive system perspective. JMIR Dermatol 2024; 7(1): 56723.
[http://dx.doi.org/10.2196/56723] [PMID: 39059000]

[102] Nelson CA, Takeshita J, Wanat KA, *et al.* Impact of store-and-forward (SAF) teledermatology on outpatient dermatologic care: A prospective study in an underserved urban primary care setting. J Am Acad Dermatol 2016; 74(3): 484-90.
[http://dx.doi.org/10.1016/j.jaad.2015.09.058] [PMID: 26679528]

[103] Coustasse A, Sarkar R, Abodunde B, Metzger BJ, Slater CM. Use of teledermatology to improve dermatological access in rural areas. Telemed J E Health 2019; 25(11): 1022-32.
[http://dx.doi.org/10.1089/tmj.2018.0130] [PMID: 30741608]

[104] Whited JD. Teledermatology. Am J Clin Dermatol 2001; 2(2): 59-64.
[http://dx.doi.org/10.2165/00128071-200102020-00001] [PMID: 11705304]

[105] Bhat KS, Jain M, Kumar N. Infrastructuring telehealth in (in) formal patient-doctor contexts. Proceedings of the ACM on Human-Computer Interaction. 1-28.
[http://dx.doi.org/10.1145/3476064]

[106] Tripathi R, Mazmudar RS, Knusel KD, Bordeaux JS, Scott JF. Big data in dermatology: Publicly available health care databases for population health research. J Am Acad Dermatol 2020; 83(5): 1546-56.
[http://dx.doi.org/10.1016/j.jaad.2020.04.145] [PMID: 32376426]

[107] Philip Chen CL, Zhang CY. Data-intensive applications, challenges, techniques and technologies: A survey on Big Data. Inf Sci 2014; 275: 314-47.
[http://dx.doi.org/10.1016/j.ins.2014.01.015]

[108] Viceconti M, Hunter P, Hose R. Big data, big knowledge: big data for personalized healthcare. IEEE J Biomed Health Inform 2015; 19(4): 1209-15.
[http://dx.doi.org/10.1109/JBHI.2015.2406883] [PMID: 26218867]

[109] Dimitrov DV. Medical internet of things and big data in healthcare. Healthc Inform Res 2016; 22(3): 156-63.
[http://dx.doi.org/10.4258/hir.2016.22.3.156] [PMID: 27525156]

[110] McNamara ME, Zisser M, Beevers CG, Shumake J. Not just "big" data: Importance of sample size, measurement error, and uninformative predictors for developing prognostic models for digital interventions. Behav Res Ther 2022; 153: 104086.

[http://dx.doi.org/10.1016/j.brat.2022.104086] [PMID: 35462242]

[111] Fan J, Han F, Liu H. Challenges of big data analysis. Natl Sci Rev 2014; 1(2): 293-314. [http://dx.doi.org/10.1093/nsr/nwt032] [PMID: 25419469]

[112] Bhadani AK, Jothimani D. Big data: challenges, opportunities, and realities. Effective Big Data Management and Opportunities for Implementation 2016; 1-24. [http://dx.doi.org/10.4018/978-1-5225-0182-4.ch001]

[113] Sagiroglu S, Sinanc D. Big data: A review. 2013 International Conference on Collaboration Technologies and Systems (CTS). 42-7. [http://dx.doi.org/10.1109/CTS.2013.6567202]

[114] National research council, division on engineering, physical sciences, board on mathematical sciences, their applications, committee on applied, theoretical statistics, committee on the analysis of massive data. Frontiers in massive data analysis. National Academies Press 2013.

[115] Lyko K, Nitzschke M, Ngonga Ngomo AC. Big data acquisition. New Horizons for a Data-Driven Economy: A Roadmap for Usage and Exploitation of Big Data in Europe 2016; 39-61. [http://dx.doi.org/10.1007/978-3-319-21569-3_4]

[116] Gudivada V, Apon A, Ding J. Data quality considerations for big data and machine learning: Going beyond data cleaning and transformations. International Journal on Advances in Software 2017; 10(1): 1-20.

[117] Nagurney JT, Brown DF, Sane S, Weiner JB, Wang AC, Chang Y. The accuracy and completeness of data collected by prospective and retrospective methods. Acad Emerg Med 2005; 12(9): 884-95. [http://dx.doi.org/10.1197/j.aem.2005.04.021] [PMID: 16141025]

[118] Gudivada V, Apon A, Ding J. Data quality considerations for big data and machine learning: Going beyond data cleaning and transformations. International Journal on Advances in Software 2017; 10(1): 1-20.

[119] Moura J, Hutchison D. Review and analysis of networking challenges in cloud computing. J Netw Comput Appl 2016; 60: 113-29. [http://dx.doi.org/10.1016/j.jnca.2015.11.015]

[120] Mishra J, Dash SK, Dash S. Mobile-cloud: A framework of cloud computing for mobile application. Advances in Computer Science and Information Technology. Computer Science and Information Technology: Second International Conference, CCSIT 2012, Bangalore, India, January 2-4, 2012. Proceedings 2012; 2(Part III): 347-56. [Springer Berlin Heidelberg.].

[121] Ayat S, Khoroushani MM. Cloud computing for providing electronic service for skin health. Journal of Automation and Control Engineering 2016; 4(4): 319-23. [http://dx.doi.org/10.18178/joace.4.4.319-323]

[122] Pulimamidi R. Leveraging IoT devices for improved healthcare accessibility in remote areas: An exploration of emerging trends. Internet of Things and Edge Computing Journal 2022; 2(1): 20-30.

[123] Blount M, Batra VM, Capella AN, *et al.* Remote health-care monitoring using Personal Care Connect. IBM Syst J 2007; 46(1): 95-113. [http://dx.doi.org/10.1147/sj.461.0095]

[124] Lakshmi GJ, Ghonge M, Obaid AJ. Cloud-based IoT smart healthcare system for remote patient monitoring. EAI Endorsed Trans Pervasive Health Technol 2021; 7(28): 4. [http://dx.doi.org/10.4108/eai.15-7-2021.170296]

[125] Rindfleisch TC. Privacy, information technology, and health care. Commun ACM 1997; 40(8): 92-100. [http://dx.doi.org/10.1145/257874.257896]

[126] Balbim GM, Marques IG, Marquez DX, *et al.* Using Fitbit as a mHealth intervention tool to promote physical activity: potential challenges and solutions. JMIR Mhealth Uhealth 2021; 9(3): 25289.

[http://dx.doi.org/10.2196/25289] [PMID: 33646135]

[127] Ali O, Shrestha A, Soar J, Wamba SF. Cloud computing-enabled healthcare opportunities, issues, and applications: A systematic review. International Journal of Information Management. 2018 Dec 1;43:146-58.

[128] Mohammed MN, Desyansah SF, Al-Zubaidi S, Yusuf E. An internet of things-based smart homes and healthcare monitoring and management system. J Phys Conf Ser. IOP Publishing. 2020; 1450: p. (1)012079.
[http://dx.doi.org/10.1088/1742-6596/1450/1/012079]

[129] Zeadally S, Bello O. Harnessing the power of Internet of Things based connectivity to improve healthcare. Internet of Things 2021; 14: 100074.
[http://dx.doi.org/10.1016/j.iot.2019.100074]

[130] Poongodi T, Rathee A, Indrakumari R, Suresh P. IoT sensing capabilities: sensor deployment and node discovery, wearable sensors, wireless body area network (WBAN), data acquisition. Principles of Internet of Things (IoT) Ecosystem: Insight Paradigm 2020; 127-51.

[131] Abdulmalek S, Nasir A, Jabbar WA, *et al.* IoT-based healthcare-monitoring system towards improving quality of life: A review. InHealthcare 2022 Oct 11. MDPI 1993; 10.

[132] Philip NY, Rodrigues JJPC, Wang H, Fong SJ, Chen J. Internet of Things for in-home health monitoring systems: Current advances, challenges, and future directions. IEEE J Sel Areas Comm 2021; 39(2): 300-10.
[http://dx.doi.org/10.1109/JSAC.2020.3042421]

[133] Faham S, Salimi A, Ghavami R. Electrochemical-based remote biomarker monitoring: Toward Internet of Wearable Things in telemedicine. Talanta 2023; 253: 123892.
[http://dx.doi.org/10.1016/j.talanta.2022.123892] [PMID: 36095939]

[134] Su M, Hua J, Sun X, Liu Z, Shi Y, Pan L. Wireless wearable devices and recent applications in health monitoring and clinical diagnosis. Biomed Mater Devices 2024; 2(2): 669-94.
[http://dx.doi.org/10.1007/s44174-023-00141-5]

[135] Aghdam ZN, Rahmani AM, Hosseinzadeh M. The role of the Internet of Things in healthcare: Future trends and challenges. Comput Methods Programs Biomed 2021; 199: 105903.
[http://dx.doi.org/10.1016/j.cmpb.2020.105903] [PMID: 33348073]

CHAPTER 5

Tele-Dermatology: Enhancing Access to Skin Cancer Experts

Sakshi Aole[1], **Safiya Bee**[1], **Taru Shrivastava**[1], **Apoorva Chourey**[2], **Ayushi Chourasia**[3] and **Shaweta Sharma**[4,*]

[1] *Mahakal Institute of Pharmaceutical Studies, Ujjain, Madhya Pradesh-456664, India*

[2] *Ujjain Institute of Pharmaceutical Sciences, Madhya Pradesh-456664, India*

[3] *Bhopal Institute of Technology & Science-Pharmacy, Bhopal-462045, India*

[4] *School of Medical and Allied Sciences, Galgotias University, Uttar Pradesh-201310, India*

Abstract: Dermatological care has been transformed by teledermatology, which has considerably improved access to skin cancer specialists. This is especially true in disadvantaged places, where there is a limited availability of specialist care resources. This chapter examines the development of teledermatology, with a focus on its techniques and the impact it has had on the treatment of skin cancer. Teledermatology makes use of both store-and-forward and real-time consultation methods, which enables the diagnosis and management of skin problems to be carried out remotely. Dermatologists can properly assess and triage patients through the use of these approaches. This allows for the early detection of skin cancers such as melanoma, basal cell carcinoma, and squamous cell carcinoma, which is essential for the survival and outcomes of patients. Recent developments in digital imaging, mobile health technologies, and the increasing use of electronic health records (EHRs) have all contributed to the acceleration of the incorporation of teledermatology into ordinary clinical practice. Furthermore, the utilization of artificial intelligence (AI) and machine learning in the field of teledermatology has resulted in an improvement in diagnosis accuracy. This has enabled assistance in the interpretation of intricate dermatological situations, hence enhancing the overall efficiency of care delivery.

The field of teledermatology, despite the many advantages it offers, is confronted with many obstacles. These obstacles include inequities in access to technology, concerns over the privacy and security of data, and the requirement for defined protocols to guarantee a uniform level of care. The legal and ethical considerations that are linked with teledermatology are also discussed in this chapter. Particular attention is paid to the issue of patient permission and the practice of medicine across jurisdictions. This chapter takes a look into the future and analyzes potential future directions in the field of teledermatology. These prospects include the possibility of deeper integration of

* **Corresponding author Shaweta Sharma:** School of Medical and Allied Sciences, Galgotias University, Uttar Pradesh-201310, India; E-mail: shawetasharma@galgotiasuniversity.edu.in

Akhil Sharma, Shaweta Sharma, Shivkanya Fuloria & Sudhir Kumar (Eds.)

artificial intelligence, the expansion of teledermatology services to other locations, and the ongoing development of innovative technology to improve patient care. Through the resolution of these problems and the utilization of the full potential of teledermatology, healthcare systems can guarantee wider and more equitable access to skin cancer expertise, which will ultimately result in improved patient outcomes internationally.

Keywords: Artificial intelligence, Dermatology, Digital health, EHR integration, Ethical considerations, Healthcare access, Melanoma, Real-time consultation, Remote consultation, Skin cancer, Teledermatology.

INTRODUCTION

Telemedicine is the practice of providing medical information and services through the utilization of various forms of telecommunication technologies. It is from the Greek root word "tele" that we get the phrase "telemedicine," which means "distant." Teledermatology is the term used to describe the practice of applying the concepts of telemedicine to the profession of dermatology. The practice of medicine at a distance is what is meant by the term "teledermatology," according to one definition. In recent years, there has been a consistent increase in the utilization of telemedicine [1]. This can be attributed to the ever-increasing affordability of emerging health and information technology, the enhancement of performance, and the growing clinical acceptability of telemedicine among both patients and medical professionals. Professionals in the field of dermatology have shown reluctance to implement telemedicine, just as they have in other medical specialties. The traditional doctor-patient connection, which has been considered the "gold standard" for a long time, is becoming more questioned [2]. On the other hand, teledermatology shows potential as an alternative method of providing medical care. Patients are increasingly expressing a desire for a change in the administration of health care. Some medical professionals, particularly those who have reservations about technology, have come to view telemedicine as a potential danger and are worried that the relationship between the physician and the patient may become more strained as a result. As a result of the elimination of traveling for patients, physicians, and nurses, teledermatology provides an obvious form of service delivery that is aimed at enhancing access and reducing costs. Radiology, psychiatry, cardiology, pathology, obstetrics, surgery, pathology, and nursing are some of the other medical specialties that have embraced and utilized the advent of telemedicine recently [3, 4].

Real-time teledermatology involves a live video consultation with the patient. In contrast, store-and-forward teledermatology involves the images of the patient being transmitted to the teleconsultant as the first step. After this, the consultant provides a relevant plan of action regarding diagnosis or management. Real-time teledermatology is a more advanced form of teledermatology. Both "real-time" and "store-and-forward" teledermatology are components that are included in hybrid teledermatology treatments. Mobile-teledermatology is the term used to describe teledermatology, which is performed utilizing mobile phones. There are a few extensions of teledermatology, such as teledermatopathology or telecytology, in which dermatopathology or cytology images are transferred, and teledermoscopy, in which physicians consult on dermoscopic images that are provided electronically [5].

Over the past two decades, teledermatology has demonstrated an increasing potential for use. The practice of dermatology is ideally suited for the application of telemedicine due to the inherent visual character of the field. Several teledermatology protocols that have been adopted for use in civilian projects were initially developed by the United States Department of Defense, which was one of the pioneers in this field [6, 7].

Systematic studies of the relevant literature have revealed that the most prevalent applications of teledermatology are for patient management, providing medical support in nursing homes and home care settings, and providing patient consultation in remote places. According to the data that has been released, the highest number of teledermatology practices are found in both North America and Europe. In terms of the practice of teledermatology, it appears that countries with a lower physician-to-patient ratio are underrepresented in the field [8, 9]. Teledermatology, a subset of telemedicine, plays a crucial role in modern healthcare by enhancing access to dermatological services, particularly for underserved populations. This innovative approach leverages technology to provide remote consultations, diagnoses, and treatments, which is especially beneficial in dermatology due to its visually dependent nature [10, 11].

Two primary categories have traditionally been used to categorize teledermatology: real-time teledermatology and store-and-forward teledermatology, which are shown in Fig. (**1**).

Importance in Modern Healthcare

Teledermatology is increasingly important in modern healthcare as it enhances access to specialized dermatological care, particularly for patients in underserved areas, as shown in Fig. (**2**). Utilizing advanced telecommunication technologies allows for timely diagnosis and management of skin conditions, ultimately improving patient outcomes and satisfaction.

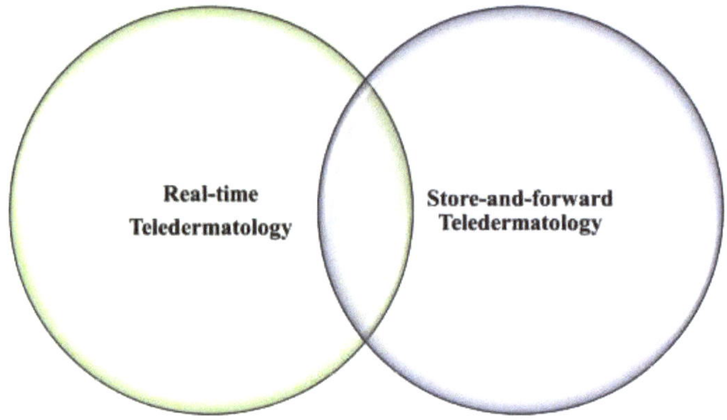

Fig. (1). Primary categories of teledermatology.

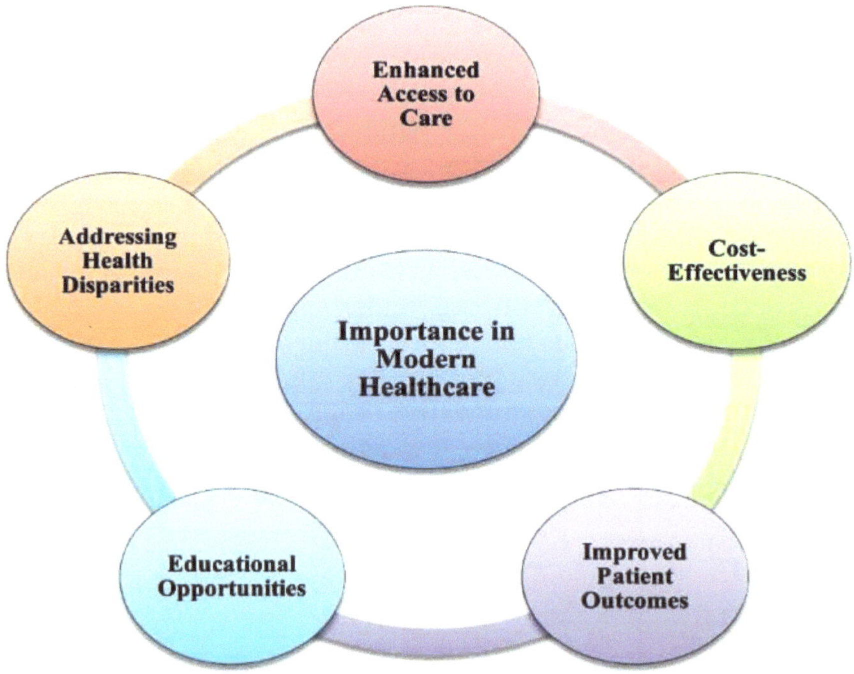

Fig. (2). Importance in modern healthcare.

Enhanced Access to Care

Patients, particularly those living in rural or disadvantaged locations, have considerably improved access to dermatological care thanks to the advent of teledermatology treatments. Because many people do not have access to dermatologists in their immediate vicinity, the diagnosis and treatment of skin problems, including skin malignancies, can be delayed. Through the utilization of teledermatology, medical professionals can access a larger patient population, hence decreasing the amount of time spent waiting for appointments and promoting prompt interventions [12, 13].

Cost-Effectiveness

The implementation of teledermatology into healthcare systems has the potential to result in significant cost reductions for healthcare providers as well as patients. Because it reduces the number of required in-person appointments, it helps patients save money on travel expenses and time away from work. The overhead costs of healthcare institutions can be reduced by the use of teledermatology, which enables these facilities to provide more efficient care to a greater number of patients [14].

Improved Patient Outcomes

There is a correlation between teledermatology and improvement in patient compliance as well as patient satisfaction. As a result of the ease of receiving care from the comfort of their own homes, patients are more likely to adhere to their treatment plans and have higher rates of follow-up appointments. Several studies have demonstrated that teledermatology is capable of achieving a high level of diagnostic accuracy. Some reports indicate that the success rate for online consultations can reach as high as 80 percent [15, 16].

Educational Opportunities

In addition, teledermatology functions as an instructional platform, offering patients and healthcare professionals access to a variety of available resources and training opportunities. By participating in remote consultations and case discussions, medical students and residents have the opportunity to get experience with a wide range of dermatological disorders. This element is of utmost significance for healthcare professionals [17, 18].

Addressing Health Disparities

Providing underprivileged groups with fair access to medical care is one of the most important contributions that teledermatology can make to the fight against health inequities. It has been demonstrated that it is beneficial to populations that have historically been subjected to obstacles in terms of accessing healthcare, such as racial minorities and individuals with lower socioeconomic positions. The use of teledermatology has the potential to enhance health outcomes in these groups by making it easier for them to obtain dermatological expertise [19, 20].

Overview of Skin Cancer

The most prevalent form of cancer in people with fair skin is skin cancer, which is found in populations all over the world. Because both the incidence and mortality rates of skin malignancies are on the rise, they pose a significant risk to the general population's health. The goal of trying to understand the etiology and pathogenesis of skin cancer is still something that healthcare systems strive to achieve. One of the most important steps in the prevention of skin cancer is to gain a better understanding of the elements that cause the disease [21]. A comprehensive examination of the factors that contribute to the development of skin cancer and the factors that cause it. The most significant contributor to the development of skin cancer is ultraviolet radiation (UV), which is emitted by the sun. The cumulative damage that is caused by sunburns and excessive exposure to the sun includes immunosuppression and the development of skin cancer. Ozone depletion, the amount of ultraviolet light, elevation, latitude, and altitude, as well as the meteorological conditions, all have an impact on the amount of ultraviolet radiation that is emitted and reaches the surface of the earth. Patients who have received organ transplants and those who have AIDS have a higher risk of developing skin cancer. Radiation therapy, phototherapy, and psoralen and long-wave ultraviolet radiation (PUVA) are all examples of treatment techniques that have the potential to increase the risk of developing skin cancer. There is a possibility that viral infections, such as the human papillomavirus, could cause squamous cell carcinomas. Those who have familial genetic disorders are more likely to develop certain types of skin cancer than the general population [22]. Many factors, including ionizing radiation, environmental contaminants, chemical carcinogens, and exposures to harmful substances, have been linked to the development of skin cancer. Attributable risks include exposure to artificial ultraviolet radiation (the kind that is found in tanning beds and lamps), aging, skin color, nutrition, and smoking. Dermatoses and various types of keratoses, wounds that are continuously wounded or take a long time to heal, and scars have all been linked to the development of skin cancer [23].

HISTORY AND EVOLUTION OF TELE-DERMATOLOGY

The exact date when telecommunications were first used in health care is unknown, but the known information is shown in Table **1**. The concept may have originated centuries ago if, for example, information about bubonic plague was transmitted across Europe by heliograph or bonfires, as was information about war and famine. It is known that the telegraph was used during the Civil War to transmit casualty lists and order medical supplies. By 1900, the telephone was in use, and physicians were among the first to adopt it. The telephone was the mainstay of medical communications for fifty years and remains a major force. At the time of World War I, radio communication was established, and by 1930, it was used in remote areas such as Alaska and Australia to transfer medical information. By the time of the Korean and Vietnam conflicts, radio communication was used regularly to dispatch medical teams and helicopters [24, 25].

Current telemedicine systems originated from developments in the operated space flight program and separately from the pioneering efforts of a few physicians using off-the-shelf commercial equipment. One of the first efforts to overcome time and distance barriers was telemetry research and development (R&D) undertaken by the National Aeronautics and Space Administration (NASA) in its operated space-flight program. Demonstrating that physiological functions for astronauts in space could be monitored successfully by physicians on Earth, NASA's scientists, engineers, and contractors developed sophisticated biomedical telemetry and telecommunications systems for biomedical applications [26]. Initially, NASA scientists were concerned with the physiological effects of zero gravity on astronauts. This concern was translated into constant monitoring of physiological functions: heart rate, blood pressure, respiration rate, and temperature. Extended flight times resulted in the development of medical support systems, including means for diagnosing and treating in-flight emergencies. NASA's experience brought into sharp focus the parallel between the needs of an earth-bound physician trying to monitor, diagnose, and treat an astronaut in space and the needs of equally earthbound physicians trying to diagnose or treat a patient in a remote location [27].

Table 1. Representation of history and evolution of tele-dermatology.

Period	Milestone/Event	Description	Reference
1970s	Early Concepts	Implementation of telemedicine ideas, with the first practice in distant consultations *via* the analog mode (*e.g.*, telephone and fax).	[33]
1980s	First Teledermatology Trials	Store-and-forward methods in early trials of teledermatology. The images were photographed, transferred to digital media, and transmitted by modem.	[34, 35]
1990s	Adoption of Digital Imaging	Advantages such as a better quality of imaging enabled by the widespread adoption of digital cameras made store-and-forward teledermatology possible.	[36]
1995	First Real-time Teledermatology Consultations	Online consultations in real-time (*via* videoconferencing): synchronous patient and doctor interaction.	[37, 38]
Late 1990s	Teledermatology in Rural Healthcare	Teledermatology services in the rural implementation of teledermatology program and remote dermatology.	[39]

(Table 1) cont.....

Period	Milestone/Event	Description	Reference
2000s	Growth of Teledermatology Networks	Creation of teledermatology networks within healthcare systems to facilitate collaboration between the dermatologist and primary care provider.	[40, 41]
2010s	Integration with Electronic Health Records (EHRs)	Uploading photos of skin conditions became the first teledermatology step integrated with EHRs, and it improved data interoperability and patient management.	[42, 43]
2010s	Mobile Teledermatology	Smartphones and mobile apps made it possible for patients to send images directly to dermatologists, which also improved the accessibility of dermatology.	[44, 45]
2015	Rise of Direct-to-Consumer Teledermatology Services	Direct-to-consumer platforms enable access to dermatology services without requiring a referral from a primary care provider.	[46, 47]
2020	COVID-19 Pandemic	Increased use of teledermatology during the pandemic, rapid uptake and use by dermatologists and patients, and greater tolerance from healthcare systems.	[48, 49]
2020s	Advanced AI and Machine Learning Integration	Integration of artificial intelligence (AI) and machine learning to aid in diagnostic accuracy, triage, and treatment recommendations within teledermatology platforms.	[50, 51]
Present and Future	Expansion of Teledermatology	Ongoing technical improvements, as well as increasing recognition of teledermatology as a routine part of the dermatologic practice (and probably, greater incorporation with AI)	[52, 53].

A second major influence on the development of telemedicine was the introduction of television. By the late 1950s, developments in closed-circuit television and video telecommunications were recognized by medical personnel, who began to use television in clinical settings. The first interactive video link was established in 1964 between the Nebraska Psychiatric Institute in Omaha and the Norfolk State Hospital, 112 miles away. The first complete telemedicine system linking paraprofessionals and physician-patient encounter settings was installed in 1967, linking the medical station at Boston's Logan Airport to Massachusetts General Hospital. During this initial stage of implementation and testing, researchers demonstrated that remote diagnosis was possible through interactive television and that X-rays, medical records, and laboratory data could be transmitted successfully [28].

During the late 1960s and early 1970s, the federal government provided funding to support the implementation of seven telemedicine research and demonstration projects. It was hoped that these projects in various settings would help determine the capabilities of the equipment and their clinical applicability, as well as the feasibility of telemedicine for solving or mitigating specific problems in medical care. Each demonstration program provided opportunities to test the capability of telemedicine to address a specific set of medical care issues, as well as opportunities for further experimentation with equipment capabilities and physical diagnosis [29].

Despite the many projects, the hoped-for definitive conclusions were not obtained. Rather, answers were found for some questions, while more research was recommended to find answers for others. The feasibility of establishing the technological base for telemedicine was verified. It was demonstrated that telecommunications could be utilized as a substitute for travel to obtain medical care, to increase coordination and extend medical and administrative functions within large institutions, and to establish a vital link in emergencies where access to a physician was difficult or impossible to arrange [30 - 32].

TYPES OF TELE-DERMATOLOGY

Teledermatology is a subfield of dermatology that utilizes telecommunications technology to facilitate the provision of healthcare in a location separate from the patient. It is mostly classified into Store-and-Forward (Asynchronous), Live Interactive (Synchronous), and Hybrid Models. Each has its processes, use cases, benefits, and challenges [54].

Store-and-Forward (Asynchronous)

Store-and-forward teledermatology refers to the process of obtaining digital images and associated medical information from the patient and sending this information for later review by a dermatologist. This approach does not need both parties to be present at the same time, so it is more flexible regarding consultations. For example, one process involves photographing skin ailments, uploading them to a digital platform securely, and then relaying the images and any relevant information to an expert who will review them and provide guidance [55, 56].

Use Cases in Skin Cancer

It is helpful in the case of skin cancer examination because this way, dermatologists can review several cases, which allows them to diagnose patients more quickly and accurately. The studies reviewed indicate that store-and-forward teledermatology is effective for triaging patients suspected of having skin malignancies and can expedite referrals to specialists when appropriate [57, 58].

Live Interactive (Synchronous)

These are teledermatological consultations that take place in real-time through video conferencing links between patients and dermatologists. In the synchronous method, healthcare providers and patients interact with each other in real-time *via* audio-visual communication tools to discuss their physical complaints, physically check on one another, and promptly prescribe or provide treatment advice [59, 60].

Use Cases in Skin Cancer

The use of live interactive consultations is an advantage for urgent cases, including potential skin cancers, in which management decisions need to be made immediately. Permitting more comfortable examinations and also the capability to talk with patients directly, this technique aids in diagnosing problems and increasing general satisfaction amongst dermatologists [59, 61].

Hybrid Models

Combining Asynchronous and Synchronous

Hybrid teledermatology integrates components of both the store-and-forward (SAF) and live interactive types of teledermatology. Asynchronous consultations can be held initially, which can then be followed by synchronous conversations if any clear clarifications or immediate interaction is required. This flexibility has the potential to improve patient care by tailoring it to differing clinical situations and patient needs [62, 63].

Benefits and Challenges

Methods of teledermatology (store-and-forward *versus* real-time [synchronous]) have their unique advantages and challenges. Store-and-forward teledermatology refers to taking and transmitting digital images of skin conditions for subsequent assessment by a dermatologist. The main advantage of this method is that it is more convenient for patients and healthcare providers; there is no need for both parties to be online at the same time to exchange information. This is particularly beneficial for rural or underserved regions, as specialists are more difficult to access. Disadvantages include the dermatologist not being able to complete an examination and relying solely on images and text, which may lead to limited diagnostic accuracy [64].

On the other hand, real-time teledermatology includes face-to-face video consultations between the patient and the dermatologist. This gives the opportunity for real-time feedback and interaction so that the dermatologist can ask questions and view the skin condition live, which is a synchronous method of teledermatology. This interconnectedness of the consultation will lead to better diagnosis and treatment plans. However, both parties need to be available at the same time, and it consumes a lot of bandwidth, requiring a significant technology infrastructure to support it (which may not be feasible in remote areas with low internet penetration). Furthermore, the quality of the video feed may sometimes also affect the overall goal of a dermatological examination [65].

Both methods achieve great advancements in dermatology care accessibility, lower travel time and costs for patients, and shorter consultative processes. On the other hand, these tools are limited in their technology and raise some privacy issues; training and guiding employees to use them well is also necessary [66].

ADVANTAGES OF TELE-DERMATOLOGY IN SKIN CANCER CARE

Teledermatology is a major innovation in the management of skin cancer, allowing for many advantages that enhance patient care and access to dermatological services [65, 67].

Improved Access to Care

Teledermatology offers a low-cost solution that does not bypass dermatologists as it expands care- any underserved or distant patient may access dermatological care directly from teledermatology. This allows for the delivery of timely skin cancer assessments and follow-ups even to patients who would otherwise find it difficult to attend in-person appointments (particularly where geographic distance or problems with gaining access to transport exist) [68].

Enhanced Diagnostic Efficiency

Teledermatology, especially with store-and-forward systems, has been shown to provide rapid diagnostics. Patients can send photographers with skin lesions to dermatologists, who will then assess them without the need for an immediate face-to-face consultation. This reduces waiting time for consultations and may lead to faster diagnosis and treatment initiation [69, 70].

High Diagnostic Concordance

Research shows that teledermatology has a similar diagnostic accuracy to standard face-to-face consultations. With teledermoscopy, we can record enhanced pictures of skin lesions, which can even give us a better diagnosis. There are many examples of this, but among the best understood are pigmented lesions and skin malignancies. As improvement in survival rates relies heavily on early detection, this reliability is crucial for the effective treatment of skin cancer [71, 72].

Cost-Effectiveness

Teledermatology can help to lower the cost of healthcare by decreasing the number of case management that need personal examination by doctors. Patients and healthcare systems also see these trips as expensive and time-consuming. Many dermatologists are now able to handle more patients with virtual consultations while still maintaining the quality of care they provide. This reality makes virtual consultations an economically viable option for skin cancer detection and management [73].

Patient Satisfaction

Often, patients show a great deal of satisfaction from receiving treatment through teledermatology. Virtual consultations provide patients with the opportunity to gain expert opinions without traveling to the consult location, thus providing a better experience for the patient overall and the people who will be best able to express satisfaction with service are the ones who, in the past, might not have made it past the door because of headaches in getting to dermatology [74].

Support for Continuous Monitoring

Teledermatology is an excellent platform for follow-up in patients with a long history of skin cancer or at high risk. Frequent virtual check-ins is equal to better long-term management outcomes. This is vital for prompt interventions and modification of treatment plans based on profiles of skin problems [75, 76].

CHALLENGES AND LIMITATIONS

Teledermatology, which has emerged in recent years, allows for really accessible and instantaneous visualization of melanomas and other skin lesions. However, apart from its advantages, it has some limitations, as shown in Fig. (**3**). In developing countries, constraints are especially associated with inadequate technological and physical infrastructure, legal restrictions, demand deficits, and restricted reimbursements. The authors from the Department of Dermatology in NY separated 5 different categories of limitations that fall under clinical, economic, technological, legal, and ethical limits. An appropriate grasp of challenges in teledermatology practice is instrumental for stakeholders (policymakers, specialists, and referring providers) to bring purposeful improvements on the ground [77, 78].

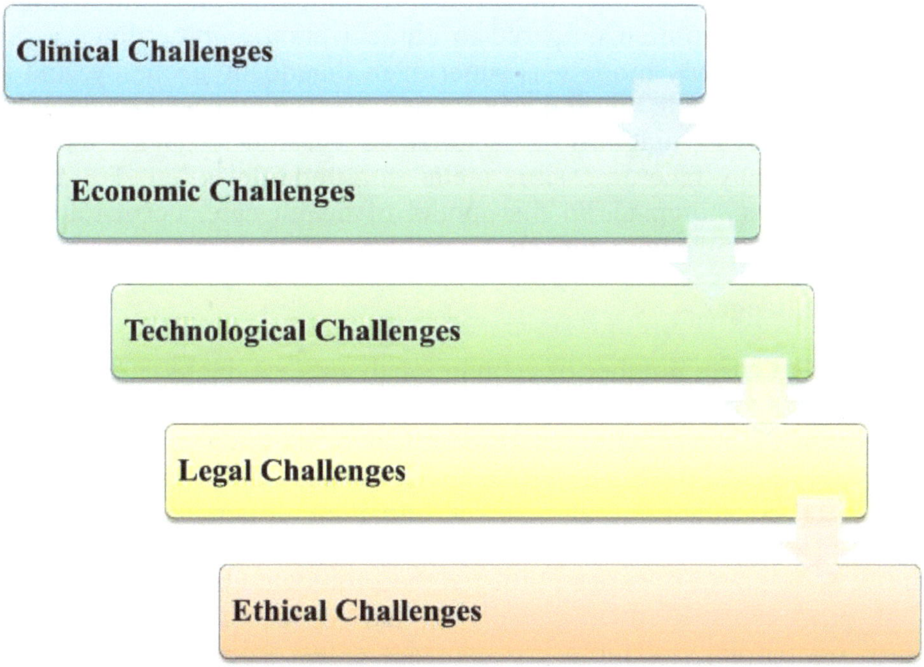

Fig. (3). Challenges and limitations of teledermatology.

Clinical Challenges

Clinical importance is strictly indicated and carries appropriate diagnosis and subsequent circumstances. For others, teledermatology accuracy might be questionable when diagnosing dermatoses like psoriasis, atopic dermatitis, and actinic keratosis. Palpation is not possible through teledermatology, although the physical examination is a precious asset during the assessment of a patient and, as such, at least equally important as visual diagnosis [79].

There are some limitations or conditions that are not ideal specifications for the store and forward model, such as when a complete body examination is required, lesions are located on hair-bearing regions, patients with naevus belonging to the high-risk group of melanoma development, or extensive medical history, which needs to be discussed in person. The store and forward model are asynchronous, which allows for the efficient practice of teledermatology, where overhead is minimized but may be less feasible in communication among referring physicians and dermatologists [80]. If patients have questions about recommendations and wish for clarification, they could very well struggle to obtain feedback. The concerns of patients regarding improper treatment and inadequate follow-up are flagged on the website, including links to reports published by MBC. This need for information exchange may hinder the development and improvement of teledermatology programs. Compared to clinical photography alone, a remote-operated teledermoscopy mode was superior in diagnostic accuracy, and paired with an in-person visit, it fell short of direct-contact (in-person) cases. Furthermore, when diagnosing pigmented lesions, GPs using only teledermatology may face a possible melanoma underdetection. To prevent the risks of unnecessary biopsies in this model of health care, dermatologists and non-dermatologists must both agree to do full-body skin examinations [81, 82].

Economic Challenges

Teledermatology has a number of economic advantages, including a decrease in the number of referrals, loss of employment, and travel time. Getting reimbursed was the most commonly identified challenge. Although this phenomenon theoretically has little basis, there is a widespread belief that teledermatology reimburses for consultations at a lower rate than in-person visits. The most frequently cited concerns are procedure refunds that can be delayed or never materialize. The possible explanation for the problems above could be the low quota of procedures in teledermatology and its newcomers. Compared to traditional dermatology, remote procedures are less known, documented, and ordered. Finally, the remuneration associated with remote consultations is also less than face-to-face contacts, which means that it may also be impossible to engage sufficient numbers of clinicians as patients in one system present for fewer follow-up visits and are also billed for fewer services per running costs of consults [83, 84].

Technological Challenges

Technological barriers are the most frequently cited challenges in teledermatology. Inefficient, costly software, billing systems integration and poor image quality are the areas in which improvement is mostly needed, as per the evidence reported. Expensive smartphones and commercially available telemedicine platforms make it difficult to produce viable, cost-effective solutions compatible with pre-existing medical record systems. The use of images taken with smartphones can be misleading, as their cameras are lower quality than professional cameras, and the healthcare workforce does not have photography training. These are all dysfunctionalities that hinder the provision of good quality and timely care [85, 86].

Legal Challenges

This is the consultative practice model of teledermatology, where practitioners make recommendations based on histories and pictures they receive. One of the most serious concerns is the security of patient information and medical data transferred electronically. According to the position statement on telemedicine from the American Academy of Dermatology Association, log notes providers must encrypt transmissions to protect health information. They should incorporate safety awareness in the consent process and keep information on servers behind firewalls. Patients ought to be fully apprised of who will have access, how information is stored, and, with it, all the benefits and challenges [87, 88].

Ethical Challenges

The support for Telemedicine is highly relevant in underserved areas. Telehealth providers and systems should give notice of the influence telehealth may have on access to health care, delivery of patient relationships, availability for equitable treatment, cost, and quality. Doctors worry that telemedicine will foster a tech-based instead of patient-centred model. And they also mention the concern that this variety of technology will never humanize medical consultations. As we tailor teledermatology to fight against patient exploitation and train doctors in rural areas, setting up the medical awareness and dermatologic understanding of those who will benefit from this service, it is still always worth keeping in mind that education remains the heart of teledermatology [89, 90].

TELE-DERMATOLOGY IN SKIN CANCER SCREENING AND DIAGNOSIS

Tele-dermatology crucially contributes to skin cancer detection, screening programs, and diagnosis.

Early Detection and Screening Programs

Teledermatology is the main digital innovation applied to skin cancer screening and diagnosis, which improves efficiency and access. It thus significantly increases the chances for early detection of skin cancer, which is pivotal for successful treatment outcomes, by enabling timely referral to experts in dermatology for dubious skin lesions. This model proves useful for areas that are more rural and may have less access to things such as specialty healthcare. Teledermatology provides a potential solution for alleviating some burden of shortages in specialists by expanding access to their clinical services by integrating with teledermoscopy and distance learning technologies, making it easier for health personnel (*e.g.*, general practitioners) trained to incorporate this information into patient care and communication without geographical barriers between them or the patients they serve [91].

This finding suggests that teledermatology is a viable way to obtain quick diagnosis and management of suspected skin cancer lesions. Both services are what is referred to as teledermatology, in which patients send in images of their undisclosed condition, and dermatologists interpret the images remotely rather than having them come into the office. This process not only speeds up diagnosis but also eases the burden on healthcare centers, enabling them to manage their resources better. Thus, teledermatology not only improves access to dermatologic care but also continues to be a critical tool for the timely diagnosis and treatment of skin cancer, which is critical in contributing to improved health outcomes [92].

AI and Machine Learning Integration

Artificial intelligence (AI) and machine learning are rapidly changing the landscape of early detection and diagnosis for diseases like skin cancer, especially actinic keratoses (AKs), which represent precancerous skin lesions that can progress to squamous cell carcinoma if untreated. AI for analyzing clinical photographs of skin lesions shows promise, and researchers are currently investigating automated detection methods. AI algorithms have been developed to detect and circumscribe AKs based on color space transforms and morphological features (detecting erythema), thus facilitating non-invasive, objective identification of AKs with a reduction in the number of biopsies required for diagnosis, improving screening efficiency [93].

Combining AI and machine learning with teledermatology has considerable promise for improving the evaluation of skin lesions in primary care. AI-enhanced teledermatology systems can offer better and more consistent evaluations of skin lesions using sophisticated image analysis methods in regions where dermatology experts are limited. Such AI-powered methodologies have demonstrated excellent sensitivity and specificity in distinguishing between benign and malignant skin lesions, including hierarchical non-invasive imaging with line-field confocal optical coherence tomography (LC-OCT) to precisely grade AKs in a non-invasive manner. AI brings automation and objectivity, which can prevent interobserver variability and make the diagnostic faster, resulting in rapid intervention and, hence, overall better patient outcomes [94, 95].

This combination of new artificial intelligence and machine-learning technologies with teledermatology will be essential for increasing rapid access to appropriate skin cancer screening, particularly where such specialist services are currently limited. With AI, healthcare will be better equipped to identify early-stage precancerous lesions and skin cancers to lower morbidity and mortality [96].

Diagnostic Accuracy

Teledermatology has been investigated extensively in terms of its accuracy and degree of agreement with an in-person dermatologist assessment, and most studies report a high level of concordance between both modalities. In particular, gigapixel teledermatology, or teledermatology combined with the interpretation of high-resolution digital images for short- and remote examination of skin lesions, is a reliable tool for diagnosing skin cancers. Studies have demonstrated high concordance (calculated by kappa statistics) between teledermatology and face-to-face assessment, and good diagnostic accuracy in clinical practice has shown that when the dermatologist is interpreting the teledermatology, it can be at least as accurate as an in-person visit for identification and classification of skin lesions [97].

It is clear from the data that the chance a teledermatologist misses a malignant skin lesion is quite low. Research indicates the misdiagnosis or missed skin cancer rates are less than 7% with teledermatology diagnosis. These features demonstrate, as teledermatology has correctly diagnosed the majority of skin cancers and early detection is critical when it comes to skin cancer treatment [98], that it has the potential to be a very good screening tool.

Please note that the diagnostic accuracy of teledermatology may differ from one study to another based on population, type of methods used in teledermatology settings, and whether dermatologists are general providers or not. The accuracy of teledermatology diagnoses depends on multiple factors such as image quality, usage of teledermoscopy, and availability of clinical history. Both studies show some significant differences in methods, and though the overall evidence points toward teledermatology being an accurate modality for diagnosing skin cancer, this is also a call to interpret results based on contexts [99, 100].

Comparison with in-Person Consultations

Teledermatology has opened up as one of the useful pieces of equipment that can deliver a potentially comparable standard of effectiveness to dermatologists' face-to-face assessments in several aspects of skin cancer management. Teledermatology has, in study after study, been shown to provide a level of diagnostic accuracy and treatment recommendations comparable to standard face-to-face consultations when conducted using appropriate protocols (for example, the use of high-quality digital imaging) and secure communication platforms. Teledermatology has one of the great benefits, which is that it can accelerate advice and management for patients presenting or referred to suspected skin cancers, dermatoses, or other dermatology diseases. Teledermatology can dramatically decrease the time interval from initial consultation to appropriate treatment/patient follow-up with telemedicine by removing the face-to-face encounter. This is especially advantageous to patients living in rural locations that have limited access to dermatology or for those with barriers to attending a physical appointment, such as transportation issues or scheduling conflicts. Teledermatology can enable resourcing around the diagnostic and management process to ensure that all patients receive care when they need it, ultimately improving outcomes for a disease where immediate treatment offers the greatest benefit [101, 102].

While this project highlights some of the benefits associated with teledermatology, it is essential to be aware of its limitations. The main limitation of teledermatology for skin cancer screening or follow-up is that it may be difficult to do a thorough total body examination on video. Without the benefit of being able to see and palpate, many skin lesions or conditions may be missed or underappreciated; that is a key advantage of an in-person dermatology exam. This can create limitations for healthcare providers as they may have to depend on images or videos provided by the patient themselves, which may not always provide them with a complete picture of what is going on with the patient's skin. For some conditions, a physical examination is required to confirm the diagnosis or identify the initial treatment plan [103]; hence, an in-person visit cannot be avoided.

The limitations related to physical examination are important. However, the advantages of teledermatology, including improved access, shorter wait times, and similar efficacy, outweigh this limitation, making it an important tool in the management of skin cancer and other dermatological conditions. With ongoing technological developments, along with the improved adaption of health systems in the face of current forces and trends, the role of teledermatology for skin cancer screening and diagnosis may become more prominent over time, resulting in better patient care free-up health resources [104].

Referral Systems and Specialist Access

Novel electronic referral systems are regarded as a paradigm shift in teledermatology, allowing for expedited diagnosis and management of skin cancer lesions. The systems, which allow general practitioners (GPs) to send digital referrals that include high-resolution photographs of skin disorders, bypass hoops around the referral process and permit dermatologists to evaluate by allowing GP Studies, for example, suggest that the mean time between referrals submitted and assessment by an expert is one day [105], which greatly shortens the diagnostic process compared to usual in-person consultations.

Teledermatology improves the timeliness of diagnosis and allows for the management of some cases to remain in primary care settings. Such an approach reduces the pressure on specialist services and enables patients to get treated promptly. Teledermatology, by its state-of-the-art geographical dispersion, also tends to desaturate the influx of dermatological consultancy requests, and reports have shown that waiting times for dermatologic appointments can be as high as weeks in some areas. Still, they are dropped down to just a few days when teledermatology is integrated into practice. Specifically, in regions where dermatologists are not available, it could increase the availability of exact diagnostics and proper management of skin lesions, which would lead to improved patient outcomes [106].

Teledermatology represents a promising strategy for increasing the capacity of healthcare provision in settings with limited dermatopathologists by making primary care the first line of defense against skin diseases while also considering alternative strategies such as providing additional services. The adoption of a more integrated model of skin cancer management resulted in deploying primary care providers with the tools and training to access teledermatology as needed. Not only does this enhance access to specialist consultations, but it also facilitates earlier detection and treatment for skin cancers, which is vital in increasing survival and mitigating the long-term healthcare burden of such malignancies [107].

IMPACT ON PATIENT OUTCOMES

Teledermatology has demonstrated significant benefits in improving patient outcomes, particularly in the context of skin cancer management. Some ways to impact patient outcomes are shown in Fig. (**4**).

Improved Survival Rates

Teledermatology can significantly improve the survival rates of skin cancers by enabling early detection, as cancers detected at an earlier stage are typically more treatable and have better prognoses. In teledermatology, patients are promptly evaluated *via* photos of suspicious lesions from dermatology experts, and they do not have to wait long for in-person referrals. Teledermatology has been shown in one significant study to reduce the time from referral to diagnosis and treatment of skin cancers compared with traditional methods. In such a study, patients have been referred to specialized units, and the waiting period to see a specialist has been reduced [108].

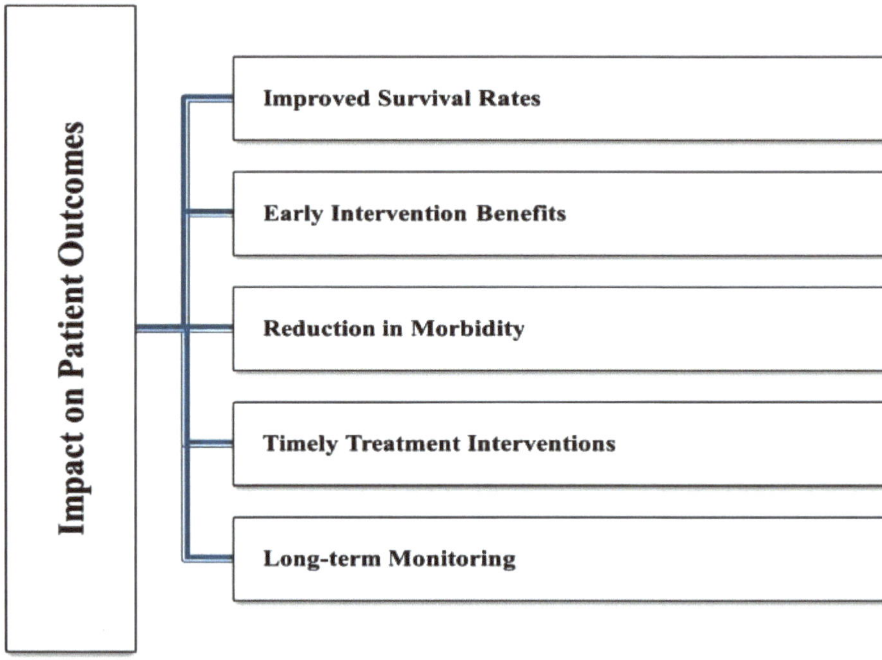

Fig. (4). Impact on patient outcomes on teledermatology.

This rapid access to professional assessment is invaluable, considering that, in the case of skin cancer, treatment times are often measured in weeks. Being able to detect skin cattle quickly and early not only gives the treatment a better success rate but also helps in reducing patient suffering. In addition, teledermatology promotes early intervention and helps avoid the progression of skin cancers to higher stages that lead to an increase in morbidity and mortality by stage. Thus, the way integration of teledermatology into healthcare systems represents a paradigm shift in skin cancer management and, consequently, improved patient-oriented outcomes and quality of life for patients with skin diseases [109].

Early Intervention Benefits

Teledermatology enables timely intervention for any suspicious lesions over the skin and accurate diagnosis followed by effective treatment of skin cancers. Teledermatology is a method of using digital technologies to provide faster access for patients than traditional methods, often enabling quicker assessment and management by dermatology specialists. Quick access is essential since early-stage skin diseases are treatable 3 orders of magnitude more easily, thus affecting patient outcome/survival [110].

In another study, patients whose diagnoses changed based on teledermatology (compared with those whose diagnoses were unchanged) had 1.97 odds of clinically improving. The added note here is that teledermatology does not just need to be a mechanism for detecting skin cancers but a means of ensuring appropriate and timely action occurs. Teledermatology helps in achieving this through an expert assessment of the diagnosis as well as a review of treatment options, leading to a more streamlined approach towards clinical management and ultimately allowing faster delivery of care to patients. Notably, through its ability to provide accurate assessments and timely interventions, the incorporation of teledermatology into skin cancer management fosters a more proactive approach toward disease treatment. It improves patient quality of care for lesions suspected to be malignant [111, 112].

Reduction in Morbidity

Early identification and management of skin cancers *via* teledermatology can help limit downstream morbidity due to advanced disease. Teledermatology provides rapid access to specialist dermatology expertise, enabling the diagnosis and prompt management of suspicious skin lesions, the latter being critical for preventing the progression of skin cancers to higher stages associated with greater morbidity and overall mortality [113].

In another study, teledermatology was integrated into the workflow of an urban safety-net hospital. It demonstrated a staggering reduction in new patient wait times from a mean of 84.6 days to 14.1 days. The significant reduction in wait times is an improvement in patient experience. Also, it means patients are receiving timely treatment, thus reducing the risk of avoidable adverse events related to dermatologically treated skin cancers. The triaging and treatment of dermatologist visits in one low-cost tool without leaving your home has an immeasurable physical and mental pillar to avoid advanced disease—something that leads to better health outcomes. Tailored to making dermatologic care available, teledermatology serves as a trickle of hope that contributes to early diagnosis and treatment of skin cancers, which leads to lower morbidity and, thus, an overall better life for the sufferer by bringing about a closer patients- to-dermatologist bridge [114].

Timely Treatment Interventions

Teledermatology can both shorten the time from presentation to diagnosis and allow for some of those cases to be treated in primary care - measures that can considerably expedite treatment compared with unmediated face-to-face encounters. Teledermatology allows dermatology specialists to rapidly assess skin lesions through the use of digital technologies, resulting in more timely diagnosis and commencement of suitable treatment regimens. This is especially useful in regions where the availability of dermatological services for patients may be delayed or not available due to some geographical difficulties, which can also prevent patients from getting treated on time, so teledermatology comes and fills up that gap and addresses timely patient care [115].

This means that some cases can be effectively treated and resolved in primary care, significantly reducing the demand for specialist services while still providing a more streamlined process for treatment. Teledermatology allows primary care providers to consult dermatologists, seek expert opinions, and put in place treatment plans for some skin diseases, thus minimizing the referrals for in-person encounters and speeding up the management of the condition by the patient overall [116].

According to the study, each additional teledermatology follow-up visit was associated with 2.06 increased odds of clinical improvement in outcomes. These findings indicate that teledermatology can improve clinical outcomes for long-term monitored skin conditions, possibly due to the timeliness of detection and prompt intervention for any treatment complications or changes. The management of skin diseases, particularly skin cancers, may be revolutionized by teledermatology to enable faster diagnosis and more efficient treatment pathways that are vital for improving outcomes and limiting morbidity from advanced disease [117, 118].

Long-term Monitoring

Teledermatology also allows for the continuous follow-up of skin lesions, which is essential for realizing early detection of changes or new injuries. This ongoing monitoring will be especially beneficial for patients with a history of skin cancer or those who are at high risk for developing skin lesions. Teledermatology permits better remote evaluation and monitoring of skin diseases, over time permitting tracking of any clinically significant changes alerting a dermatologist for early intervention optimizing results. Such a proactive effort can contribute to not just improving patient safety but also providing relief for anyone worried about the state of their skin [119].

Incorporating teledermatology services also addresses the issue of gaining new patients for already existing healthcare practices and patient health quality outcomes from existing affecting patients will improve as well. The biggest benefit of offering teledermatology is that it saves potential patients with previously identified barriers to dermatological access — long waiting times and geographical limitations aside. The addition of services will result in greater patient engagement and satisfaction as the receiving parties have been pleased with the convenience and access received from utilizing a teledermatology platform [120].

Adding teledermatology does not interfere with combined care for established patients. It does not compromise on the quality of service. Instead, it reflects in the overall delivery of the service as workflows are streamlined and healthcare providers can now accommodate a larger number of cases efficiently. With teledermatology, practices can be resource-efficient and deliver effective care to both new and existing patients promptly. This dual advantage of not only converting patients but also providing a great quality of care is the positivity behind teledermatology in modern healthcare delivery, especially dermatology [119].

FUTURE DIRECTIONS AND INNOVATIONS

The future of teledermatology will see significant advancements as new technology continues to emerge and different strategies are adopted to enhance patient care and access. Among the most promising advances is 5G technology, which allows for more real-time video consultations as well as remote monitoring of skin diseases at much higher resolutions. This technology offers fast data transmission and low latency, bringing the possibility of remote monitoring of skin diseases. Thanks to this innovation, there will be much faster interaction between patients and dermatologists; the advantage is even greater in geographically isolated areas with few specialists. Moreover, within this scope, adding wearable devices with sensors that monitor the skin condition continuously could lead to early recognition of rapid changes, favoring a prompt accomplishment of therapeutic interventions [120].

In teledermatology, the application of AI and ML is going to revolutionize diagnosis with regard to precision as well as speed. These technologies can analyze large amounts of data from patient images to assist in assessing skin lesions and predicting likely complications. With the aid of AI algorithms, improved diagnostic tools will increase dermatologists' decision-making powers and produce better patient outcomes. Also, predictive analytics help identify at-risk patients and tailor preventive measures, which leads to enhanced overall effectiveness of dermatological treatment [121].

The teledermatology domain continues to thrive, and legislative and regulatory modifications are imperative to stimulate its growth further. Funding parity for telehealth services (as we learned during the COVID-19 pandemic) will provide even more incentives for doctors to incorporate teledermatology processes. The formulation of international standards and guidelines to ensure uniformity and quality of teledermatology services across different regions and systems of healthcare is also going to be crucial [122].

The integration of teledermatology into the telemedicine networks and multi-disciplinary care model would facilitate comprehensive management of patients. Dermatologists, therefore, have the potential to provide more comprehensive care alongside primary care physicians and physicians from other specialties. This collective approach will not only increase the accessibility of dermatology services but also increase the quality of care, making faster and more effective treatment for patients suffering from skin disorders more likely [123].

CONCLUSION

There is no doubt that teledermatology has emerged as a game-changer modality in the realm of skin cancer care, particularly for enabling early identification of potentially malignant skin lesions, timely diagnosis, and successful treatment of these conditions. One of its defining characteristics is the ability to rapidly deliver dermatological expertise, especially in rural and underserved areas. A further highlight is its adoption of emerging technologies such as AI and ML (which enhance diagnostic accuracy and patient outcomes). Furthermore, effective implementation of teledermatology programs has been associated with increased patient satisfaction and decreased waiting times, highlighting this modality's delivery of timely care.

The future of teledermatology in managing skin cancer is optimistic. The optimism comes with the advancements in telecommunication technology, mainly 5G, alongside the increasing availability of wearable devices to monitor skin diseases anywhere and at any time. Predictive analytics and better diagnostic tools will also allow practitioners to deliver care that is more personalized and preventative. Changes in policies and regulations will also be integral in enabling the expansion of telehealth services to ensure equitable access to dermatological care for patients.

In summary, improving access to teledermatology is essential for enhancing a health outcome and reducing inequities regarding skin cancer treatment. This growth of teledermatology receives momentum from modern technologies as well as its supportive collaboration in the healthcare system. That will ultimately enable it to deliver speed, efficacy, and adequacy in terms of delivery for a patient's skin health needs. In the future, stakeholders must prioritize the integration of teledermatology into standard practice. So that all patients benefit from the innovations that can be made in this extremely important area.

REFERENCES

[1] Kahen N, Colavincenzo M. Procedures in cosmetic dermatology 1-Medical workup for hair loss. 2024. Available from: https://www.sciencedirect.com/science/article/abs/pii/B978032382921200010X

[2] Yadav S, Yadav S, Chaturvedi V, Verma P, Rajput A, Chaubey R. Telemedicine and its role in innovating the provision of healthcare. 2022; pp. 1-11. [http://dx.doi.org/10.1007/978-3-030-99457-0_1]

[3] Kaliyadan F, Amin TT, Kuruvilla J, Ali WHAB. Mobile teledermatology – patient satisfaction, diagnostic and management concordance, and factors affecting patient refusal to participate in Saudi Arabia. J Telemed Telecare 2013; 19(6): 315-9. [http://dx.doi.org/10.1177/1357633X13501778] [PMID: 24163295]

[4] Brinker TJ, Hekler A, Von Kalle C, Schadendorf D, Esser S, Berking C, *et al.* Teledermatology: Comparison of store-and-forward versus live interactive video conferencing. J Med Internet Res. JMIR Publications Inc. 2018; 20.

[5] Clark AK, Bosanac S, Ho B, Sivamani RK. A systematic review of mobile phone-based teledermatology. Arch Dermatol Res. Springer Verlag 2018; 310: pp. 675-89. [http://dx.doi.org/10.1007/s00403-018-1862-4]

[6] Giansanti D. Advancing dermatological care: A comprehensive narrative review of tele-dermatology and mHealth for bridging gaps and expanding opportunities beyond the COVID-19 pandemic. Healthcare (Switzerland). Multidisciplinary Digital Publishing Institute (MDPI) 2023; 11.

[7] van der Heijden JP, Spuls PI, Voorbraak FP, de Keizer NF, Witkamp L, Bos JD. Tertiary teledermatology: a systematic review. Telemed J E Health 2010; 16(1): 56-62. [http://dx.doi.org/10.1089/tmj.2009.0020] [PMID: 20064068]

[8] Barcaui CB, Lima PMO. Application of teledermoscopy in the diagnosis of pigmented lesions. Int J Telemed Appl 2018. [http://dx.doi.org/10.1155/2018/1624073]

[9] Kaliyadan F, Venkitakrishnan S. Teledermatology: Clinical case profiles and practical issues. Indian J Dermatol Venereol Leprol 2009; 75(1): 32-5. [http://dx.doi.org/10.4103/0378-6323.45217] [PMID: 19172028]

[10] Bashshur RL, Howell JD, Krupinski EA, Harms KM, Bashshur N, Doarn CR. The empirical foundations of telemedicine interventions in primary care. Telemed J E Health 2016; 22(5): 342-75. [http://dx.doi.org/10.1089/tmj.2016.0045] [PMID: 27128779]

[11] Petretto DR, Carrogu GP, Gaviano L, *et al.* Telemedicine, e-Health, and Digital Health Equity: A Scoping Review. Clin Pract Epidemiol Ment Health 2024; 20(1): 17450179279732. [http://dx.doi.org/10.2174/0117450179279732231211110248] [PMID: 38660571]

[12] Khodadad-Saryazdi A. Exploring the telemedicine implementation challenges through the process innovation approach: A case study research in the French healthcare sector 2021. [http://dx.doi.org/10.1016/j.technovation.2021.102273]

[13] Haleem A, Javaid M, Singh RP, Suman R. Telemedicine for healthcare: Capabilities, features, barriers, and applications. Sensors International. KeAi Communications Co. 2021; 2.

[14] Haimi M. The tragic paradoxical effect of telemedicine on healthcare disparities- a time for redemption: a narrative review. BMC Medical Informatics and Decision Making. BioMed Central Ltd 2023; 23.

[15] Santiago S, Lu J. Patient and provider satisfaction with teledermatology. Telemed e-Health. 2017; 23: pp. (8)684-90.

[16] Marchell R, Locatis C, Burgess G, Maisiak R, Liu WL, Ackerman M. Patient and provider satisfaction with teledermatology. Telemed J E Health 2017; 23(8): 684-90. [http://dx.doi.org/10.1089/tmj.2016.0192] [PMID: 28375822]

[17] Boyers LN, Schultz A, Baceviciene R, *et al.* Teledermatology as an educational tool for teaching dermatology to residents and medical students. Telemed J E Health 2015; 21(4): 312-4. [http://dx.doi.org/10.1089/tmj.2014.0101] [PMID: 25635528]

[18] Lam M, Doiron PR. The use of teledermatology in medical education. Med Sci Educ. Springer 2022; 32: pp. 243-6.

[19] Maddukuri S, Patel J, Lipoff JB. Teledermatology addressing disparities in health care access: a review. Curr Dermatol Rep. Springer 2021; 10: pp. 40-7. [http://dx.doi.org/10.1007/s13671-021-00329-2]

[20] Davis CM, Apter AJ, Casillas A, *et al.* Health disparities in allergic and immunologic conditions in racial and ethnic underserved populations: A Work Group Report of the AAAAI Committee on the Underserved. J Allergy Clin Immunol 2021; 147(5): 1579-93. [http://dx.doi.org/10.1016/j.jaci.2021.02.034] [PMID: 33713767]

[21] Roky AH, Islam MM, Ahasan AMF, *et al.* Overview of skin cancer types and prevalence rates across continents. Cancer Pathogenesis and Therapy 2024. Available from: https://linkinghub.elsevier.com/retrieve/pii/S2949713224000582

[22] Hasan N, Nadaf A, Imran M, Jiba U, Sheikh A, Almalki WH, *et al.* Skin cancer: understanding the journey of transformation from conventional to advanced treatment approaches. Molecular Cancer. BioMed Central Ltd 2023; 22. [http://dx.doi.org/10.1186/s12943-023-01854-3]

[23] Mall J, Haider MF, Naseem N, Rahman MA, Ahmad I. Lipid-based nanocarriers in combination chemotherapy: a promising strategy for advanced skin cancer management. Naunyn-Schmiedeberg's Arch Pharmacol. 2025; pp. 1-29. [http://dx.doi.org/10.1007/s00210-025-04431-1]

[24] Torisk E. Technological change and the practice of healthcare communication: Implications for patient-centered care, from a communication: Implications for patient-centered care, From a communication ethics perspective communication ethics perspective. 2021. Available from: https://dsc.duq.edu/etd

[25] Tensen E, van der Heijden JP, Jaspers MWM, Witkamp L. Two decades of teledermatology: Current status and integration in national healthcare systems. Vol. 5, Current Dermatology Reports. Current Medicine Group LLC 2016; 1: 96-104.

[26] Brown JHU. Management in health care systems. CRC Press 2018.

[27] Demontis GC, Germani MM, Caiani EG, Barravecchia I, Passino C, Angeloni D. Human pathophysiological adaptations to the space environment. Frontiers in Physiology. Frontiers Media S.A. 2017; 8.

[28] Vernice NA, Meydan C, Afshinnekoo E, Mason CE. Long-term spaceflight and the cardiovascular system. Precis Clin Med 2020; 3(4): 284-91. [http://dx.doi.org/10.1093/pcmedi/pbaa022] [PMID: 33391848]

[29] Baran R, Marchal S, Campos SG, Rehnberg E, Tabury K, Baselet B, *et al.* The Cardiovascular System in Space: Focus on *in vivo* and *in vitro* Studies. Biomedicines MDPI. 2022; 10.

[30] Scott RT, Antonsen EL, Sanders LM, Hastings JJ. Park S min, Mackintosh G, *et al.* Beyond Low Earth Orbit: Biomonitoring. Artificial Intelligence, and Precision Space Health. 2021.

[31] Kollias J, Van Derveer D, Dorchak KJ, Greenleaf JE. Physiologic responses to water immersion in man: A compendium of research 1976.

[32] Clément GR, Boyle RD, George KA, *et al.* Challenges to the central nervous system during human spaceflight missions to Mars. J Neurophysiol 2020; 123(5): 2037-63. [http://dx.doi.org/10.1152/jn.00476.2019] [PMID: 32292116]

[33] Shirzadfar H. The Evolution and Transformation of Telemedicine. Int J Biosens Bioelectron 2017;

3(4).
[http://dx.doi.org/10.15406/ijbsbe.2017.03.00070]

[34] Dasgupta A, Deb S. Telemedicine: A new horizon in public health in India. Indian J Community Med 2008; 33 Available from: http://journals.lww.com/ijcm

[35] Eedy DJ, Wootton R. Teledermatology: a review. Br J Dermatol 2001; 144(4): 696-707.
[http://dx.doi.org/10.1046/j.1365-2133.2001.04124.x] [PMID: 11298526]

[36] Tynes D. The Aquila Digital Community. The diffusion of telehealth: System-level conditions for the diffusion of telehealth: System-level conditions for successful adoption successful adoption. 2019. Available from: https://aquila.usm.edu/dissertations

[37] Mounessa JS, Chapman S, Braunberger T, *et al.* A systematic review of satisfaction with teledermatology. J Telemed Telecare 2018; 24(4): 263-70.
[http://dx.doi.org/10.1177/1357633X17696587] [PMID: 28350281]

[38] Rajda J, Seraly MP, Fernandes J, Niejadlik K, Wei H, Fox K, Steinberg G, Paz HL. Impact of direct to consumer store-and-forward teledermatology on access to care, satisfaction, utilization, and costs in a commercial health plan population. Telemedicine and e-Health. 2018;24(2):166-9.

[39] Blashki Kathy. Isaias Pedro Handbook of research on human-computer interfaces and new modes of interactivity. Engineering Science Reference, an imprint of IGI Global 2020.

[40] Maddukuri S, Patel J, Lipoff JB. Teledermatology addressing disparities in health care access: A review 2021.
[http://dx.doi.org/10.1007/s13671-021-00329-2]

[41] Campagna M, Naka F, Lu J. Teledermatology: An updated overview of clinical applications and reimbursement policies. Int J Women's Dermatol. Elsevier Inc. 2017; 3: pp. 176-9.

[42] Ehrenstein V, Kharrazi H, Lehmann H, Taylor CO. A service of the National Library of Medicine. National Institutes of Health 2019. Available from: https://www.ncbi.nlm.nih.gov/books/NBK551878/

[43] Evans RS. Electronic health records: Then, now, and in the future. Yearb Med Inform 2016; 25(S 01) (Suppl. 1): S48-61.
[http://dx.doi.org/10.15265/IYS-2016-s006] [PMID: 27199197]

[44] Kochmann M, Locatis C. Direct to consumer mobile teledermatology apps: An exploratory study. Telemed J E Health 2016; 22(8): 689-93.
[http://dx.doi.org/10.1089/tmj.2015.0189] [PMID: 26960113]

[45] Brewer AC, Endly DC, Henley J, *et al.* Mobile applications in dermatology. JAMA Dermatol 2013; 149(11): 1300-4.
[http://dx.doi.org/10.1001/jamadermatol.2013.5517] [PMID: 24067948]

[46] Wongvibulsin S, Yan MJ, Pahalyants V, Murphy W, Daneshjou R, Rotemberg V. Current state of dermatology mobile applications with artificial intelligence features. JAMA dermatology. 2024 Jun 1;160(6):646-50.

[47] Ranpariya V, Kats D, Lipoff JB. Direct-to-consumer teledermatology growth: A review and outlook for the future. Cutis. Frontline Medical Communications Inc 2022; 109: pp. 211-7.

[48] Ibrahim AE, Magdy M, Khalaf EM, Mostafa A, Arafa A. Teledermatology in the time of COVID-19. Int J Clin Pract 2021; 75(12): 15000.
[http://dx.doi.org/10.1111/ijcp.15000] [PMID: 34714575]

[49] Bhargava S, Negbenebor N, Sadoughifar R, Ahmad S, Kroumpouzos G. Global impact on dermatology practice due to the COVID-19 pandemic. Clin Dermatol 2021; 39(3): 479-87.
[http://dx.doi.org/10.1016/j.clindermatol.2021.01.017] [PMID: 34518007]

[50] Tak A. Artificial intelligence and machine learning in diagnostics and treatment planning. J Artif Intell Cloud Comput 2023; 1-6.
[http://dx.doi.org/10.47363/JAICC/2023(2)150]

[51] Giansanti D. The artificial intelligence in teledermatology: A narrative review on opportunities, perspectives, and bottlenecks. International Journal of Environmental Research and Public Health. MDPI 2023; 20.

[52] Tommasino N, Megna M, Cacciapuoti S, Villani A, Martora F, Ruggiero A, *et al.* The past, the present and the future of teledermatology: A narrative review. Clin Cosmet Investig Dermatol. Dove Medical Press Ltd 2024; 17: pp. 717-23.

[53] Tognetti L, Fiorani D, Russo F, Lazzeri L, Trovato E, Flori ML, Moscarella E, Cinotti E, Rubegni P. Teledermatology in 2020: past, present and future perspectives. Italian Journal of Dermatology and Venereology. 2021;156(2):198-212.

[54] Pasquali P, Sonthalia S, Moreno-Ramirez D, *et al.* Teledermatology and its current perspective. Indian Dermatol Online J 2020; 11(1): 12-20.
[http://dx.doi.org/10.4103/idoj.IDOJ_241_19] [PMID: 32055502]

[55] Romero G, Garrido JA, García-Arpa M. Telemedicina y teledermatología (I): concepto y aplicaciones. Actas Dermosifiliogr 2008; 99(7): 506-22.
[http://dx.doi.org/10.1016/S0001-7310(08)74735-5] [PMID: 18682163]

[56] Kantharaj GR, *et al.* Store and forward teledermatology 2007.
[http://dx.doi.org/10.4103/0378-6323.30643]

[57] Nikolakis G, Vaiopoulos AG, Georgopoulos I, Papakonstantinou E, Gaitanis G, Zouboulis CC. Insights, advantages, and barriers of teledermatology *vs.* face-to-face dermatology for the diagnosis and follow-up of non-melanoma skin cancer: A systematic review. Cancers. Multidisciplinary Digital Publishing Institute (MDPI) 2024; 16.

[58] Mashoudy KD, Perez SM, Nouri K. From diagnosis to intervention: a review of telemedicine's role in skin cancer care. Arch Dermatol Res. Springer Nature 2024; 316.

[59] Kanthraj G. Newer insights in teledermatology practice. Indian J Dermatol Venereol Leprol 2011; 77(3): 276-87.
[http://dx.doi.org/10.4103/0378-6323.79696] [PMID: 21508565]

[60] Pearlman RL, Le PB, Brodell RT, Nahar VK. Evaluation of patient attitudes towards the technical experience of synchronous teledermatology in the era of COVID-19. Arch Dermatol Res 2021; 313(9): 769-72.
[http://dx.doi.org/10.1007/s00403-020-02170-2] [PMID: 33403572]

[61] Janda M, Horsham C, Vagenas D, *et al.* Accuracy of mobile digital teledermoscopy for skin self-examinations in adults at high risk of skin cancer: an open-label, randomised controlled trial. Lancet Digit Health 2020; 2(3): 129-e137.
[http://dx.doi.org/10.1016/S2589-7500(20)30001-7] [PMID: 33334577]

[62] Tracy J. Telemedicine technical assistance documents A guide to getting started in telemedicine 2004.

[63] Wang RH, Barbieri JS, Kovarik CL, Lipoff JB. Synchronous and asynchronous teledermatology: A narrative review of strengths and limitations. J Telemed Telecare 2022; 28(7): 533-8.
[http://dx.doi.org/10.1177/1357633X221074504] [PMID: 35108130]

[64] Paudel V. Patterns and barriers of teledermatology in resource-limited settings in COVID-19 pandemic: A descriptive cross-sectional survey of Nepalese dermatologists. JAAD Int 2022; 7: 62-6.
[http://dx.doi.org/10.1016/j.jdin.2022.02.011] [PMID: 35281323]

[65] Kanthraj GR. Patient-assisted teledermatology practice: What is it? When, where, and how it is applied?. Indian J Dermatol Venereol Leprol 2015; 81: 136-43.

[66] Kozera EK, Yang A, Murrell DF. Patient and practitioner satisfaction with tele-dermatology including Australia's indigenous population: A systematic review of the literature. Int J Womens Dermatol 2016; 2(3): 70-3.
[http://dx.doi.org/10.1016/j.ijwd.2016.06.004] [PMID: 28492013]

[67] Peracca SB, Jackson GL, Weinstock MA, Oh DH. Implementation of teledermatology: Theory and practice. Vol. 8, Current Dermatology Reports. Current Medicine Group LLC 2019; 1: 35-45.

[68] Delans K, Goldstein E, Grichnik JM, Goldstein B, Goldstein AO. Teledermoscopy – An emerging technology for skin cancer detection. Telehealth and Medicine Today. Partners in Digital Health 2023; 8.

[69] Jiang SW, Flynn MS, Kwock JT, Nicholas MW. Store-and-forward images in teledermatology: Narrative literature review. JMIR Dermatol. JMIR Publications Inc. 2022; 5.

[70] Beer J, Hadeler E, Calume A, Gitlow H, Nouri K. Teledermatology: Current indications and considerations for future use. Arch Dermatol Res. Springer science and business media deutschland GmbH 2021; 313: pp. 11-5.

[71] Marwaha SS, Fevrier H, Alexeeff S, Crowley E, Haiman M, Pham N, Tuerk MJ, Wukda D, Hartmann M, Herrinton LJ. Comparative effectiveness study of face-to-face and teledermatology workflows for diagnosing skin cancer. Journal of the American Academy of Dermatology. 2019 Nov 1;81(5):1099-106.

[72] Preclaro IAC, Gulmatico-Flores Z, Tianco EAV. Concordance and accuracy of teledermatology using mobile phones in the outpatient clinic of Jose R Reyes memorial medical center: Cross-sectional study. JMIR Dermatol 2022; 5(4): 32546.
[http://dx.doi.org/10.2196/32546] [PMID: 37632883]

[73] López-Liria R, Valverde-Martínez MÁ, López-Villegas A, Bautista-Mesa RJ, Vega-Ramírez FA, Peiró S, *et al.* Teledermatology versus face-to-face dermatology: An analysis of cost-effectiveness from eight studies from Europe and the United States. International Journal of Environmental Research and Public Health. MDPI 2022; 19.
[http://dx.doi.org/10.3390/ijerph19052534]

[74] Yadav D, Bhatia S, Ramam M, *et al.* Patient perception and satisfaction with a smartphone-based teledermatology service initiated during the COVID-19 pandemic at a tertiary care hospital in North India. Indian J Dermatol Venereol Leprol 2022; 88(5): 623-32.
[http://dx.doi.org/10.25259/IJDVL_608_2021] [PMID: 35389031]

[75] Drabarek D, Habgood E, Janda M, *et al.* Experiences of patient-led surveillance, including patient-performed teledermoscopy, in the MEL-SELF pilot randomized controlled trial: Qualitative interview study. JMIR Dermatol 2022; 5(3): 35916.
[http://dx.doi.org/10.2196/35916] [PMID: 37632893]

[76] Young AT, Vora NB, Cortez J, Tam A, Yeniay Y, Afifi L, *et al.* The role of technology in melanoma screening and diagnosis. Pigment Cell Melanoma Res. Blackwell Publishing Ltd 2021; 34: pp. 288-300.
[http://dx.doi.org/10.1111/pcmr.12907]

[77] Mahmoud NM, Soliman AM. Early automated detection system for skin cancer diagnosis using artificial intelligent techniques. Sci Rep 2024; 14(1): 9749.
[http://dx.doi.org/10.1038/s41598-024-59783-0] [PMID: 38679633]

[78] Pala P, Bergler-Czop BS, Gwiżdż JM. Teledermatology: Idea, benefits, and risks of the modern age – a systematic review based on melanoma. Postepy Dermatol Alergol. Termedia Publishing House Ltd. 2020; 37: pp. 159-67.

[79] Shah A, Shah M, Pandya A, Sushra R, Sushra R, Mehta M, Patel K, Patel K. A comprehensive study on skin cancer detection using artificial neural network (ANN) and convolutional neural network (CNN). Clinical eHealth. 2023;6:76-84.

[80] Giavina-Bianchi M, Sousa R, Cordioli E. Part I: Accuracy of teledermatology in inflammatory dermatoses. Front Med (Lausanne) 2020; 7: 585792.
[http://dx.doi.org/10.3389/fmed.2020.585792] [PMID: 33195344]

[81] Giavina-Bianchi M, Santos AP, Cordioli E. Teledermatology reduces dermatology referrals and

improves access to specialists. EClinicalMedicine 2020; 29-30: 100641. [http://dx.doi.org/10.1016/j.eclinm.2020.100641] [PMID: 33437950]

[82] Bashshur RL, Shannon GW, Tejasvi T, Kvedar JC, Gates M. The empirical foundations of teledermatology: A review of the research evidence. Telemed J E Health 2015; 21(12): 953-79. [http://dx.doi.org/10.1089/tmj.2015.0146] [PMID: 26394022]

[83] Wang RH, Barbieri JS, Nguyen HP, *et al.* Clinical effectiveness and cost-effectiveness of teledermatology: Where are we now, and what are the barriers to adoption?. J Am Acad Dermatol 2020; 83(1): 299-307. [http://dx.doi.org/10.1016/j.jaad.2020.01.065] [PMID: 32035106]

[84] Beck J, Goncalves De Lira R, Maul LV, *et al.* Teledermatological services at a Swiss university hospital-evaluation of patient benefits and economic impact. J Dermatol Treat 2025; 36(1): 2555189. [http://dx.doi.org/10.1080/09546634.2025.2555189]

[85] Armstrong AW, Kwong MW, Ledo L, Nesbitt TS, Shewry SL. Practice models and challenges in teledermatology: a study of collective experiences from teledermatologists. PLoS One 2011; 6(12): 28687. [http://dx.doi.org/10.1371/journal.pone.0028687] [PMID: 22194887]

[86] Trettel A, Eissing L, Augustin M. Telemedicine in dermatology: findings and experiences worldwide–a systematic literature review. Journal of the European Academy of Dermatology and Venereology. 2018;32(2):215-24.

[87] Arimany-Manso J, Pujol RM, García-Patos V, Saigí U, Martin-Fumadó C. Medicolegal aspects of teledermatology 2020. [http://dx.doi.org/10.1016/j.adengl.2020.08.014]

[88] Abbott LM, Miller R, Janda M, *et al.* Practice guidelines for teledermatology in Australia. Australas J Dermatol 2020; 61(3): 293-e302. [http://dx.doi.org/10.1111/ajd.13301] [PMID: 32363572]

[89] Keenan AJ, Tsourtos G, Tieman J. Promise and peril-defining ethical telehealth practice from the clinician and patient perspective: A qualitative study. Digit Health 2022; 8. [http://dx.doi.org/10.1177/20552076211070394] [PMID: 35024158]

[90] Anawade PA, Sharma D, Gahane S. A comprehensive review on exploring the impact of telemedicine on healthcare accessibility. Cureus 2024; 16(3): 55996. [http://dx.doi.org/10.7759/cureus.55996] [PMID: 38618307]

[91] Jones Charindu K. I Ranmuthu Per N Hall Garth Funston Fiona M Walter OT, Jones OT, Funston Á F M Walter ÁG, I Ranmuthu CK, Hall PN. Recognizing Skin Cancer in Primary Care 2019.

[92] Coustasse A, Sarkar R, Abodunde B, Metzger BJ, Slater CM. Use of teledermatology to improve dermatological access in rural areas. Telemed J E Health 2019; 25(11): 1022-32. [http://dx.doi.org/10.1089/tmj.2018.0130] [PMID: 30741608]

[93] Reddy S, Giri D, Patel R. Artificial intelligence-based distinction of actinic keratosis and seborrheic keratosis. Cureus 2024; 16(4): 58692. [http://dx.doi.org/10.7759/cureus.58692] [PMID: 38774175]

[94] Melarkode N, Srinivasan K, Qaisar SM, Plawiak P. AI-powered diagnosis of skin cancer: A contemporary review, open challenges and future research directions. Cancers. MDPI 2023; 15.

[95] Debelee TG. Skin lesion classification and detection using machine learning techniques: A systematic review. Diagnostics. Multidisciplinary Digital Publishing Institute (MDPI) 2023; 13.

[96] Safa G, Djebbar A, Farida H, Merouani D, Gasmi S. Advancing skin cancer research with machine learning and deep learning models: A systematic review. J Pak Assoc Dermatol 2024; 34 Available from: https://www.researchgate.net/publication/381741764

[97] Bourkas AN, Barone N, Bourkas MEC, *et al.* Diagnostic reliability in teledermatology: a systematic

review and a meta-analysis. BMJ Open 2023; 13(8): 068207.
[http://dx.doi.org/10.1136/bmjopen-2022-068207] [PMID: 37567745]

[98] Giavina-Bianchi M, Azevedo MFD, Sousa RM, Cordioli E. Part II: Accuracy of Teledermatology in Skin Neoplasms. Front Med (Lausanne) 2020; 7: 598903.
[http://dx.doi.org/10.3389/fmed.2020.598903] [PMID: 33330564]

[99] Kanthraj GR. Teledermatology: Case selection and consultation "Technology is best when it brings patient–Physician together." Clinical Dermatology Review 2023; 7(1): 3-9.
[http://dx.doi.org/10.4103/cdr.cdr_23_22]

[100] Patel N, Aboukhatwah N, Esdaile B. Effectiveness and diagnostic accuracy of teledermatology for the assessment of skin conditions. Australas J Dermatol 2024; 65(4): 342-9.
[http://dx.doi.org/10.1111/ajd.14239] [PMID: 38421885]

[101] Lee KJ, Finnane A, Soyer HP. Recent trends in teledermatology and teledermoscopy. Dermatology practical & conceptual. 2018;8(3):214.

[102] Bastola M, Locatis C, Fontelo P. Diagnostic reliability of in-person *versus* remote dermatology: a meta-analysis. Telemedicine and e-Health. 2021 Mar 1;27(3):247-50.

[103] Pathipati A, Armstrong A. Teledermatology: Outcomes and economic considerations. Telemedicine Techniques and Applications. InTech 2011.

[104] Jones LK, Oakley A. Store-and-forward teledermatology for assessing skin cancer in 2023: Literature review. JMIR Dermatol 2023; 6: 43395.
[http://dx.doi.org/10.2196/43395] [PMID: 37632914]

[105] Gao JL, Oakley A. Teledermatology for enhancing skin cancer diagnosis and management: Retrospective chart review. JMIR Dermatol 2023; 6: 45430.
[http://dx.doi.org/10.2196/45430] [PMID: 37632911]

[106] Jones L, Jameson M, Oakley A. Remote skin cancer diagnosis: Adding images to electronic referrals is more efficient than wait-listing for a nurse-led imaging clinic. Cancers (Basel) 2021; 13(22): 5828.
[http://dx.doi.org/10.3390/cancers13225828] [PMID: 34830982]

[107] Afroj S. E-learning and teledermatology: Are web-based images good enough for learning? 2014.

[108] Susan J. White Early detection, improved treatments for skin cancer _ Endeavor Health 2024.

[109] Stratigos AJ, Katsambas AD. The value of screening in melanoma. Clin Dermatol 2009; 27(1): 10-25.
[http://dx.doi.org/10.1016/j.clindermatol.2008.09.002] [PMID: 19095150]

[110] Panagoulias DP, Tsoureli-Nikita E, Virvou M, Tsihrintzis GA. Dermacen analytica: A novel methodology integrating multi-modal large language models with machine learning in tele-dermatology. 2024. Available from: http://arxiv.org/abs/2403.14243

[111] Panagoulias DP, Tsoureli-Nikita E, Virvou M, Tsihrintzis GA. Dermacen analytica: A novel methodology integrating multi-modal large language models with machine learning in dermatology. International Journal of Medical Informatics. 2025 Jul 1;199:105898.

[112] Yotsu RR, Almamy D, Vagamon B, *et al.* An mHealth app (eSkinHealth) for detecting and managing skin diseases in resource-limited settings: Mixed methods pilot study. JMIR Dermatol 2023; 6: 46295.
[http://dx.doi.org/10.2196/46295] [PMID: 37632977]

[113] Pala P, Bergler-Czop BS, Gwiżdż JM. Teledermatology: Idea, benefits and risks of modern age – a systematic review based on melanoma. Postepy Dermatol Alergol. Termedia Publishing House Ltd. 2020; 37: pp. 159-67.

[114] Funkhouser CH, Funkhouser ME, Wolverton JE, Maurer T. Teledermatology consults in a county hospital setting: retrospective analysis. JMIR dermatology. 2021;4(2):e30530.

[115] Maita KC, Maniaci MJ, Haider CR, *et al.* The impact of digital health solutions on bridging the health care gap in rural areas: a scoping review. Perman J. 2024; 28: p. (3)130.

[http://dx.doi.org/10.7812/TPP/23.134]

[116] Finnane A, Dallest K, Janda M, Soyer HP. Teledermatology for the diagnosis and management of skin cancer: a systematic review. JAMA dermatology. 2017;153(3):319-27.

[117] Marwaha SS, Fevrier H, Alexeeff S, Crowley E, Haiman M, Pham N, Tuerk MJ, Wukda D, Hartmann M, Herrinton LJ. Comparative effectiveness study of face-to-face and teledermatology workflows for diagnosing skin cancer. Journal of the American Academy of Dermatology. 2019 Nov 1;81(5):1099-106.

[118] Rangineni S, Bhanushali A, Suryadevara M, Venkata S, Peddireddy K. A Review on enhancing data quality for optimal data analytics performance. International Journal of Computer Sciences and Engineering. 2023;11(10):51-8.

[119] Andrees V, Klein TM, Augustin M, Otten M. Live interactive teledermatology compared to in-person care - a systematic review. J Eur Acad Dermatol Venereol. 2020 Apr; 34(4): 733-745. doi: 10.1111/jdv.16070. Epub 2020 Jan 29. PMID: 31715035.

[120] Ahuja S, Briggs SM, Collier SM. Teledermatology in rural, underserved, and isolated environments: a review. Current dermatology reports. 2022;11(4):328-35.

[121] Mbunge E, Muchemwa B, Jiyane S, Batani J. Sensors and healthcare 50: transformative shift in virtual care through emerging digital health technologies. Global Health Journal. KeAi Communications Co. 2021; 5: pp. 169-77.

[122] Murugan Vignesh. Telemedicine: Transforming patient-provider relationships in the digital age. JCHM 2024.

[123] Ahmed S, Irfan S, Kiran N, Masood N, Anjum N, Ramzan N. Remote health monitoring systems for elderly people: a survey. Sensors. 2023 Aug 10;23(16):7095.

CHAPTER 6

Digital Dermoscopy: Advancements in Visualizing Skin Lesions

Ashish Verma[1], **Sunita**[2], **Akhil Sharma**[2], **Shaweta Sharma**[3], **Shilpa Thukral**[4] and **Akanksha Sharma**[2,*]

[1] *Mangalmay Pharmacy College, Greater Noida, Uttar Pradesh-201306, India*

[2] *R. J. College of Pharmacy, Raipur, Uttar Pradesh - 202165, India*

[3] *School of Medical and Allied Sciences, Galgotias University, Uttar Pradesh-201310, India*

[4] *Dnyan Ganga College of Pharmacy, Thane, Maharashtra-400615, India*

Abstract: Digital dermoscopy is an emerging novel advancement in dermatology that has transformed the assessment and diagnosis of skin lesions. Although effective, traditional skin inspection techniques depend on interpreting dermatologists, so there might be variations in diagnosis. Digital dermoscopy is a high-resolution imaging technology that has transformed how we examine lesions, making it possible to detect melanoma and non-melanoma skin cancers more objectively, accurately, and at an early stage. There have been developments in digital dermoscopy with the integration of artificial intelligence (AI) and machine learning algorithms, which help in analyzing skin lesions by detecting patterns and distinguishing between benign and malignant lesions more accurately. Artificial intelligence-driven systems can minimize human error and improve diagnosis accuracy in essential care settings, where access to the dermatologist could be challenging. These systems are useful in diagnostic support and improve the possibility of training for health care providers. Furthermore, teledermoscopy, a digital dermoscopy subset, has improved access to dermatologic care. When combined with telemedicine platforms, patients can be consulted digitally, and skin lesions can be monitored longitudinally using dermoscopic images. This can be especially beneficial in areas with few dermatologic services, such as rural regions. This is particularly valuable in rural or underserved regions with limited dermatological services. Digital dermoscopy also enables the storage and comparison of images over time, facilitating better monitoring of lesion evolution. This functionality is especially important for patients with a history of skin cancer or high-risk patients, allowing the identification of subtle changes that may suggest malignant potential. In conclusion, digital dermoscopy will be a cornerstone of dermatology in the future because it provides better diagnosis as well as accessibility and outcomes for patients. With continued advancements, it would be able to lower the number of cases of skin cancer deaths and could change the standard for how skin disease is detected early on.

* **Corresponding author Akanksha Sharma:** R. J. College of Pharmacy, Raipur, Uttar Pradesh - 202165, India; E-mail: akankshasona012@gmail.com

Akhil Sharma, Shaweta Sharma, Shivkanya Fuloria & Sudhir Kumar (Eds.)

Keywords: Biopsy, Cancer, Cryotherapy, Dermatology, Digital dermoscopy, Skin lesions, Teledermoscopy.

INTRODUCTION

Dermoscopy, also known as dermatoscopy and chemiluminescence microscopy) is a non-invasive diagnostic method for studying skin lesions. It uses a special device called a dermatoscope with a good quality magnifying lens and a light source that enables viewing structures within the skin not seen by the naked eye. Dermoscopy is a non-invasive tool that is predominantly used to evaluate pigmented lesions. It also assists in diagnosing other conditions, including melanoma, basal cell carcinoma (BCC), and other skin malignancies. Dermatologists can more precisely discriminate between benign and neoplastic lesions based on characteristics such as pigmentation, color, and structure (symmetry and border shape) than with visual inspection [1 - 3].

A clear gel may be applied to the skin to help visualize the surface during a dermoscopy exam, but newer models of dermatoscopes typically do not require this. A device is then mounted over the lesion, enabling the clinician to view the skin in-depth, free from surface reflections. It greatly increases diagnostic specificity (and sensitivity, particularly for melanoma) and reduces surgical excisions of benign lesions. It is also helpful for tracking changes in known moles and diagnosing dermatologic diseases other than skin cancer, including inflammatory and infectious skin conditions [4 - 6].

Digital dermoscopy, also known as sequential digital dermoscopy (SDI) or digital dermoscopic monitoring, refers to capturing, storing, and comparing successive dermoscopic images of skin lesions over time. This sensitivity is helpful when analyzing small variations in lesions that can announce the onset of melanoma or another type of skin cancer. Visual inspection alone has a lower accuracy in early melanoma detection, which is improved by digital dermoscopy and computerized methods of analysis. It also allows observation of lesions for changes over time, which is critical for detecting melanoma at an early stage. It establishes a standardized method for comparing images taken of the same image by different cameras, even within a facility. Also, it supports whole-body mapping and tracking of multiple lesions per patient, particularly in the high-risk population [7, 8].

Different types of equipment are used to perform digital dermoscopy. Handheld dermatoscopes with smartphone attachments or built-in photography systems dedicated digital chemiluminescence systems or videodermatoscopes in major centers, and smartphone-compatible dermatoscopy apps can be used for image capture and storage. Best practices suggest guidelines for image orientation, resolution, scale, focus, and color to anchor consistency. It is important to keep these parameters standardized in order to evaluate lesions correctly over time [9, 10].

Full-body mapping and subsequent follow-up are time-consuming, particularly in the presence of multiple lesions. Using different devices for sequential imaging at a single facility may introduce heterogeneity in image quality and characteristics. No incumbent binding standards in digital dermoscopy image quality can lead to poor clinical images. Patients transfer from one facility to another, so continuous tracking is challenging. Digital dermoscopy is one of the beneficial applications for early detection and longitudinal monitoring of melanoma and other skin cancers. Dermatologists use images captured at risk points to compare and identify minor changes that could indicate malignancy, leading to earlier diagnoses and improved patient outcomes [11, 12].

Development in Digital Dermatology

Advancements in dermatology due to increasing digital relevance, especially in teledermatology and AI incorporation for diagnoses, highlight the need for attention to this emerging aspect of dermatology and skin cancer detection. Fig. (**1**) summarizes the relevance of digital dermatology in skin cancer detection.

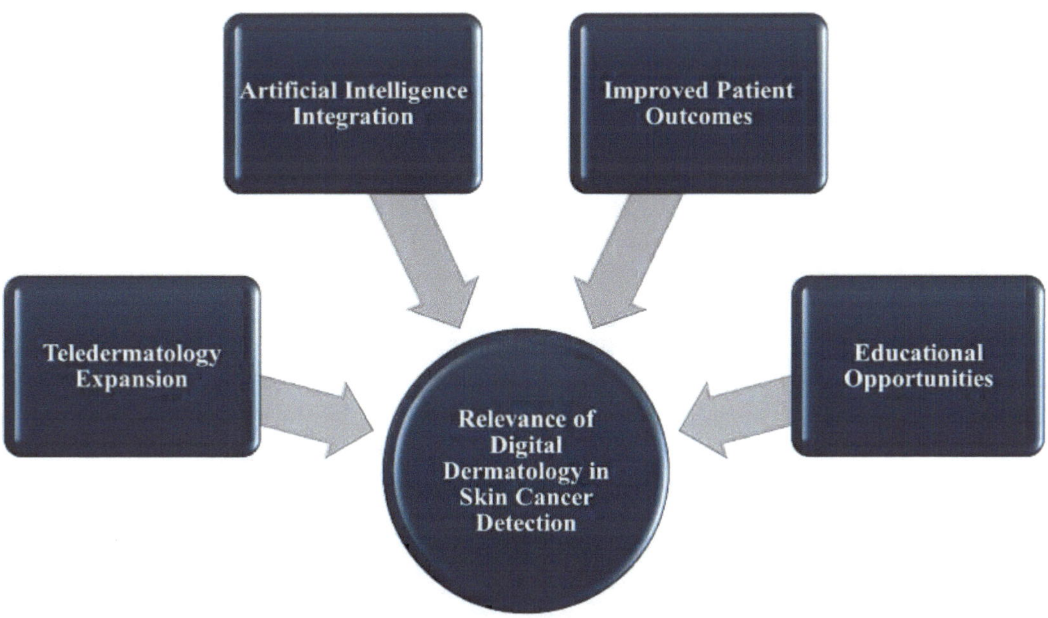

Fig. (1). Relevance of digital dermatology in skin cancer detection.

Teledermatology Expansion

Teledermatology enables virtual consultations where dermatologists can assess skin lesions *via* digital images. While this strategy increases access to dermatological services, especially in underserved populations, it also provides more accurate diagnoses (*e.g.*, melanoma and basal cell carcinoma). This has demonstrated decreasing wait times, redundant excisions, and positive, timely referrals to specialists [13].

Artificial Intelligence Integration

AI has been successfully applied to dermatoscopic images, particularly convolutional neural networks (CNNs). They have shown the potential for classifying skin lesions with accuracies close to those of experienced dermatologists. AI can aid in automating the diagnostic process and enabling clinicians to make more informed decisions [14].

Improved Patient Outcomes

Digital dermatology tools, such as smartphone applications and teledermatology systems involving video consultations, have been shown to improve patient satisfaction with accelerated access to dermatological evaluation. They can be used for self-detection and early process intervention, both important for treating skin cancer [15].

Educational Opportunities

Digital platforms are also used for dermatology education to fill the training void among healthcare workers. It is especially critical as telemedicine permeates dermatology practice to ensure the skills and competencies required from practitioners, enabling effective utilization of these technologies [16].

Digital dermatology is changing the landscape by providing improved access to care, increasing diagnostic accuracy, and supporting ongoing education and monitoring. These improvements are also particularly important in early skin cancer detection and vital for effective treatment and overall patient outcomes [17].

TRADITIONAL METHODS OF SKIN LESION DIAGNOSIS

Skin lesion diagnosis is conventionally performed by manual and visual examination, which, however, can generate misdiagnosis or delay in skin cancer detection. The main traditional methods used in dermatology are discussed below and summarized in Fig. (**2**).

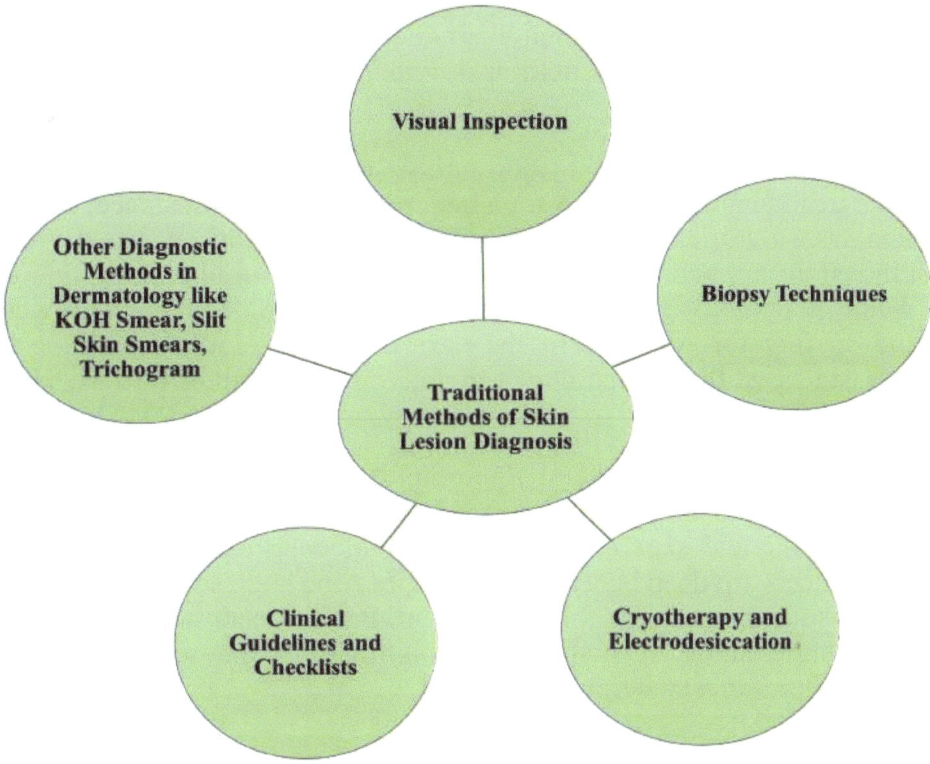

Fig. (2). Traditional methods of skin lesion diagnosis.

Visual Inspection

Visual inspection is the basis of dermatologists' method to evaluate skin lesions. This initial assessment is critical for diagnosing skin lesions, including benign and malignant lesions like melanoma. The dermatologist often obtains a comprehensive patient history prior to the examination, including any past skin disorders the individual has experienced, any family background of skin cancer, and whether there have been changes in existing lesions or any new lesions formed. The skin exam is thorough and generally very systematic to ensure that no areas of the body are overlooked. This could include the entire body, including patches often not exposed to sunlight like the scalp, between toes and armpits [18, 19].

Clinically, lesions are assessed on various major features, including the general appearance of the lesion (texture and surface characteristics). Different colors are used for the lesion, including brown, black, red, or white. Characteristics of the lesion (*e.g.*, larger lesions are often considered suspicious because they may be malignant; typically, any lesion greater than 6 mm in size is suspicious). Irregular shapes and poorly defined edges may raise concerns. Dermatologists tend to record their observations in detailed charts describing each lesion's features and course over time. This documentation is important for tracking lesions during follow-up visits [20, 21].

Skin cancers, when visualized thoroughly, can be detected early so that appropriate treatment can be given for a better prognosis. For instance, early-stage melanoma has a significantly better survival rate than advanced stages. Although most skin lesions are benign, visual inspection is useful in identifying innocuous moles *versus* potentially malignant proliferation; the avoided biopsies lower both costs and anxiety for patients. In the case of a suspicious lesion, the visual inspection can assist the dermatologist in determining whether further diagnostic methods should be performed (*e.g.*, dermoscopy or biopsy) [22, 23].

Though visual inspection is an important step in skin diagnosis, it has disadvantages. For example, the correctness of the diagnosis relies on the clinician's training and experience, resulting in inconsistency among arguments. Some skin cancers are deep beneath normal-appearing skin, so other tools, such as dermoscopy, must be used for full assessment. Practitioners with less experience may miss subtle signs of malignancy, highlighting the need for continual education and training in dermatology [24].

Biopsy Techniques

A biopsy is generally done to confirm a suspected lesion histopathologically. Numerous biopsy types exist, each with indications and techniques described below.

Excisional Biopsy

An excisional biopsy is a surgical procedure that consists of removing, along with some normal or healthy skin, a single appearing lesion. The method is used to achieve a definitive diagnosis and to treat in a single procedure. Excisional biopsies are typically carried out in the following situations. They are frequently indicated when melanoma or other skin cancers are suspected because they enable a simultaneous diagnostic and therapeutic approach. It is an important procedure to evaluate the depth of tumors, which helps in staging and prognostication. Excisions can also be performed for benign lesions needing removal for cosmetic or symptomatic reasons [25, 26].

An excisional biopsy procedure typically follows these steps. The patient is laid down comfortably, and the lesion site is sterilized to reduce the chances of infection. Local anesthesia is administered to numb the region around the lesion so that the patient does not feel pain during the procedure. Using a scalpel, the surgeon cuts around the lesion and includes an area of normal tissue in the sample to ensure healthy cells are also part of it. The margin size may vary depending on the suspicion of malignancy. The full lesion is excised together with the surrounding tissue. This might include slicing into several layers of epidermis based on the thickness of the cavity. The incision is then sutured and closed after the lesion is removed. The size and location of the biopsy may determine the type of sutures used. The excised tissue is sent to a pathology laboratory for histological examination. A pathologist then examines the tissue, confirming the diagnosis and determining the presence of any malignancy [27, 28].

A definite diagnosis can be made through histopathological assessment of the sample; hence, appropriate treatment strategies can be formulated. This allows the lesion to be removed and, simultaneously, can be diagnosed in one procedure instead of multiple procedures. Though it has some limitations, this is an invasive process and may require local anesthesia, which can be painful. Potential complications may be associated with this procedure, such as infection, bleeding, scarring, and changes in skin sensation at the biopsy site. This can excise more healthy tissue than needed, which can lead to cosmetic concerns [29].

Excisional biopsy remains a useful diagnostic and therapeutic modality in dermatology, especially for evaluating suspicious skin lesions. Excisional biopsies are important in skin cancer and dermatologic disease management as they provide a definitive diagnosis and allow the excision of all potentially malignant tissue [30].

Incisional Biopsy

An incisional biopsy is a surgical procedure to remove only a part of the skin lesion for histopathological examination. Such a technique is commonly used for large lesions that cannot be fully excised due to the importance of preserving surrounding healthy tissue. In the case of a large lesion, an incisional biopsy is preferable as it provides sufficient tissue to make a diagnosis and allows for planning the future surgical removal. An incisional biopsy may be performed initially if complete excision is not possible in cases of suspected melanoma. This enables a diagnosis to be made while sparing the surrounding tissue for further therapy planning. Incisional biopsy is commonly used when lesions are in an anatomically critical area or it is important to preserve surrounding normal tissue [31, 32].

Like excisional biopsies, a local anesthetic is placed, and part of the lesion is removed. This sample is subject to histological analysis. This type of biopsy preserves the adjacent normal tissue, especially in areas where maximal cosmetic preservation is needed or if complete excision may not be possible at the primary surgery. This method allows the diagnosis of large skin lesions that cannot be fully excised in one procedure. There are some limitations, such as part of the lesion being removed and sampling error, as it may not represent the whole lesion. Sometimes, definitive treatment involves the diagnostic incisional biopsy and a complete excision of the lesion (sometimes necessitating multiple procedures) [33 - 35].

Punch Biopsy

A punch biopsy is a minimally invasive procedure that employs a circular tool to extract a small, cylindrical core of skin containing the epidermis and part of the dermis. This small skin operation is often used as a landscape sample for diagnosis. A punch biopsy is much more frequently used to obtain a specimen of several inflammatory disorders affecting the skin, including lichen planus, sarcoidosis, and vasculitis, in which a representative sample of the affected skin is necessary. Punch biopsies are ideal for sampling small skin lesions like nevi or pimples that would be difficult to excise completely. A punch biopsy is a quick and minimally invasive method for obtaining a tissue sample when a rapid diagnosis is needed. Punch biopsies tend to be preferable as they leave relatively small scars (compared with excisional or incisional biopsies). They may be better suited for cosmetically sensitive locations or where scarring is a concern [36, 37].

The punch biopsy process includes these steps: the patient is placed for comfort, and the area used to collect tissue is secured and sanitized. Local anesthesia is given to numb the area, thus minimizing discomfort that may be caused during the procedure. This involves pressing a circular punch tool at right angles into the skin, usually between 2 to 6 mm in diameter. So, the tool is rotated to penetrate the epidermis and dermis, and, as such, portions of a cylindrical core are cut out. The punch is removed, and the biopsy sample is nibbled to be withdrawn with forceps. Bleeding is controlled with pressure; if needed, a styptic agent may be used at the biopsy site. Depending on how large a punch is used, either one or multiple stitches are placed to close the biopsy site. In certain situations, the location may be allowed to heal by secondary intention. The tissue sample is sent to a pathology lab for histological examination and diagnosis [38, 39].

Punch biopsies are less invasive than excisional or incisional; therefore, they provide smaller scars and quicker healing times. A punch biopsy will quickly allow the healthcare professional to confirm a diagnosis by taking some of the tissue from the patient. In some cases, the small size of the tissue sampled with a punch biopsy may not allow for an evaluation of the entire lesion or make it difficult to arrive at a definitive diagnosis. As with other biopsy techniques, there is a risk of sampling error, where the biopsy may not accurately reflect the entire lesion [40 - 42].

Cryotherapy and Electrodesiccation

Cryotherapy and electrodesiccation are skin lesion treatment modalities, especially for pre-cancerous lesions such as actinic keratosis. Though they may sometimes be useful for initial diagnostic purposes, their predominant use is therapeutic and not diagnostic.

Cryotherapy

Cryotherapy involves freezing lesions with liquid nitrogen, leading to cell death through cryo-injury. This procedure is efficient for treating superficial lesions since it induces necrosis. It is commonly used for seborrheic keratosis, actinic keratosis, and other benign lesions [43].

Electrodesiccation

Electrodesiccation utilizes heat produced by current to conduct tissue destruction. Through thermal energy, this technique evaporates and ablates the lesion. It is commonly applied for superficial skin lesions, such as warts, basal cell carcinomas, and other benign lesions.

Both processes are simple, and many do not require more than an office visit to perform, so it allows both patients and healthcare providers the convenience of being in their routine environment. These laser procedures are more effective for certain benign or surface lesions and can result in rapid resolution, equating to very little leftover skin damage. However, these are unsuitable for deeper lesions or those where malignancy is suspected as they do not provide any histopathological sample. These techniques preclude confirming a diagnosis by laboratory analysis because no tissue sample is preserved. It is particularly important for lesions requiring further investigation to exclude malignancy [44, 45].

Cryotherapy and electrodesiccation are important adjunctive tools in dermatology that are typically used for therapy rather than as diagnostic procedures. Although they provide fast and efficient treatments for specific skin lesions, the fact that they do not allow histological examination of tissue specimens raises some caution, at least in case of suspected lesions. However, they keep the traditional methods of getting an accurate diagnosis, such as excisional or incisional biopsies, which are essential for correct diagnosis, especially regarding skin cancers [46].

Clinical Guidelines and Checklists (ABCDE Criteria)

Dermatologists visually evaluate skin lesions using standardized guidelines, such as the ABCDE criteria, to find early signs of melanoma. The ABCDE system offers a simple and systematic way to examine moles and other skin lesions based on five important features. Asymmetry indicates that one half of the lesion is a different shape than the other, and border irregularity emphasizes uneven, notched, or blurred borders that can signify malignancy. Microscopic coloration is another warning sign; if a single lesion has several shades of brown, black, red, white, or blue, it is in trouble. The diameter principle holds that lesions greater than 6mm, about the size of a pencil eraser, are suspect and should be examined closely, though smaller lesions can still be problematic. Lastly, evolving means that changes in size, shape, color, and symptoms (such as itching or bleeding) change over time [47 - 49].

ABCD criteria are a noninvasive, simple, and practical method of monitoring skin lesions by dermatologists and patients to detect melanoma at an early stage. This approach minimizes the chances of diagnosis in later stages by promoting seeking medical advice when a suspicious change occurs. Finally, the ABCDE approach is easily implemented without special equipment and is scalable to any clinical setting [50].

However, the ABCDE criteria are also limited. This method may be subjective as it depends widely on the dermatologist's interpretation of the characteristics of the lesion. However, some melanomas, such as nodular melanoma, do not have all of the ABCDE features and can be missed. Moreover, non-malignant lesions like seborrheic keratosis can occasionally fulfill at least one or more of the ABCDE criteria, resulting in unwarranted biopsies. The ABCDE framework is undoubtedly a less-than-perfect tool in the skin cancer screening and early detection toolbox, even with its limitations [51].

Other Diagnostic Methods in Dermatology

Dermatologists may also conduct traditional assessments to consider skin conditions besides visual exams and biopsies. They may assist in determining infections, inflammatory diseases, and other dermatological problems. Some of the key techniques are as follows:

KOH Smear

A KOH smear is a test to diagnose fungal disease of the skin, hair, or nails. This involves taking a skin, hair, or nail sample, which is then put on a glass slide. A KOH (potassium hydroxide) solution is then placed on top of the sample, removing keratin and other material debris and making the fungal elements more easily visible. The slide is then viewed in a microscope to identify if any fungal hyphae or spores are present. This test is mainly applied in diagnosing tinea (ringworm), candidiasis, and superficial fungal infections [52, 53].

Slit Skin Smears

Slit skin smears are useful for diagnosing leprosy (also Hansen's disease) and some other infectious diseases of the skin. The skin is washed, and a small incision (or slit) is created on the skin, usually over a lesion. It collects and spreads the fluid from the slit onto a glass slide. This smear is then stained (mostly with Ziehl-Neelsen stain) and observed under the microscope for Mycobacterium leprae or other pathogens. This approach is important in diagnosing leprosy since it helps identify the etiological agent and classify the disease severity [54, 55].

Trichogram

A trigram is a test in which the expert examines hair samples under a microscope, primarily used to check the reason for hair loss. Takes a couple of hairs from the scalp or affected area but is intact with roots. The hairs that are collected are placed on a microscope slide and reviewed in detail for different characteristics like the morphology of the hair shaft or any abnormalities of the hair follicle. It helps diagnose telogen effluvium, alopecia areata and other hair loss conditions. It helps assess if the hair loss is due to a growth cycle problem, fungal infection, or other causes [56, 57].

ADVANCEMENTS IN DIGITAL DERMOSCOPY

Recent advancements in digital dermoscopy have improved the ability of dermatologists to diagnose and monitor skin lesions.

Enhanced Imaging Technologies

Transition to Digital Dermoscopy

Digital dermoscopy improves conventional dermoscopy with high-resolution digital imaging and analytic software to improve skin lesion analysis. This step enables the visualization of skin microstructures that cannot be seen with the naked eye and effectively bridges clinical observation and histopathological examination. Digital dermoscopy, the *in vivo* examination of skin lesions, enables dermatologists to capture subtle changes in the lesion over time and enhances diagnostic performance [58, 59].

This rapid evolution in digital dermoscopy, especially the shift towards high-resolution imaging and intelligent software applications, has changed the face of dermatological diagnostics. These technologies increase the precision of skin lesion assessments and improve the capacity to assess temporal changes on diseased skin, ultimately providing better clinical implications in the early identification and treatment of cutaneous disorders [60, 61].

Videodermoscopy

Videodermoscopy is an innovative approach that enhances traditional dermoscopy, enabling multiple physicians to observe and discuss high-magnification dermoscopic images in real-time. This technique is a great learning aid and enhances the capabilities of dermatology diagnosis. Videodermoscopy provides an interactive learning experience in which the instructor and trainees can view dermoscopic features in real time together. Videodermoscopy provides high-resolution images that reveal intricate details of skin lesions, aiding in accurately diagnosing conditions such as melanoma and other skin cancers [62, 63].

This is useful for dermatology training programs and teaches residents and trainees multiple dermoscopic features to improve their diagnostic skills. Fluorescence-advanced videodermoscopy is a novel form of videodermoscopy that utilizes monochromatic light to interact with selective skin molecules (melanin and hemoglobin) that emit fluorescence. It is helpful in the differentiation of benign and malignant melanocytic tumors and the evaluation of hair and scalp and disorders. The videodermoscopy portability makes it easier for telemedicine users to use, and dermatologists can visit remotely. Images can be obtained and forwarded for interpretation, thus increasing access to dermatological services, especially in rural or underserved regions [64 - 66].

Videodermoscopy represents a significant advancement in dermatological practice, enhancing diagnostic accuracy and educational opportunities. By facilitating real-time collaboration and providing high-resolution imaging, this technique improves the ability to evaluate skin lesions effectively. As technology evolves, video dermoscopy will likely play an increasingly important role in clinical practice and dermatology education [67].

Fluorescence-Advanced Videodermoscopy

Fluorescence-advanced video dermoscopy (FAV) is a novel, non-invasive imaging that improves skin lesion assessment using fluorescence to capture deeper information on skin structures at the cellular level. FAV employs a monochromatic light source with a wavelength of approximately 405 nm. Certain molecules in the skin (like hemoglobin or melanin) will absorb and re-emit it as fluorescence at that particular wavelength. This property makes it feasible to visualize skin lesions better [68].

It offers a main magnification of 12-fold, which allows dermatologists to visualize details of the epidermis and dermis needed for proper diagnosis. With FAV, you can focus on skin at different depths sequentially (35–50 µm or deeper, depending on the technique), visualizing structures at different layers of skin. The following features may come in handy for evaluating different skin troubles [69].

FAV is a promising tool for evaluating melanocytic lesions (moles and melanoma) and vascular lesions, helping to distinguish malignant from benign growths. The method has been used in trichoscopy (the dermatoscopic study of hair and scalp), which shows a higher resolution of healthy scalp architecture and alopecic lesions to facilitate diagnostic interpretation. Research has shown that FAV has a higher resolution than regular trichoscopy. FAV is a non-invasive technique for the *in vivo* diagnosis of several dermatoses, including parasitic infections, because it provides insights regarding the visualization and assessment of lesions without invasive procedures [70, 71].

FAV is a patient-friendly option for skin evaluation that minimizes the need for invasive diagnostic measures. Finally, its high magnification and fluorescence detection properties increase the chance of detecting early tedious variations in skin lesions, which may contribute to an earlier diagnosis. By adding more information to traditional techniques like trichoscopy, FAV can complement classical methods in an ideal setting, increasing confidence in our diagnosis and decreasing biopsies [72].

Fluorescence-advanced video dermoscopy is an important step in the evolution of skin imaging. It provides a high-resolution, noninvasive assessment of skin lesions. Particularly for melanocytic and vascular lesions and hair and scalp assessments, its detailed visualization of skin microstructures adds value to the diagnosis. With time and progress in this technology, it could serve as a novel login tool in dermatology, enabling better patient care and outcomes [73].

Integration with Artificial Intelligence (AI)

AI-Assisted Diagnosis

The development of artificial intelligence (AI) and machine learning (ML) in digital dermoscopy has made breakthroughs in dermatology, especially in skin lesion diagnosis. Computer-aided diagnosis (CAD) systems use these technologies to interpret dermoscopic images, improving skin cancer detection.

Artificial Intelligence (AI) has been developed to analyze dermoscopic images and recognize specific patterns associated with malignancy. Training on large labeled datasets allows these systems to learn subtle pathological features distinguishing benign from malignant lesions [74, 75].

It uses deep learning algorithms, particularly Convolutional Neural Networks (CNNs), to work directly with images. The ability of these algorithms to automatically perform feature extraction on dermoscopic images, whether without requiring manual feature selection, can optimize diagnostic performance. Research has demonstrated that AI-assisted diagnosis can achieve dermatologist-level diagnostic accuracy compared to experienced dermatologists. AI has found applications in numerous medical fields, and some models have achieved sensitivity and specificity values exceeding those of human observers, especially for melanoma detection [76, 77].

AI systems can analyze dermoscopic images much faster than human clinicians, significantly reducing the time required for diagnosis. In skin cancer, the ability to quickly analyze tissue so treatment can be started promptly is invaluable. The development of AI systems continuously increases their efficiency through learning new data. Increasing the number of images in the training datasets allows for improved pattern recognition by the algorithms, which can result in better diagnostic accuracy as time progresses [78, 79].

AI-aided diagnosis has been particularly promising in the early detection of melanoma (where treating as early as possible is crucial). Other applications include analyzing dermoscopic images with AI systems to detect new signs of melanoma that could be missed with visual inspection. AI can also support dermatology in the longitudinal monitoring of old lesions, precisely evaluating whether a lesion is stable or evolving into malignancy. This feature is indispensable for patients with several moles or a previous history of melanoma [80, 81].

AI-assisted diagnosis in digital dermoscopy is an innovative tool for skin cancer detection. Using deep learning algorithms and pattern recognition, these systems can assist the dermatologist in improving patient outcomes through early diagnosis and timely intervention. Nevertheless, data quality, interpretability, and integration issues must be addressed to facilitate the successful adoption of AI into clinical practice. Technology continues to evolve, and AI is set to contribute a vital role in the future of dermatological care [82, 83].

Smartphone Compatibility

The most important digital dermoscopy innovations are smartphone-compatible devices, which have improved access to care. Most dermatoscopes are made to attach to smartphones or tablets, so dermatologists have a powerful tool for imaging and documentation. Modern dermatoscopes with smartphone attachments enable high-resolution imaging of skin lesions. Such imaging capabilities are crucial for accurately diagnosing and monitoring skin diseases like melanoma and other skin cancers [84].

Smartphones are compact and can easily be carried anywhere, so dermatologists can perform the examination anywhere, including in clinics, patients' houses, or remote areas. Such portability is especially advantageous in underdeveloped areas where the availability of dermatological support is low. The smartphone alignment makes patient cases easy to document. Images may be stored, annotated, and organized directly on the device, simplifying record-keeping and follow-up assessments. This efficiency enhances the overall workflow for dermatologists [85].

Using smartphone technology in dermoscopy allows teledermatology to support consultations between dermatologists and patients at a distance. Patients can send photos of their skin lesions through secure portals, and a dermatologist can assess the image to diagnose the condition without seeing the patient in person. Such ability broadens the scope of treatment options for patients in distant or rural areas. They also help improve patient engagement because you can start monitoring your skin with a smartphone. Patients can take photos of their lesions, follow along as they change, and send this information to healthcare providers for a collaborative care approach [86].

Smartphone-compatible dermatoscopes allow dermatologists to hold remote consultations, assess skin conditions, and recommend treatment without patients needing to travel. Dermatology trainees can use smartphone technology to obtain images to comment on and discuss such images with their peers. This improves the process of learning and saves healthcare professionals from sharing knowledge. The quality of images is easy to capture and share and is essential for research data collection in dermatology. Collecting big data sets on skin lesions allows research into prevalence, treatment outcomes, and diagnostic accuracy [87 - 89].

Improved Diagnostic Accuracy and Workflow

Increased Sensitivity and Specificity

Digital dermoscopy has been recognized as a helpful method in dermatology, increasing the sensitivity of melanoma and other skin cancer diagnoses. Studies have shown that digital dermoscopy can improve diagnostic sensitivity and specificity by up to 35% compared to manual visual examination. Such advancement is essential to promote early detection and treatment of skin cancers, thus potentiating an impact on the patient's prognosis [90].

With digital dermoscopy, skin lesions are imaged at high resolution, offering dermatologists microscopic images of the epidermis and, in some cases, papillary dermis. It provides better visualization of slight characteristics that can suggest malignancy (irregular borders, color variations, and patterns specific to melanoma). Digital dermoscopy utilizes advanced algorithms for complex pattern recognition in skin lesions. This has led to using some algorithms that can detect certain features in dermoscopic images relevant to malignant lesions for optimal differentiation between benign and malignant growths [91, 92].

Digital dermoscopy eliminates the subjectivity of visual inspection. Dermatologists can use more objective and visual evidence to support their decision-making on whether further investigation or intervention is needed. It allows the progression of skin lesions with multiple images to be monitored, documented, and archived over time. Dermatologists can look for changes in current images compared to past ones that might signal malignant disease so they can intervene early. Dermatologists can compare current images with previous ones to detect changes that may indicate malignancy, leading to timely interventions [93].

The prognosis of melanoma is much better if the disease is detected at an early stage. Melanoma discovered early in its development (*in situ* or localized) has a nearly 100% five-year survival rate, but that drops significantly for more advanced-stage melanomas. Digital dermoscopy can reduce unnecessary biopsies and excisions by accurately identifying benign lesions. This not only reduces pain to the patient but also saves healthcare costs for unnecessary investigations [94].

This further increases the sensitivity and specificity of digital dermoscopy, which is an important step towards more effective melanoma and skin cancer detection and treatment. Digital dermoscopy improves dermatologists' diagnostic accuracy by offering detailed visualization, objective assessment, and comprehensive monitoring capabilities. This enhancement can significantly impact patient outcomes and their possible treatment success by enabling timely interventions.

With the rapid development of technology, digital dermoscopy will be a more important weapon to combat skin cancer [95].

Total Body Imaging

Digital dermoscopy, specifically total body imaging, is a technique that enables dermatologists to photograph all skin lesions on the patient's surface. This systematic approach is very useful, especially when the patient has many moles, previous skin cancer, or an elevated risk of skin cancer. It allows dermatologists to map the entire surface of a patient's skin visually. The mapping incorporates high-resolution photos of each lesion and mole, creating a baseline for future reference [96].

Dermatologists can use captured images of the entire body to monitor changes over time in existing lesions. Such a longitudinal approach is critical to detecting any changing features that may reflect malignancy, including size, shape, or color changes. The systematic monitoring enabled by total body imaging improves the diagnosis of skin cancers at their furthest upstage. Identifying the signs early helps provide effective treatment and greatly increases the chances of survival [97].

Total body imaging can serve as an educational tool for the patient. Dermatologists can show patients what their skin looks like so they may better appreciate why they should check their neutrals and when changes might need checking out. These detailed photographic records are useful documentation in clinical decision-making. Compared with prior images, dermatologists can evaluate changes and determine if biopsies or other interventions are necessary [98].

Total body imaging can also be performed on patients with a family history of melanoma, large numbers of atypical moles (dysplastic nevi), or a history of skin cancer. Regular monitoring can lead to timely interventions for these patients. The systematic collection of total body images can contribute to research efforts to understand the epidemiology of skin cancer and evaluate the effectiveness of screening programs [99].

Total body imaging supported by digital dermoscopy is a paradigm shift in how dermatologists can now monitor skin lesions through systematic examination. It increases early detection of skin cancer in this population and improves patient outcomes, particularly for those at higher risk. Through thorough documentation and the ability to educate patients, total body imaging is important in preventing skin health. With ongoing technological development, total body imaging will likely be performed more often in routine dermatology practice, with constant further improvement of care quality in dermatology [100, 101].

Remote Monitoring of Skin Lesions

Remote monitoring of skin lesions is a new tool in dermatology that uses technology to help patients and healthcare systems monitor the evolution of skin disorders over time, albeit with fewer face-to-face contacts. Patients can take images of their skin lesions in the home setting and upload these *via* mobile applications, specialized dermatoscopy, and high-resolution imaging systems. Dermatologists evaluate these images and can assess the changes in lesion size, shape, or color promptly before providing instructions for further actions [102, 103].

It is especially helpful for those with many moles or prior skin cancer or who live in rural areas where skin services are difficult to access. For instance, continuous observation by remote monitoring could detect malignant transformations early on, thus decreasing the probability of an advanced-stage diagnosis. It also allows more individualized follow-up schedules, where patients with stable lesions avoid unnecessary visits to the clinician, and patients with changing or suspected lesions are flagged for urgent attention [104].

Remote monitoring has numerous advantages, such as ease of access and possibly reducing healthcare system costs by decreasing in-person visits. It helps patients take charge of their skin health and allows for prompt action if a change could suggest malignancy. Additionally, AI-driven tools are increasing the precision of telediagnosis by helping dermatologists detect otherwise inadequately visible changes in lesions [105].

However, remote monitoring is not without its challenges. Image quality and consistency depend on patient exercise and the devices used, and vital signals can be missed without an experienced expert. To address these limitations, however, remote monitoring is evolving to enhance skin lesion management and remote access to dermatological care [106].

BENEFITS OF DIGITAL DERMOSCOPY

Digital dermoscopy offers several significant benefits in detecting and managing skin lesions, improving both patient experience and clinical outcomes. These are discussed below and summarized in Fig. (**3**).

Non-Invasive and Pain-Free Procedures

This non-invasive approach is advantageous for patients with many moles or lesions because it minimizes unnecessary biopsies and invasive procedures (that are uncomfortable and can be a stressful experience for the patient). Digital dermoscopy reduces the risk of complications with invasive diagnosis (*e.g.*, surgery-related infection, scarring, or bleeding) as there is absolutely no need for surgical intervention [107, 108].

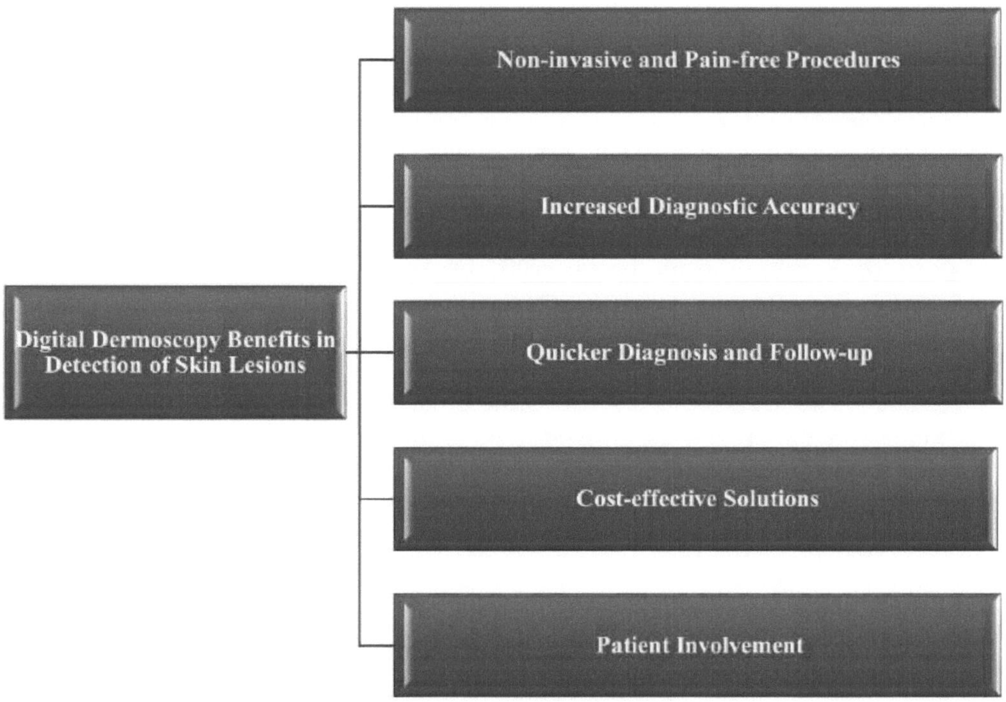

Fig. (3). Digital dermoscopy benefits in the detection of skin lesions.

Digital dermoscopy is also painless, which drives more patients to seek early referrals for dermatological treatment, especially when they normally avoid medical care due to fear of pain. In the early detection of skin cancer like melanoma, this can be particularly crucial, as successful treatments are dependent on early intervention. Digital dermoscopy provides a reproducible, quantitative, and precise approach to noninvasively monitoring skin changes over time and detecting subtle pathological features simply through imaging without needing additional invasive testing on patients or the need for biopsies [109].

Digital dermoscopy is noninvasive and facilitates real-time in-office assessments, significantly reducing the delay in receiving biopsy results and immediate consultations. This leads to better patient satisfaction since patients can obtain a total skin assessment quickly, safely, and without the anxiety often provided by conventional diagnostic procedures [110].

Increased Diagnostic Accuracy

Determining subsurface structures such as pigment networks, vascular patterns, and asymmetries enhances the dermatologist's diagnostic accuracy by improving their ability to differentiate between benign and malignant lesions. These high-resolution images are critical in recognizing the early signs of skin cancers, where hints of melanoma phenotypes can be quite subtle visually and would escape notice without magnification [111, 112].

Digital dermoscopy also enables saving and comparing images, which aids dermatologists in monitoring changes in lesions over time. This is essential to establish the suspect evolution of a mole or lesion, for example, regarding size, shape, or color changes, all indicators of malignancy [113].

Moreover, AI tools enable more accurate diagnostics. Dermatologists can be helped by AI algorithms trained on vast datasets of skin lesion images that accurately recognize patterns and irregularities. This minimizes the opportunity for human error, especially in complicated matters. The improved imaging and automated AI-assisted nature of digital dermoscopy greatly improves contour accuracy and empowers early diagnosis and treatment of skin cancers and other dermatological conditions [114].

Quicker Diagnosis and Follow-up

It allows dermatologists to obtain high-resolution images of lesions at the office visit itself to accurately decide the facial features associated with benign *versus* possibly malignant nature. Such an early assessment assists in spotting suspicious lesions for additional imaging or immediate therapy and decreases the time from detection to treatment [115, 116].

Digital dermoscopy also facilitates the follow-up process. Images can be stored for comparison over time, making it easier for dermatologists to precisely monitor changes in lesions over time. This would reduce the need to return in person unless a lesion changes, allowing for remote surveillance. This reduces time spent by patients and providers and allows for more targeted follow-up care [117].

Integrating AI into the workflow accelerates the diagnosis process even more and aids in pattern recognition for early identification of malignant signs, improving speed and accuracy. Digital dermoscopy provides more rapid diagnosis and clinical follow-up possibilities, leading to better patient outcomes, cost-effectiveness of healthcare provision, and less diagnostic anxiety among patients [118].

Patient Involvement

The diagnostic process has been made much clearer for patients, who can view high-resolution images of their skin lesions through digital platforms. A visual representation of their condition helps patients understand the nature of their skin conditions. It builds confidence that the dermatologist has diagnosed them appropriately and recommended a proper treatment plan. Patients can better see changes in size, shape, or color, all particular signals of malignancy [119, 120].

Additionally, most digital dermoscopy systems have a remote monitoring function that allows patients to send images of their lesions from home *via* a mobile app or dedicated device. This enhances patient convenience by minimizing the frequency of physical examinations and promoting self-examinations for suspicious changes in their skin, enabling timely intervention [121].

With patients being more engaged in their care, there is a higher likelihood of compliance with follow-up recommendations and empowerment to report any issues proactively. Patients become more aware of changes in their skin, so this engagement may lead to earlier detection and improved overall outcomes. Digital dermoscopy improves patient engagement by facilitating the cooperation between patients and healthcare providers [122].

Cost-Effective Solutions

Existing techniques for diagnosing skin lesions, including biopsies and surgical excisions, are costly because they require additional specialized procedures, pathology services, and follow-up treatments. Digital dermoscopy is a useful tool that decreases this noninvasive cost because it provides quick and efficient evaluation of skin lesions without surgical manipulation or tissue removal [123].

The high-resolution imaging of lesions allows dermatologists to provide more upfront accurate diagnoses, which can minimize the need for unnecessary biopsies or surgeries. This reduces not only the expense of the medical procedure but also discomfort and recovery time for patients. Digital dermoscopy promotes safe follow-up instead of immediate excision for benign lesions, further decreasing unnecessary surgeries and their costs [124].

Efficient follow-up of these patients and comparison between digital images can also be done over time. This allows patients with stable lesions to be monitored remotely and avoids the time and cost of travel and consultation fees, as well as taking time off work by attending multiple in-person visits. This can be especially useful for people living in rural or underserved areas with less access to dermatology services [125].

Moreover, AI advances in digital dermoscopy improve the accuracy of diagnosis and avoid misdiagnoses with possible expensive delays or overtreatment. Melanoma and many other skin cancers can be treated very successfully if detected early, making early intervention both a lifesaver and a money saver (treatment of early-stage cancer is much less cost expensive than treatment of later stages). Thus, digital dermoscopy represents a cost-effective strategy for dealing with skin lesions, optimizing healthcare resources, and improving patient outcomes [126].

ROLE OF AI IN DIGITAL DERMOSCOPY

AI is a breakthrough technology that has recently shown promise in classifying skin lesions and differentiating between benign and malignant entities using digital dermoscopy. The deep learning algorithms are AI technologies integrated into dermatology practices, enabling accurate and efficient diagnosis.

Deep Learning Algorithms

Convolutional Neural Networks (CNNs), a deep learning algorithm, are some of the most advanced AI tools in digital dermoscopy. These algorithms allow automatic feature extraction from dermoscopic images without any prior manual feature selection, meaning they can learn complex patterns corresponding to different skin lesions. AI systems examine extensive databases of dermatoscopic photographs, detecting features that might signify malignancy. Research has proven that some of these algorithms can be as diagnostically similar to an experienced dermatologist (and with overall accuracy rates up to 92% for both the classification of benign and malignant lesions). Recently, hybrid models have been designed to fuse features of two or more algorithms to improve diagnostic performance. These models can exploit the advantages of various methods and enhance lesion classification robustness [127, 128].

How AI Enhances Lesion Classification

The instant attention, especially in AI algorithms, is capable of image processing and analysis, which would provide dermatologists with immediate feedback regarding the probability of malignancy. This is important for making quick decisions in the clinical setting. AI systems can reduce human evaluator variability by consistently assessing skin lesions. This is especially helpful in cases when lesions have ambiguous characteristics. Most AI uses self-learning functionality to improve diagnosis over time based on the data they process. This continual learning process improves the adaptation of algorithms to differences in presentations of lesions and enhances classification results [129, 130].

Continuous Improvement in Diagnostic Capabilities

The performance of AI in dermoscopy is contingent on the quality and diversity of the training datasets. Efforts such as the International Skin Imaging Collaboration (ISIC) offer large, publicly accessible datasets to train and validate AI algorithms such that these algorithms generalize well in practice. The increasing evolution of AI-related technology has made integration into routine dermatological work evermore possible. AI-assisted tools can help dermatologists in lesion triage by prioritizing urgent cases and enhancing the overall management of patients [131, 132].

Limitations of AI in Digital Dermoscopy

Despite the promising advancements, AI has several limitations in digital dermoscopy. AI algorithms should be an aid to dermatologists rather than a replacement. Even the AI-generated assessment must be confirmed by a trained expert so we do not make any wrong clinical decisions. Misdiagnosis due to false positives or negatives produced by AI systems. This risk highlights the necessity of constant validation and fine-tuning processes to reduce errors in classification. The effectiveness of AI algorithms depends on the quality and representativity of training datasets. If the datasets are biased, wrong diagnoses will undoubtedly occur, underscoring diversity and inclusive data sets [133, 134].

CHALLENGES AND LIMITATIONS OF AI IN DIGITAL DERMOSCOPY

The challenges and limitations of AI in digital dermoscopy are summarized in Table **1**.

FUTURE DIRECTIONS IN DIGITAL DERMATOLOGY

The evolution of AI will explain lesion classification and diagnosis with growing precision. Given improvements in AI technology, future systems will use more advanced deep learning algorithms, as well as greater sizes and varieties of datasets for training. This would enhance diagnostic accuracy, allowing AI to detect minute changes more reliably and predict results. AI-assisted live diagnostics and on-the-spot treatment planning based on the latest assessments of lesions could facilitate personalized patient management [142, 143].

Another key trend is telemedicine expansion assistance. More telemedicine means easier access to dermatological care, especially in remote or underserved areas. With telemedicine platforms becoming increasingly popular for consultations, digital dermoscopy can integrate into these platforms to provide remote consultation and follow-up services, expanding the reach of specialized dermatology care to patients who otherwise had little access to this type of care [144].

Table 1. Challenges and limitations of AI in digital dermoscopy.

Challenge/Limitations	Impact
Data quality and variability	This can lead to decreased accuracy and reliability of AI systems [135].
Generalization across populations	This may result in biased or less effective diagnoses for underrepresented groups [136].
Interpretability	Understanding how decisions are made can hinder trust and clinical adoption [137].
Integration with clinical workflows	It can be challenging and require significant adjustments to current practices [138].
Over-reliance on AI	Potential for missed diagnoses if AI fails or provides inaccurate results [139].
Continuous learning and adaptation	Maintenance of AI systems can be complex and resource-demanding [140].
Limited contextual understanding	This can lead to incomplete or suboptimal diagnostic recommendations [141].

This led to a fundamental change in access to dermatology care, especially for the underserved population. Telemedicine and remote monitoring would enable access to dermatological care delivery for underserved populations in rural or low socioeconomic regions. This expanded access means more people get necessary assessments and treatment faster, thus addressing inequities in healthcare access [145].

Secure data management with blockchain: This is a monumental development for patient data security. Blockchain technology could guarantee the transparent sharing of dermoscopic images and other patient information. Ultimately, this decentralization of data management provides improved security, integrity, and patient agency over their medical records, which reinforces trust in both the patients themselves and between the patients and providers/researchers [146].

CONCLUSION

The advances in digital dermoscopy have revolutionized the ability to detect skin conditions early on and have widely improved patient outcomes. Advancements in high-resolution imaging coupled with deep learning have revolutionized diagnosis. It helps to visualize the skin lesions in detail, enabling dermatologists to find even subtle changes that indicate malignancy. Advanced AI features take diagnostic precision a step higher by leveraging enormous datasets to identify patterns and abnormalities that traditional methods would miss. Real-time analysis of data from various internal and external sources by AI makes diagnosing diseases faster and developing more personalized treatment plans, making healthcare much better. This has immense ramifications for early detection. In recent years, wearable devices and mobile applications have allowed for continuous skin disease monitoring, enabling patients and doctors to assess changes in lesions over time and leading to earlier treatment when needed. This preventive measure has been proven to dramatically ameliorate prognosis by catching melanomas and other skin tumors at earlier, more treatable stages. Digital dermoscopy has great promise for future advancements in dermatology. Telemedicine will broaden access to dermatology services, including through remote consultations and follow-up visits, greatly improving the ability of patients in underserved areas to receive care. Blockchain Integration: A prospective approach to securing, protecting, and maintaining the privacy of patient data by sharing the information securely using distributed ledger technology. Moreover, further AI developments could result in more accurate diagnostics tools, permitting better-tailored and effective treatment approaches. In summary, the advancements in digital dermoscopy have already transformed skin lesion diagnosis and management, and ongoing innovations promise to enhance further early detection, patient outcomes, and overall dermatological care.

REFERENCES

[1] Weber P, Tschandl P, Sinz C, Kittler H. Dermatoscopy of neoplastic skin lesions: recent advances, updates, and revisions. Curr Treat Options Oncol 2018; 19(11): 56. [http://dx.doi.org/10.1007/s11864-018-0573-6] [PMID: 30238167]

[2] Arige S, Atmakuri LR, Shaik R, Gude M, Ghanta VK, Alluri R. Digital Dermoscopy: Advancements in Skin Cancer Diagnosis and Monitoring. Biomed Pharmacol J 2025; 18(March Spl Edition): 33-43. [http://dx.doi.org/10.13005/bpj/3071]

[3] Rao BK, Ahn CS. Dermatoscopy for melanoma and pigmented lesions. Dermatol Clin 2012; 30(3): 413-34. [http://dx.doi.org/10.1016/j.det.2012.04.005] [PMID: 22800549]

[4] Alsararatee HH. Diagnostic tools and methods for dermatological assessment. Br J Nurs 2025; 34(10): 502-12. [http://dx.doi.org/10.12968/bjon.2024.0383]

[5] Mahajan VK, Handa S. Diagnosis of skin diseases. Atlas of dermatology, dermatopathology and venereology: Cutaneous anatomy, biology and inherited disorders and general dermatologic concepts 2021; 45-107.

[6] Young AT, Vora NB, Cortez J, *et al.* The role of technology in melanoma screening and diagnosis. Pigment Cell Melanoma Res 2021; 34(2): 288-300. [http://dx.doi.org/10.1111/pcmr.12907] [PMID: 32558281]

[7] Sonthalia S, Pasquali P, Agrawal M, *et al.* Dermoscopy update: Review of its extra diagnostic and expanding indications and prospects. Dermatol Pract Concept 2019; 9(4): 253-64. [http://dx.doi.org/10.5826/dpc.0904a02] [PMID: 31723457]

[8] Pagliarello C, Stanganelli I, Fabrizi G, Feliciani C, Nuzzo S. Digital dermoscopy monitoring: is it time to define a quality standard. Acta Derm Venereol 2017; 97(7): 864-5.
[http://dx.doi.org/10.2340/00015555-2663] [PMID: 28358167]

[9] Sinz C, Tschandl P, Rosendahl C, *et al.* Accuracy of dermatoscopy for the diagnosis of nonpigmented cancers of the skin. Journal of the American Academy of Dermatology. 2017;77(6):1100-9.

[10] Borroni R, Panasiti V, Valenti M, *et al.* Long-term sequential digital dermoscopy of low-risk patients may not improve early diagnosis of melanoma compared to periodical handheld dermoscopy. Cancers (Basel) 2023; 15(4): 1129.
[http://dx.doi.org/10.3390/cancers15041129] [PMID: 36831472]

[11] Korotkov K, Quintana J, Puig S, Malvehy J, Garcia R. A new total body scanning system for automatic change detection in multiple pigmented skin lesions. IEEE Trans Med Imaging 2015; 34(1): 317-38.
[http://dx.doi.org/10.1109/TMI.2014.2357715] [PMID: 25222947]

[12] Jaffray DA. Image-guided radiotherapy: from current concept to future perspectives. Nat Rev Clin Oncol 2012; 9(12): 688-99.
[http://dx.doi.org/10.1038/nrclinonc.2012.194] [PMID: 23165124]

[13] Coustasse A, Sarkar R, Abodunde B, Metzger BJ, Slater CM. Use of teledermatology to improve dermatological access in rural areas. Telemed J E Health 2019; 25(11): 1022-32.
[http://dx.doi.org/10.1089/tmj.2018.0130] [PMID: 30741608]

[14] Aractingi S, Pellacani G. Computational neural network in melanocytic lesions diagnosis: artificial intelligence to improve diagnosis in dermatology?. Eur J Dermatol 2019; 29(S1): 4-7.
[http://dx.doi.org/10.1684/ejd.2019.3538] [PMID: 31017580]

[15] Ahuja S, Briggs SM, Collier SM. Teledermatology in rural, underserved, and isolated environments: a review. Current dermatology reports. 2022;11(4):328-35.

[16] Sohail N, Puyana C, Zimmerman L, Tsoukas MM. Artificial intelligence in dermatology: Bridging the gap in patient care and education. Clin Dermatol 2024; 42(5): 434-6.
[http://dx.doi.org/10.1016/j.clindermatol.2024.06.009] [PMID: 38936639]

[17] Glines KR, Haidari W, Ramani L, Akkurt ZM, Feldman SR. Digital future of dermatology. Dermatol Online J 2020; 26(10)
[http://dx.doi.org/10.5070/D32610050455] [PMID: 33147661]

[18] Jones OT, Ranmuthu CKI, Hall PN, Funston G, Walter FM. Recognising skin cancer in primary care. Adv Ther 2020; 37(1): 603-16.
[http://dx.doi.org/10.1007/s12325-019-01130-1] [PMID: 31734824]

[19] Dinnes J, Deeks JJ, Chuchu N, *et al.* Dermoscopy, with and without visual inspection, is used to diagnose melanoma in adults. Cochrane Database Syst Rev 2018; 2018.

[20] Sáez A, Acha B, Serrano A, Serrano C. Statistical detection of colors in dermoscopic images with a texton-based estimation of probabilities. IEEE J Biomed Health Inform 2019; 23(2): 560-9.
[http://dx.doi.org/10.1109/JBHI.2018.2823499] [PMID: 29993674]

[21] Catalano O, Varelli C, Sbordone C, *et al.* A bump: what to do next? Ultrasound imaging of superficial soft-tissue palpable lesions. J Ultrasound 2020; 23(3): 287-300.
[http://dx.doi.org/10.1007/s40477-019-00415-z] [PMID: 31786796]

[22] Gardner LJ, Strunck JL, Wu YP, Grossman D. Current controversies in early-stage melanoma. J Am Acad Dermatol 2019; 80(1): 1-12.
[http://dx.doi.org/10.1016/j.jaad.2018.03.053] [PMID: 30553298]

[23] Lyons F, Ousley LE. Dermatology for the advanced practice nurse 2014.
[http://dx.doi.org/10.1891/9780826136442]

[24] Sortino AM, Abdalla CM, Abdalla BM, *et al.* Ancillary tools for dermatological skin assessment:

Dermoscopy, reflectance confocal microscopy and optical coherence tomography. Oncodermatology: An evidence-based, multidisciplinary approach to best practices 2023; 69-151.

[25] Harvey NT, Chan J, Wood BA. Skin biopsy in the diagnosis of neoplastic skin disease. Aust Fam Physician 2017; 46(5): 289-94.
[PMID: 28472574]

[26] Sisik A, Kilic A, Kilic A, Kivanc AE. Biopsy techniques for skin disease and skin cancer: A new approach. J Cutan Aesthet Surg 2020; 13(3): 251-4.
[http://dx.doi.org/10.4103/JCAS.JCAS_173_19] [PMID: 33209007]

[27] Dockery GD. Aseptic techniques. Lower extremity soft tissue & cutaneous plastic surgery 2012; 53-68.
[http://dx.doi.org/10.1016/B978-0-7020-3136-6.00007-2]

[28] Ehrhart N, Culp WT. Principles of surgical oncology. Veterinary surgical oncology 2012; 3-13.
[http://dx.doi.org/10.1002/9781118729038.ch1]

[29] Romano A, Di Stasio D, Petruzzi M, *et al.* Noninvasive imaging methods to improve the diagnosis of oral carcinoma and its precursors: State of the art and proposal of a three-step diagnostic process. Cancers (Basel) 2021; 13(12): 2864.
[http://dx.doi.org/10.3390/cancers13122864] [PMID: 34201237]

[30] Dobre eg, Surcel M, Constantin C, *et al.* Skin cancer pathobiology at a glance: a focus on imaging techniques and their potential for improved diagnosis and surveillance in clinical cohorts. Int J Mol Sci 2023; 24(2): 1079.
[http://dx.doi.org/10.3390/ijms24021079] [PMID: 36674595]

[31] Ponnarasu S, Schmieder GJ. Excisional biopsy. StatPearls 2022.

[32] Smith N, Johnson TM, Kelly JW, Sober AJ, Bichakjian C. Biopsy of suspected melanoma. Cutaneous melanoma 2020; 195-203.
[http://dx.doi.org/10.1007/978-3-030-05070-2_10]

[33] Greenwood JD, Merry SP, Boswell CL. Skin biopsy techniques. Prim Care 2022; 49(1): 1-22.
[http://dx.doi.org/10.1016/j.pop.2021.10.001] [PMID: 35125151]

[34] Abdalla BM, Filho RT. Biopsy Techniques. Oncodermatology: An evidence-based, multidisciplinary approach to best practices 2023; 171-8.
[http://dx.doi.org/10.1007/978-3-031-29277-4_8]

[35] Pugliese S, Nino T, Torres A. Skin biopsy techniques. Practical dermatologic surgery 2021; 41-6.
[http://dx.doi.org/10.1201/9781003052432-5]

[36] AlGhamdi KM, AlEnazi MM. Versatile punch surgery. J Cutan Med Surg 2011; 15(2): 87-96.
[http://dx.doi.org/10.2310/7750.2011.10002] [PMID: 21477556]

[37] Fung MA, Awasthi S, Hwang ST, Lee JS. Skin biopsies: their utility to allergists and immunologists. Allergic and Immunologic Diseases 2022; 543-78.
[http://dx.doi.org/10.1016/B978-0-323-95061-9.00019-9]

[38] Sturgess J, Crawley F, Kirollos R, Cattle K. Applied anatomy for clinical procedures at a glance. John Wiley & Sons 2020.

[39] Masterson BJ. Manual of gynecologic surgery. Springer Science & Business Media 2012.

[40] Alguire PC, Mathes BM, Gurnee E, Miller SJ. Skin biopsy techniques. Primary care: Clinics in office practice. 2022; 49: pp. (1)1-22.

[41] Sleiman R, Kurban M, Abbas O. Maximizing diagnostic outcomes of skin biopsy specimens. Int J Dermatol 2013; 52(1): 72-8.
[http://dx.doi.org/10.1111/j.1365-4632.2012.05731.x] [PMID: 23278612]

[42] Stevenson P, Rodins K. Improving diagnostic accuracy of skin biopsies. Aust J Gen Pract 2018; 47(4):

216-20.
[http://dx.doi.org/10.31128/AFP-10-17-4376] [PMID: 29621863]

[43] Robilotto AT, Baust JM, Van Buskirk RG, Baust JG. Models and mechanisms of tissue injury in cryosurgery. Theory and Applications of Heat Transfer in Humans 2018; 2: 591-617.
[http://dx.doi.org/10.1002/9781119127420.ch27]

[44] Shitzer A. Temperature fields and lesion sizes in electrosurgery and induction LAT. Heat transfer in medicine and biology: Analysis and Applications 2012; 2: 55.

[45] Winkelmann RR, Desai TD, Farsi M, Torres A. Topical therapies for nonmelanoma skin cancers. Skin cancer management: A practical approach. Cham: Springer International Publishing 2021; pp. 9-30.
[http://dx.doi.org/10.1007/978-3-030-50593-6_2]

[46] Rezakovic S, Zuzul K, Kostovic K. Basal cell carcinoma: a review of treatment modalities. J Dermatolog Clin Res 2014; 2(5): 1035.

[47] Okuboyejo DA, Olugbara OO. A review of prevalent methods for automatic skin lesion diagnosis. Open Dermatol J 2018; 12(1): 14-53.
[http://dx.doi.org/10.2174/1874372201812010014]

[48] Jaworek-Korjakowska J. Novel method for border irregularity assessment in dermoscopic color images. Comput Math Methods Med 2015; 2015(1): 1-11.
[http://dx.doi.org/10.1155/2015/496202] [PMID: 26604980]

[49] Kalkhoran S, Milne O, Zalaudek I, *et al.* Historical, clinical, and dermoscopic characteristics of thin nodular melanoma. Arch Dermatol 2010; 146(3): 311-8.
[http://dx.doi.org/10.1001/archdermatol.2009.369] [PMID: 20231503]

[50] Garrison ZR, Hall CM, Fey RM, *et al.* Advances in early detection of melanoma and the future of at-home testing. Life (Basel) 2023; 13(4): 974.
[http://dx.doi.org/10.3390/life13040974] [PMID: 37109503]

[51] Robinson MT. Melanoma and people of color: The role of physical therapists. Rehabil Oncol 2024; 42(3): 130-7.
[http://dx.doi.org/10.1097/01.REO.0000000000000368]

[52] Atzori L, Pizzatti L, Pau M, Aste N. Mycological examination. European handbook of dermatological treatments 2023; 1351-75.
[http://dx.doi.org/10.1007/978-3-031-15130-9_123]

[53] Jaishi VL, Parajuli R, Dahal P, Maharjan R. Prevalence and risk factors of superficial fungal infection among patients attending a tertiary care hospital in central Nepal. Interdiscip Perspect Infect Dis 2022; 2022(1): 1-10.
[http://dx.doi.org/10.1155/2022/3088681] [PMID: 36247346]

[54] Sehcal VN, Joginder . Slit-skin smear in leprosy. Int J Dermatol 1990; 29(1): 9-16.
[http://dx.doi.org/10.1111/j.1365-4362.1990.tb03746.x] [PMID: 1691740]

[55] Ranjitha ML. A Prospective Study of Fluorescent Microscopy in Detection of Mycobacterium Leprae Bacilli in Skin Biopsy Specimens of Leprosy Patients November 2015 to. (Doctoral dissertation, Rajiv Gandhi University of Health Sciences (India)). 2017.

[56] Shapiro J, Sicco KL, Otberg N, Cummins D, Tuan HH, Eds. Hair loss and restoration. CRC Press 2024.
[http://dx.doi.org/10.1201/9781003344384]

[57] Kumar MA. The skin. Techniques in small animal wound management 2024; 1-1.

[58] El-Shafai W, El-Fattah IA, Taha TE. Advancements in non-invasive optical imaging techniques for precise diagnosis of skin disorders. Opt Quantum Electron 2024; 56(7): 1112.
[http://dx.doi.org/10.1007/s11082-024-06823-8]

[59] Chen X, Lu Q, Chen C, Jiang G. Recent developments in dermoscopy for dermatology. J Cosmet

Dermatol 2021; 20(6): 1611-7.
[http://dx.doi.org/10.1111/jocd.13846] [PMID: 33197276]

[60] Zareen SS, Hossain MS, Wang J, Kang Y. Recent innovations in machine learning for skin cancer lesion analysis and classification: A comprehensive analysis of computer-aided diagnosis. Precis Med Sci 2025 Mar; 14(1): 15-40.
[http://dx.doi.org/10.1002/prm2.12156]

[61] Soenksen LR, Kassis T, Conover ST, *et al.* Using deep learning for dermatologist-level detection of suspicious pigmented skin lesions from wide-field images. Sci Transl Med 2021; 13(581): abb3652.
[http://dx.doi.org/10.1126/scitranslmed.abb3652] [PMID: 33597262]

[62] Chiu LW, Hu SCS. Recent advances in noninvasive imaging of the skin – dermoscopy and optical coherence tomography. Zhonghua Pifuke Yixue Zazhi 2021; 39(3): 115-7.
[http://dx.doi.org/10.4103/ds.ds_36_21]

[63] Soglia S, Pérez-Anker J, Lobos Guede N, Giavedoni P, Puig S, Malvehy J. Diagnostics using non-invasive technologies in dermatological oncology. Cancers (Basel) 2022; 14(23): 5886.
[http://dx.doi.org/10.3390/cancers14235886] [PMID: 36497368]

[64] Forsea AM, Tschandl P, Zalaudek I, *et al.* The impact of dermoscopy on melanoma detection in the practice of dermatologists in Europe: results of a pan-European survey. J Eur Acad Dermatol Venereol 2017; 31(7): 1148-56.
[http://dx.doi.org/10.1111/jdv.14129] [PMID: 28109068]

[65] Scarfì F, Trane L, Maio V, *et al.* Fluorescence-advanced videodermatoscopy (FAV) for the differential diagnosis of suspicious facial lesions: A single-centre experience with pattern analysis and histopathological correlation. Photodermatol Photoimmunol Photomed 2022; 38(3): 266-76.
[http://dx.doi.org/10.1111/phpp.12748] [PMID: 34713502]

[66] Singh SR, Meka AP, Nguyen G, Tejasvi T. Teledermoscopy for Teledermatology. Curr Dermatol Rep 2016; 5(2): 71-6.
[http://dx.doi.org/10.1007/s13671-016-0133-x]

[67] Micali G, Lacarrubba F, Eds. Dermatoscopy in clinical practice: beyond pigmented lesions. CRC Press 2018.
[http://dx.doi.org/10.1201/9781315372358]

[68] Alsayyah A. Differentiating between early melanomas and melanocytic nevi: A state-of-the-art review. Pathol Res Pract 2023; 249: 154734.
[http://dx.doi.org/10.1016/j.prp.2023.154734] [PMID: 37573619]

[69] Sanlorenzo M, Vujic I, De Giorgi V, *et al.* Fluorescence-advanced videodermatoscopy: a new method for *in vivo* skin evaluation. Br J Dermatol 2017; 177(5): 209-e210.
[http://dx.doi.org/10.1111/bjd.15594] [PMID: 28421598]

[70] Scarfì F, Trane L, Maio V, *et al.* Fluorescence-advanced videodermatoscopy (FAV) for the differential diagnosis of suspicious facial lesions: A single-centre experience with pattern analysis and histopathological correlation. Photodermatol Photoimmunol Photomed 2022; 38(3): 266-76.
[http://dx.doi.org/10.1111/phpp.12748]

[71] Varma K, Singh U, Kataria M. Trichoscopy in common scalp alopecia: an observational study. International Journal of Research in Dermatology 2020; 6(3): 361.
[http://dx.doi.org/10.18203/issn.2455-4529.IntJResDermatol20201581]

[72] Ramondetta A, Ribero S, Quaglino P, Broganelli P. *in vivo* observation of cutaneous larva migrans by fluorescence-advanced videodermatoscopy. Emerg Infect Dis 2021; 27(1): 281-3.
[http://dx.doi.org/10.3201/eid2701.203137] [PMID: 33350908]

[73] Taylor MA. Development and evaluation of a nurse practitioner-directed dermoscopy program in an outpatient dermatology practice. Delaware: Wilmington University 2023.

[74] Mahmood F, Bendayan S, Ghazawi FM, Litvinov IV. The emerging role of artificial intelligence in

dermatology. Front Med (Lausanne) 2021; 8: 751649.
[http://dx.doi.org/10.3389/fmed.2021.751649] [PMID: 34869445]

[75] Senan EM, Jadhav ME. Classification of dermoscopy images for early detection of skin cancer–a review. Int J Comput Appl 2019; 975: 8887.

[76] Bernal J, Kushibar K, Asfaw DS, *et al.* Deep convolutional neural networks for brain image analysis on magnetic resonance imaging: a review. Artif Intell Med 2019; 95: 64-81.
[http://dx.doi.org/10.1016/j.artmed.2018.08.008] [PMID: 30195984]

[77] Li Z, Koban KC, Schenck TL, Giunta RE, Li Q, Sun Y. Artificial intelligence in dermatology image analysis: current developments and future trends. J Clin Med 2022; 11(22): 6826.
[http://dx.doi.org/10.3390/jcm11226826] [PMID: 36431301]

[78] Patel S, Wang JV, Motaparthi K, Lee JB. Artificial intelligence in dermatology for the clinician. Clin Dermatol 2021; 39(4): 667-72.
[http://dx.doi.org/10.1016/j.clindermatol.2021.03.012] [PMID: 34809771]

[79] Pianykh OS, Langs G, Dewey M, *et al.* Continuous learning AI in radiology: implementation principles and early applications. Radiology 2020; 297(1): 6-14.
[http://dx.doi.org/10.1148/radiol.2020200038] [PMID: 32840473]

[80] Patel RH, Foltz EA, Witkowski A, Ludzik J. Analysis of artificial intelligence-based approaches applied to non-invasive imaging for early detection of melanoma: a systematic review. Cancers (Basel) 2023; 15(19): 4694.
[http://dx.doi.org/10.3390/cancers15194694] [PMID: 37835388]

[81] Metta C, Beretta A, Guidotti R, *et al.* Advancing dermatological diagnostics: Interpretable AI for enhanced skin lesion classification. Diagnostics (Basel) 2024; 14(7): 753.
[http://dx.doi.org/10.3390/diagnostics14070753] [PMID: 38611666]

[82] Semerci ZM, Toru HS, Çobankent Aytekin E, *et al.* The role of artificial intelligence in early diagnosis and molecular classification of head and neck skin cancers: A multidisciplinary approach. Diagnostics (Basel) 2024; 14(14): 1477.
[http://dx.doi.org/10.3390/diagnostics14141477] [PMID: 39061614]

[83] Kelly CJ, Karthikesalingam A, Suleyman M, Corrado G, King D. Key challenges for delivering clinical impact with artificial intelligence. BMC Med 2019; 17(1): 195.
[http://dx.doi.org/10.1186/s12916-019-1426-2] [PMID: 31665002]

[84] Ouellette S, Rao BK. The usefulness of smartphones in dermatology: a US-based review. Int J Environ Res Public Health 2022; 19(6): 3553.
[http://dx.doi.org/10.3390/ijerph19063553] [PMID: 35329240]

[85] Lofgreen SJ, Ashack K, Burton KA, Dellavalle RP. Mobile device use in dermatologic patient care. Curr Dermatol Rep 2016; 5(2): 77-82.
[http://dx.doi.org/10.1007/s13671-016-0132-y]

[86] Giavina-Bianchi M, Santos AP, Cordioli E. Teledermatology reduces dermatology referrals and improves access to specialists. EClinicalMedicine 2020; 29-30: 100641.
[http://dx.doi.org/10.1016/j.eclinm.2020.100641]

[87] No 13, p. Giansanti D. Advancing dermatological care: a comprehensive narrative review of teledermatology and mHealth for bridging gaps and expanding opportunities beyond the COVID-19 pandemic. InHealthcare 2023 Jul 1. MDPI 1911; 11.

[88] Shahriari N, Grant-Kels J, Murphy MJ. Dermatopathology education in the era of modern technology. J Cutan Pathol 2017; 44(9): 763-71.
[http://dx.doi.org/10.1111/cup.12980] [PMID: 28612388]

[89] Gençoğlu Ş. Analysis of skin health management through telemedicine and mobile health in dermatology in the post-COVID era. The European Research Journal ; 1-0.

[90] Heibel HD, Hooey L, Cockerell CJ. A review of noninvasive techniques for skin cancer detection in dermatology. Am J Clin Dermatol 2020; 21(4): 513-24.
[http://dx.doi.org/10.1007/s40257-020-00517-z] [PMID: 32383142]

[91] Lovatto L, Carrera C, Salerni G, Alós L, Malvehy J, Puig S. *in vivo* reflectance confocal microscopy of equivocal melanocytic lesions detected by digital dermoscopy follow-up. J Eur Acad Dermatol Venereol 2015; 29(10): 1918-25.
[http://dx.doi.org/10.1111/jdv.13067] [PMID: 25752663]

[92] Pathan S, Prabhu KG, Siddalingaswamy PC. Techniques and algorithms for computer aided diagnosis of pigmented skin lesions—A review. Biomed Signal Process Control 2018; 39: 237-62.
[http://dx.doi.org/10.1016/j.bspc.2017.07.010]

[93] Fried L, Tan A, Bajaj S, Liebman TN, Polsky D, Stein JA. Technological advances for the detection of melanoma. J Am Acad Dermatol 2020; 83(4): 983-92.
[http://dx.doi.org/10.1016/j.jaad.2020.03.121] [PMID: 32348823]

[94] Gong HZ, Zheng HY, Li J. Amelanotic melanoma. Melanoma Res 2019; 29(3): 221-30.
[http://dx.doi.org/10.1097/CMR.0000000000000571] [PMID: 30672881]

[95] Thomas L, Puig S. Dermoscopy, Digital Dermoscopy and Other Diagnostic Tools in the Early Detection of Melanoma and Follow-up of High-risk Skin Cancer Patients. Acta Derm Venereol 2017; (Suppl. 218)0.
[http://dx.doi.org/10.2340/00015555-2719] [PMID: 28676882]

[96] Salerni G, Carrera C, Lovatto L, *et al.* Benefits of total body photography and digital dermatoscopy ("two-step method of digital follow-up") in the early diagnosis of melanoma in patients at high risk for melanoma. J Am Acad Dermatol 2012; 67(1): 17-e27.
[http://dx.doi.org/10.1016/j.jaad.2011.04.008] [PMID: 21683472]

[97] Freeman K, Dinnes J, Chuchu N, *et al.* Algorithm-based smartphone apps to assess the risk of skin cancer in adults: a systematic review of diagnostic accuracy studies. BMJ 2020; 368

[98] Musthaq S, Sahu A, Rotemberg V. Dermatologic Imaging for Immunosuppressed Patients. Dermatology and Solid Organ Transplantation 2021; 36-50.
[http://dx.doi.org/10.1201/9781003001461-3]

[99] Rameshkumar AP. The Role of Total Body Photography in Early Melanoma Detection. PQDT-Global 2020.

[100] Ahmedt-Aristizabal D, Nguyen C, Tychsen-Smith L, *et al.* Monitoring of pigmented skin lesions using 3D whole body imaging. Comput Methods Programs Biomed 2023; 232: 107451.
[http://dx.doi.org/10.1016/j.cmpb.2023.107451] [PMID: 36893580]

[101] Navarrete-Dechent C, Liopyris K, Rishpon A, Marghoob NG, Monnier J, Marghoob AA. Total body photography as an aid for the early detection of skin cancer. Photography in Clinical Medicine 2020; pp. 253-69.
[http://dx.doi.org/10.1007/978-3-030-24544-3_18]

[102] Wongvibulsin S, Frech TM, Chren MM, Tkaczyk ER. Expanding personalized, data-driven dermatology: leveraging digital health technology and machine learning to improve patient outcomes. JID Innov 2022; 2(3): 100105.
[http://dx.doi.org/10.1016/j.xjidi.2022.100105] [PMID: 35462957]

[103] Modaragama S. Decision intelligence: Transformational developments in skin cancer screening using mobile applications. SSRN 3687522.2023; .

[104] Drabarek D, Habgood E, Ackermann D, *et al.* Perspectives and experiences of patient-led melanoma surveillance using digital technologies from clinicians involved in the MEL-SELF pilot randomized controlled trial: a qualitative interview study. JMIR Dermatol 2022; 5(4): 40623.
[http://dx.doi.org/10.2196/40623] [PMID: 37632906]

[105] Luo N, Zhong X, Su L, Cheng Z, Ma W, Hao P. Artificial intelligence-assisted dermatology diagnosis: From unimodal to multimodal. Comput Biol Med 2023; 165: 107413.
[http://dx.doi.org/10.1016/j.compbiomed.2023.107413] [PMID: 37703714]

[106] Virginia Anikwe C, Friday Nweke H, Chukwu Ikegwu A, *et al.* Mobile and wearable sensors for data-driven health monitoring system: State-of-the-art and future prospect. Expert Syst Appl 2022; 202: 117362.
[http://dx.doi.org/10.1016/j.eswa.2022.117362]

[107] Alzahrani S. Artificial Intelligence for skin lesion analysis based on computer vision and deep learning. United Kingdom: The University of Liverpool 2023.

[108] Jung JM, Cho JY, Lee WJ, Chang SE, Lee MW, Won CH. Emerging minimally invasive technologies for the detection of skin cancer. J Pers Med 2021; 11(10): 951.
[http://dx.doi.org/10.3390/jpm11100951] [PMID: 34683091]

[109] Weller RB, Hunter HJ, Mann MW. Clinical dermatology 2015.

[110] Foltz EA, Ludzik J, Leachman S, *et al.* Revolutionizing skin cancer triage: The role of patient-initiated teledermoscopy in remote diagnosis. Cancers (Basel) 2024; 16(14): 2565.
[http://dx.doi.org/10.3390/cancers16142565] [PMID: 39061204]

[111] Dick V, Sinz C, Mittlböck M, Kittler H, Tschandl P. Accuracy of computer-aided diagnosis of melanoma: a meta-analysis. JAMA Dermatol 2019; 155(11): 1291-9.
[http://dx.doi.org/10.1001/jamadermatol.2019.1375] [PMID: 31215969]

[112] Ring C, Cox N, Lee JB. Dermatoscopy. Clin Dermatol 2021; 39(4): 635-42.
[http://dx.doi.org/10.1016/j.clindermatol.2021.03.009] [PMID: 34809768]

[113] Malvehy J, Puig S. Follow-up of melanocytic skin lesions with digital total-body photography and digital dermoscopy: a two-step method. Clin Dermatol 2002; 20(3): 297-304.
[http://dx.doi.org/10.1016/S0738-081X(02)00220-1] [PMID: 12074871]

[114] Goyal M, Knackstedt T, Yan S, Hassanpour S. Artificial intelligence-based image classification methods for skin cancer diagnosis: Challenges and opportunities. Comput Biol Med 2020; 127: 104065.
[http://dx.doi.org/10.1016/j.compbiomed.2020.104065] [PMID: 33246265]

[115] Bakos RM, Blumetti TP, Roldán-Marín R, Salerni G. Noninvasive imaging tools in diagnosing and treating skin cancers. Am J Clin Dermatol 2018; 19(S1) (Suppl. 1): 3-14.
[http://dx.doi.org/10.1007/s40257-018-0367-4] [PMID: 30374899]

[116] Mashoudy KD, Perez SM, Nouri K. From diagnosis to intervention: a review of telemedicine's role in skin cancer care. Arch Dermatol Res 2024; 316(5): 139.
[http://dx.doi.org/10.1007/s00403-024-02884-7] [PMID: 38696032]

[117] Stanganelli I, Longo C, Mazzoni L, *et al.* Integration of reflectance confocal microscopy in sequential dermoscopy follow-up improves melanoma detection accuracy. Br J Dermatol 2015; 172(2): 365-71.
[http://dx.doi.org/10.1111/bjd.13373] [PMID: 25154446]

[118] Mun SK, Wong KH, Lo SCB, Li Y, Bayarsaikhan S. Artificial intelligence for the future radiology diagnostic service. Front Mol Biosci 2021; 7: 614258.
[http://dx.doi.org/10.3389/fmolb.2020.614258] [PMID: 33585563]

[119] Goulart JM, Malvehy J, Puig S, Martin G, Marghoob AA. Dermoscopy in skin self-examination: A useful tool for select patients. Arch Dermatol 2011; 147(1): 53-8.
[http://dx.doi.org/10.1001/archdermatol.2010.387] [PMID: 21242394]

[120] Nie Y, Sommella P, Carratu M, Ferro M, O'Nils M, Lundgren J. Recent advances in the diagnosis of skin lesions using dermoscopic images based on deep learning. IEEE Access 2022; 10: 95716-47.
[http://dx.doi.org/10.1109/ACCESS.2022.3199613]

[121] Marin-Gomez FX, Vidal-Alaball J, Poch PR, Sariola CJ, Ferrer RT, Peña JM. Diagnosis of skin

lesions using photographs taken with a mobile phone: an online survey of primary care physicians. J Prim Care Community Health 2020; 11
[http://dx.doi.org/10.1177/2150132720937831] [PMID: 32590923]

[122] Janda M, Horsham C, Koh U, *et al.* Evaluating healthcare practitioners' views on store-and-forward teledermoscopy services for the diagnosis of skin cancer. Digit Health 2019; 5
[http://dx.doi.org/10.1177/2055207619828225] [PMID: 30792879]

[123] Zakaria A, Amerson EH. Teledermatology: Economics and cost-effectiveness. Teledermatology: A comprehensive overview 2023; 49-57.

[124] Khattab SY, Hijaz BA, Semenov YR. Cutaneous imaging techniques 2024.
[http://dx.doi.org/10.1016/j.hoc.2024.05.011]

[125] Evers EC, Fritz SA, Colditz GA, Burnham JP. Perceptions of telemedicine and costs incurred by a visit to a general infectious diseases clinic: a survey. Open Forum Infectious Diseases. US: Oxford University Press. 2022; 9: p. (3)661.
[http://dx.doi.org/10.1093/ofid/ofab661]

[126] Atkins MB, Curiel-Lewandrowski C, Fisher DE, *et al.* The state of melanoma: emergent challenges and opportunities. Clin Cancer Res 2021; 27(10): 2678-97.
[http://dx.doi.org/10.1158/1078-0432.CCR-20-4092] [PMID: 33414132]

[127] Yee J, Rosendahl C, Aoude LG. The role of artificial intelligence and convolutional neural networks in the management of melanoma: a clinical, pathological, and radiological perspective. Melanoma Res 2024; 34(2): 96-104.
[http://dx.doi.org/10.1097/CMR.0000000000000951] [PMID: 38141179]

[128] Balasubramaniam V. Artificial intelligence algorithm with SVM classification using dermascopic images for melanoma diagnosis. Journal of Artificial Intelligence and Capsule Networks 2021; 3(1): 34-42.
[http://dx.doi.org/10.36548/jaicn.2021.1.003]

[129] Du-Harpur X, Watt FM, Luscombe NM, Lynch MD. What is AI? Applications of artificial intelligence to dermatology. Br J Dermatol 2020; 183(3): 423-30.
[http://dx.doi.org/10.1111/bjd.18880] [PMID: 31960407]

[130] Anisuzzaman DM, Wang C, Rostami B, Gopalakrishnan S, Niezgoda J, Yu Z. Image-based artificial intelligence in wound assessment: a systematic review. Adv Wound Care (New Rochelle) 2022; 11(12): 687-709.
[http://dx.doi.org/10.1089/wound.2021.0091] [PMID: 34544270]

[131] Combalia M, Codella N, Rotemberg V, *et al.* Validation of artificial intelligence prediction models for skin cancer diagnosis using dermoscopy images: the 2019 International Skin Imaging Collaboration Grand Challenge. Lancet Digit Health 2022; 4(5): 330-e339.
[http://dx.doi.org/10.1016/S2589-7500(22)00021-8] [PMID: 35461690]

[132] Smith MP, Schulman JM. Emerging applications of artificial intelligence in dermatopathology. Curr Dermatol Rep 2024; 13(3): 133-40.
[http://dx.doi.org/10.1007/s13671-024-00431-1]

[133] Goktas P, Gulseren D, Tobin AM. Large Language and Vision Assistant in dermatology: a game changer or just hype?. Clin Exp Dermatol 2024; 49(8): 783-92.
[http://dx.doi.org/10.1093/ced/llae119] [PMID: 38570376]

[134] Fatima M, Pachauri P, Akram W, Parvez M, Ahmad S, Yahya Z. Enhancing retinal disease diagnosis through AI: Evaluating performance, ethical considerations, and clinical implementation. Informatics and Health 2024; 1(2): 57-69.
[http://dx.doi.org/10.1016/j.infoh.2024.05.003]

[135] Groh M, Harris C, Daneshjou R, Badri O, Koochek A. Towards transparency in dermatology image datasets with skin tone annotations by experts, crowds, and an algorithm. Proceedings of the ACM on

Human-Computer Interaction. 1-26.
[http://dx.doi.org/10.1145/3555634]

[136] Rezk E, Eltorki M, El-Dakhakhni W. Leveraging artificial intelligence to improve the diversity of dermatological skin color pathology: protocol for an algorithm development and validation study. JMIR Res Protoc 2022; 11(3): 34896.
[http://dx.doi.org/10.2196/34896] [PMID: 34983017]

[137] Manole I, Tiplica GS. Integrating Artificial Intelligence in dermatology: progress, challenges and perspectives. Romanian Medical Journal 2024; 71(2).
[http://dx.doi.org/10.37897/RMJ.2024.2.5]

[138] Herrick G, Mukarram M, Li V, Skemp E, Mounger R. Integrating deep learning with dermoscopic imaging for enhanced melanoma detection. Ameri J Clin Med Re 2024.

[139] Chan S, Reddy V, Myers B, Thibodeaux Q, Brownstone N, Liao W. Machine learning in dermatology: current applications, opportunities, and limitations. Dermatol Ther (Heidelb) 2020; 10(3): 365-86.
[http://dx.doi.org/10.1007/s13555-020-00372-0] [PMID: 32253623]

[140] Munoz MA, Tromp JG, Zhushun C. Review of virtual reality evaluation methods and psychophysiological measurement tools. Emerging Technologies for Health and Medicine 2018; 69-86.
[http://dx.doi.org/10.1002/9781119509875.ch6]

[141] Sriram T, Wafra MR, Fernando TJ, Mohottiarachchi MA. Intelligent system for skin disease prediction. European journal of science. Innovation and Technology 2024; 4(3): 422-43.

[142] Garg S, Williams NL, Ip A, Dicker AP. Clinical integration of digital solutions in health care: an overview of the current landscape of digital technologies in cancer care. JCO Clin Cancer Inform 2018; 2(2): 1-9.
[http://dx.doi.org/10.1200/CCI.17.00159] [PMID: 30652580]

[143] Lepakshi VA. Machine learning and deep learning based AI tools for development of diagnostic tools. Computational Approaches for Novel Therapeutic and Diagnostic Designing to Mitigate SARS-CoV-2 Infection 2022; 399-420.
[http://dx.doi.org/10.1016/B978-0-323-91172-6.00011-X]

[144] Colven R, Shim MHM, Brock D, Todd G. Dermatological diagnostic acumen improves with use of a simple telemedicine system for underserved areas of South Africa. Telemed J E Health 2011; 17(5): 363-9.
[http://dx.doi.org/10.1089/tmj.2010.0163] [PMID: 21599529]

[145] Maddukuri S, Patel J, Lipoff JB. Teledermatology addressing disparities in health care access: a review. Curr Dermatol Rep 2021; 10(2): 40-7.
[http://dx.doi.org/10.1007/s13671-021-00329-2] [PMID: 33747638]

[146] Naveen VE, Dhivya S, Jenefa A. DenseNet melanoma classification in blockchain-driven healthcare. Blockchain for biomedical research and healthcare: Concept, trends, and future implications 2024; 99-122.
[http://dx.doi.org/10.1007/978-981-97-4268-4_5]

CHAPTER 7

Machine Learning Algorithms for Dermatopathology Analysis

Akanksha Sharma[1], **Ashish Verma**[2], **Sunita**[1], **Akhil Sharma**[1], **Shivkanya Fuloria**[3] and **Shaweta Sharma**[4,*]

[1] *R. J. College of Pharmacy, Raipur, Uttar Pradesh - 202165, India*

[2] *Mangalmay Pharmacy College, Greater Noida, Uttar Pradesh-201306, India*

[3] *Faculty of Pharmacy, AIMST University, Semeling Campus, Bedong - 08100, Kedah, Malaysia*

[4] *School of Medical and Allied Sciences, Galgotias University, Uttar Pradesh-201310, India*

Abstract: Dermatopathology is a sub-specialty of dermatology that involves microscopic examination of skin biopsy information for clinical diagnosis. While knowledge of disease and skill in diagnosis have improved with advances in technology and science, the amount of clinical information and the quality of biopsy specimens remains a challenge. Typically, the specimens are biopsied, and the analyses are pathologic, serving a supportive or confirming role in the diagnostic algorithm. Automation and artificial intelligence in dermatopathology provide lower human mistakes, higher efficiency and productivity, improved traceability, uptake of digital pathology, and cost savings. Machine learning algorithms essentially fall into three categories: supervised learning algorithms, unsupervised learning algorithms, and semi-supervised learning algorithms. Regression algorithms discover the connection between target output variables and input features to predict output for new instances. In dermatology, AI can be used to detect skin cancer, especially melanoma. AI models can then accurately learn all the patterns and features that are indicative of malignancy from a large dataset of labelled skin lesion images. However, the implementation of such systems utilising artificial intelligence is wholly dependent on the availability of high-quality and diverse training data. By applying advanced neural architectures to clinical, dermoscopic secretions, or histopathological features, AI models may stratify patients with melanoma into high- and low-risk cohorts and tailor management and surveillance accordingly. Image preprocessing is a crucial step in the dermatopathology pipeline to guarantee high image quality and uniformity. One of the most important strategies in dermatopathology is data augmentation, which expands the data without further image acquisition. We can also include advanced augmentation techniques that can vary skin lesions with rotation, flipping and scaling. Annotation and labelling are needed for crafting a machine learning model, but they are impossible to avoid, as they

* **Corresponding author Shaweta Sharma:** School of Medical and Allied Sciences, Galgotias University, Uttar Pradesh-201310, India; E-mail: shawetasharma@galgotiasuniversity.edu.in

Akhil Sharma, Shaweta Sharma, Shivkanya Fuloria & Sudhir Kumar (Eds.)

provide such models with the essential nature of the image. Techniques, as you might have seen, oversampling or undersampling the dataset, are pretty useful because we want our model to have enough exposure to less frequent cases present in a balanced dataset to ensure the models that we build are robust ones. Statistical approaches involving cross-validation and hyperparameter tuning can be used to estimate the skill of machine learning models. There are many evaluation metrics based on which your machine learning models are trained, such as accuracy, precision, recall, F1 score, ROC-AUC, *etc*., which are all short to better understand your ML models.

Keywords: Clinical practice integration, Convolutional neural networks (CNNs), Dermatopathology, Machine learning, Predictive analytics, Random forests, Support vector machines (SVMs).

INTRODUCTION

Dermatopathology is an increasingly rising sub-specialty of dermatology. This subspecialty of dermatology and pathology is directed at the linking of clinical data and microscopic findings of skin biopsies to supply diagnostic information to the doctor who is caring for the patient.

It evolved to find not just very novel qualities but plenty of considerable ground over its development. Diagnostic ability and an understanding of the pathogenesis of these disorders have been tremendously enhanced with the development of new techniques for their study, such as electron and immunofluorescence microscopy and immunohistochemistry. While scientific and technological progress has been made, the plenty of biopsy specimens and the clinical information linked with them remain a significant challenge for dermatopathologists in their work as a diagnostician. Like dermatology, dermatopathology is a discipline best learned by observing hundreds of cases and histopathology slides, in addition to conceptually understanding the disease process [1, 2].

Pathologic examination of the biopsy material is often at least an ancillary or confirming part of the diagnosis. Until recently, the diagnosis of disease by histopathology depended on the examination of hematoxylin and eosin (H&E)-stained slides with the help of some histochemical stains. However, there are many methodologies based on immunohistochemistry and molecular biology that will aid in the identification of infections. H&E-stained slides mostly diagnose dermatological inflammatory diseases. On the other hand, infectious diseases are diagnosed through the use of histochemical stains. Immunohistochemistry, an ancillary method in histopathological diagnosis, is a highly valuable instrument. Nonetheless, the traditional perspective gained over many years is that dermatopathology involves both macroscopic and microscopic skin pathology and that even dermatoscopic analysis is an integral part of the pathologic diagnosis [3, 4].

One of the most dynamic fields of dermatology in terms of diagnostic tools and techniques is a perfect example of the continued quest for precision in studying and treating skin diseases. The ability of dermatologists and dermatopathologists to diagnose skin disorders has undergone great advancements over the lifespan of their careers, from visual inspection to the use of advanced microscopy and molecular analysis. In this rapidly evolving technological landscape, large language models (LLMs), which are a kind of artificial intelligence that is widely used for text recognition and generation, are emerging as powerful aids for improving diagnostic sensitivity and accuracy [5]. AI is commonly used for text identification and generation. Deep learning and artificial intelligence flatten the details of skin-based pathology with the performance of algorithms trained on data to reproduce and produce human-similar text for a new paradigm shift in dermatopathology. They are rapidly transforming the landscape of clinical pathology itself, including dermatopathology (DP, the histopathological diagnosis of skin diseases), as we explored in this chapter. This is achieved through the historical development of diagnostic modalities in this niche, as well as an overview of the benefits of implementation of LLM in dermatopathology and opisthosoma cases of this technology in practice. Further, challenges to the deployment of this technology are reviewed to contextualise the applicability of its potential use cases [6, 7].

BENEFITS OF AUTOMATION IN DERMATOPATHOLOGY

Automation in dermatopathology offers several advantages that can improve patient outcomes and streamline laboratory processes, as shown in Fig. (**1**).

Reduced Human Errors

Automated systems reduce the possibility of human errors in sample preparation and staining, for instance. It can result in more precise and consistent outcomes, eliminating under- or over-diagnosing [8].

Automation enables laboratories to process their samples faster and more efficiently, leading to shorter turnaround times and increased throughput. In high-amount environments, analysis of this sort can take time and require many human resources [9]. Thus, this is especially useful.

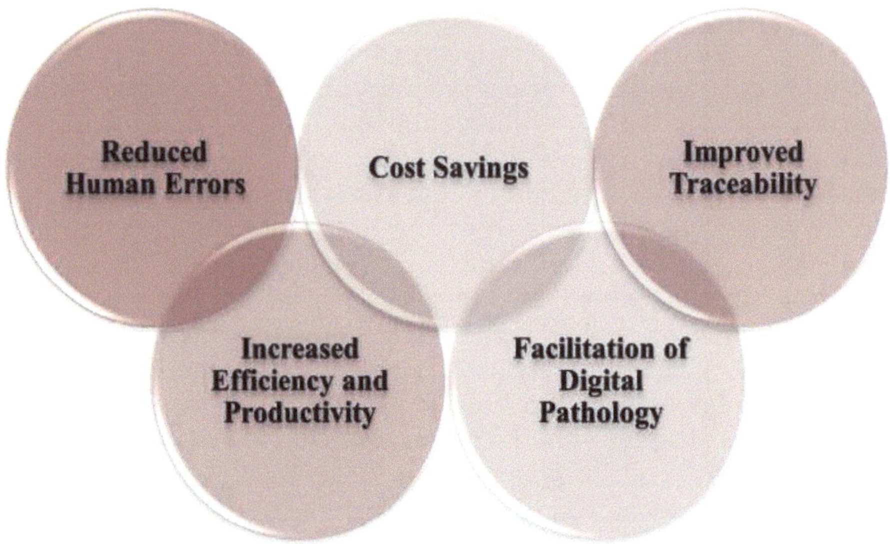

Fig. (1). Benefits of automation in dermatopathology.

Improved Traceability

Unlike an automatic process, where the traceability of your samples throughout the workflow is more detailed. Digital technologies for bar-coding and tracking systems ensure the identification and traceability of samples, improving the quality of the process [10].

Enabling Digital Pathology

The emergence of automation is enabling digital pathology where digitalising glass slides into high-resolution digital images are captured. This can facilitate the distant dormant interpretation, consultation, and computer-based image analysis, realising the potential for better patient care [11].

Cost Savings

Automation can help dermatopathology laboratories save thousands of dollars by minimising errors, maximising efficiency, and optimising workflows. It is estimated that when automation is implemented, savings in materials and labour of $2.50 to $3.00 per case can be expected [12].

TYPES OF MACHINE LEARNING ALGORITHMS

The selection of appropriate machine learning algorithms is quite tedious and time-consuming, as there are a variety of machine learning algorithms available. These algorithms can be classified into two types [13]. They are categorised first according to their learning pattern, and second, a similarity in their function is explained in Fig. (**2**).

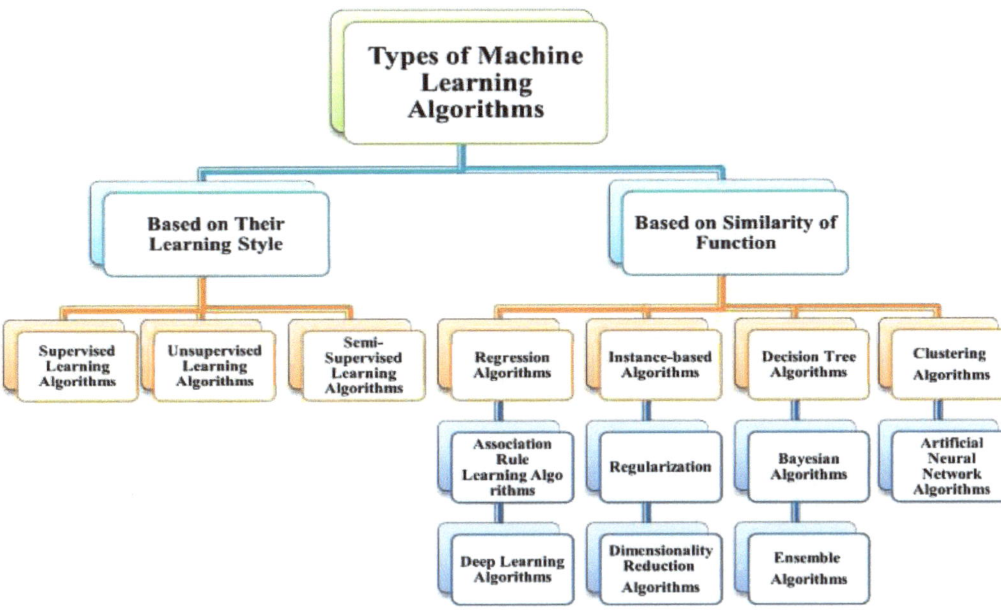

Fig. (2). Types of machine learning algorithms.

Based on their Learning Style

Supervised Learning Algorithms

The training data comes with a label that says how the training must be processed. The model is trained to a certain point where accuracy meets the acceptable level using the training data. These problem types include those such as classification and regression. The algorithms used are Logistic Regression, Nearest Neighbor, Naive Bayes, Decision Trees, Linear Regression, Support Vector Machines (SVM), and Neural Networks [14, 15].

Unsupervised Learning Algorithms

There is no label attached to the input data. The input data comes with patterns, and we capture those patterns while preparing the model. Clustering, dimensionality reduction, and association rule learning are examples of this kind of problem. Examples of algorithms that are used for these kinds of problems are the Apriori algorithm and Associations Rules, K-Means [16, 17].

Semi-Supervised Learning Algorithms

Labelling the data is very costly as it involves skilled human experts. The mix of both label data and unlabeled data. It learns the underlying patterns itself and makes predictions accordingly. It is a hybrid problem, half classification and half clustering [18, 19].

Based on the Similarity of Function

Regression Algorithms

One type of supervised learning is regression, which is the analysis of a relationship between one or more independent input features and the target output variables to be predicted on the new data points. Some of the common types of regression algorithms are: 1) Simple Linear Regression, 2) Lasso Regression, 3) Logistic regression, 4) Multivariate Regression algorithm, and 5) Multiple Regression Algorithm [20, 21].

Instance-based Algorithms

They are from the family of learning that compares new examples of the problem to those in the training set to identify the best match, then makes a prediction based on the matched neighbours. We can list the most popular instance-based algorithms as follows: k-nearest Neighbor, Learning Vector Quantization, Self-Organizing Map, Locally Weighted Learning, and Support Vector Machines [22, 23].

Regularisation

Regularisation is the method of regularising the learning process from a specific pool of features. It normalises and moderates. Normalised weights are attached to the features that inhibit some features dominating the prediction process. It avoids the overfitting issue in a machine-learning way. Other Regularization Algorithms: Ridge regression, LASSO (least absolute shrinkage and selection operator), and LARS (least-angle regression) [24].

Decision Tree Algorithms

These approaches create a tree-based model built on the decisions based on the values of the attributes. Decision trees are applicable for classification and regression tasks. Below are some of the popular decision tree algorithms: Classification and Regression Tree (C4. 5, and C5. 0), Conditional Decision Trees, Chi-squared Automatic Interaction Detection, and Decision Stump [25, 26].

Bayesian Algorithms

These algorithms utilise the Bayes theorem for class or regression problems. These are Naive Bayes (NB), Gaussian NB, Multinomial NB, Bayesian Belief Network, Bayes Net, and Averaged One Dependence Estimators [27, 28].

Clustering Algorithms

The respective groups having similar data points concerning data distribution are called clusters. All the data points in the same group are similar, whereas the data points belonging to separate groups are very dissimilar. Clustering is a type of unsupervised learning and is commonly used for statistical data analysis in various domains. This includes algorithms such as k-means, k-medians, Expectation Maximization, Hierarchical Clustering, and Density-Based Spatial Clustering of Applications with Noise [29, 30].

Association Rule Learning Algorithms

Association rule learning is a very large dataset rule-based learning method to their relations between variables. We use Association Rule learning mainly in market basket analysis. The two predominated are the Apriori algorithm and the Eclat algorithm [31, 32].

Artificial Neural Network Algorithms

Artificial neural network algorithms use bits from biological neurons in human brains. They come under the category of nonlinear pattern matching and predicting methods in the context of classification and regression problems. Perceptrons, Multilayer Perceptrons, back–Propagation, Stochastic Gradient Descent, Radial Basis Function Networks, and Hopfield Networks are some of the most popular artificial neural network algorithms [33, 34].

Deep Learning Algorithms

These are updated examples of artificial neural networks that can operate on enormous and multifarious labelled databases. The deep learning process is optimised for textual, visual, and auditory data. Deep learning employs self-delivered learning frameworks with an increased number of hidden layers to manage big data and is accompanied by more advanced computing hardware. The leading deep learning methods include Convolutional Neural Networks, Recurrent Neural Networks, Deep Boltzmann Machines, Auto-Encoders Deep Belief Networks, and Long Short-Term Memory Networks [35, 36].

Dimensionality Reduction Algorithms

Dimensionality Reduction algorithms take advantage of the inner nature of data using an unsupervised fashion to represent data by smaller information sets. High-dimensional data is represented in a lower dimension that can be used in the place of supervised learning methods such as classification and regression. Popular Dimensionality Reduction algorithms are Principal Component Analysis, Principal Component Regression, Linear Discriminant Analysis, Quadratic Discriminant Analysis, Mixture Discriminant Analysis, Flexible Discriminant Analysis, and Sammon Mapping [37, 38].

Ensemble Algorithms

Ensemble methods are models that consist of multiple weaker models trained in isolation and whose individual predictions are decided through some method to get the final prediction. The output quality depends on the strategy used to merge the individual outcomes. Some of the common methods include Random Forest, Boosting, Bootstrapped Aggregation, AdaBoost, Stacked Generalization, Gradient Boosting Machines, Gradient Boosted Regression Trees, and Weighted Average [37, 39].

APPLICATIONS IN DERMATOPATHOLOGY

Skin Cancer Detection

Among the non-genetic aspects, AI algorithms analyse dermoscopic or histopathological images to identify the presence of skin cancer, particularly melanoma. AI models can learn to recognise patterns and features that are indicative of malignancy from a large dataset of photos of skin lesions that have already been labelled as benign or malignant, producing diagnoses significantly faster and more accurately than dermatologists through traditional methods of visual examination. AI can help save lives by facilitating early intervention and treatment of skin cancer; it may prove especially effective in areas that may lack access to specialist care.

A wide variety of skin lesion images, labelled by expert dermatologists, are collected and preprocessed to train deep learning models (mostly convolutional neural networks (CNNs)) that can automatically extract visual features often related to the difference between benign and malignant lesions. To identify predictive features of melanoma like asymmetries, border irregularities, colour, and diameter, such models are then fit to assist in the classification of darts they have not previously observed. After training, these models can act as decision support systems for dermatologists or even have the ability to be used as screening devices in rural and remote areas, maintaining a diagnostic performance close to or superior to humans but faster and more consistent. However, the arbitrary nature of training data can lead to disastrous performance of these AI systems; for instance, if certain skin types or lesional types are rare (or even missing) from the dataset, then they are unlikely to be classified well in practice. These and some other such challenges, such as dataset bias and poor interpretability, have motivated continuous research to improve the robustness and generalizability of AI-based skin cancer detection systems [40 - 42].

Classification of Skin Lesions

Skin lesion classification *via* artificial intelligence and its interpretation (Benign nevi, melanoma, basal cell carcinoma, and squamous cell carcinoma). Such classification is critical for differential diagnosis and providing appropriate treatment. Artificial intelligence algorithms have been adapted to dermatology and improve the accuracy of diagnosis by analysing dermoscopic and histopathologic images to identify dozens of features of various skin lesions. Several studies have shown that trained artificial intelligence models can match or even outperform dermatologists in diagnosing skin cancer when trained on datasets of varying types. These types of models are only as good as their training datasets. Many existing datasets have been flagged for possible gaps in the representation of skin types and lesions as they pertain to persons with skin of colour, possibly leading to inequalities in diagnosis. Current research challenges these limitations through the development of more representative corpora and greater interpretability of AI systems. This will ultimately lead to improving the applicability of AI systems in the clinical context and eliminating, to some extent, the disparities in skin cancer detection and treatment [43, 44].

Histopathological Image Analysis

Advanced image analysis and machine learning techniques initially developed for engineering applications are now being adapted for quantitative diagnosis, prognosis, and digital pathology to meet the demands of increasingly complex diseases, especially cancer, which arise from vast amounts of histopathology data employing whole-slide digital scanners. It includes preprocessing images to standardise colour and extract regions of interest, feature extraction using either traditional descriptors or deep learning approaches, and classification with machine learning algorithms or Convolutional Neural Networks (CNNs), classifying images into benign or malignant states. However, Histopathological images are more challenging to analyse, as the diverse appearances, inconsistent staining, and overlapping nuclei make histopathology a complex task. The main obstacles to the widespread implementation of histopathological image analysis have been authority and high throughput. Still, it has been used for Computer-Assisted Diagnosis (CAD) systems, which can help in creating diagnostic tools that enable pathologists to tackle one side of the problems in disease detection and prognosis prediction and for slide-based analysis approaches such as HipoMap, which transformed the whole-slide images into organised representation and classification and survival analyses. Efforts are underway to enhance the robustness and generalizability of these techniques, with a focus on improving diagnostic performance, ultimately assisting pathologists in their decision-making [45, 46].

Prediction of Disease Progression

Melanoma progression or recurrence risk could be estimated based on a quantitative integration of clinical, dermoscopic, and histopathological features. AI models could provide personalised risk stratification and management. These models utilise extensive databases to detect patterns and correlations where data might overlap or yield insight out of information on a patient demographic, lesion characteristic, or prior treatment history, provided that they pass clinical accreditation and verification. The combination of multiple types of data results in a complete representation of each patient and allows ML algorithms to examine critical characteristics (*e.g*., tumour thickness, ulceration status, mitotic rate, and unique dermoscopic features) associated with the risk of disease progression. This ability to predict enables healthcare providers to customise surveillance and treatment plans, providing more intensive monitoring and intervention for those patients at the highest risk. Additionally, AI algorithms can be updated as new data is obtained, allowing them to be fine-tuned to be more accurate in predicting prognosis as our understanding of melanoma progression evolves. In summary, AI paradigms for predicting melanoma progression might facilitate clinical decision-making, enable personalised treatment pathways for patients and better management of melanoma and other skin cancers, and ultimately enhance the clinical outcomes and survival of patients [47 - 49].

Feature Extraction and Segmentation

Deep learning is a form of AI that has changed how skin lesion images are analysed, allowing for the automatic extraction of relevant features (*e.g.*, colour, texture, and morphology) needed to diagnose skin lesions accurately, such as melanoma and other skin cancers. Using convolutional neural networks (CNNs), AI can be trained to recognise complex features in the images that correlate with malignancy, potentially minimising the need for manual dermatological assessment. Apart from feature extraction, these AI algorithms can accurately segment cnSk from the surrounding normal skin with exact delineation of the edges of a lesion, thus allowing for the exact measurement of the size and shape of a lesion. The described segmentation process provides quantitative metrics that contribute to the clinical evaluation of lesion characteristics, which is crucial for diagnosis and treatment planning. Automatic feature extraction and segmentation capability improves diagnostic accuracy and efficiency, allowing dermatologists to make clinical decisions based on comprehensive data analytics. Thus, AI-based feature extraction and segmentation are promising advances in dermatology and a step toward patient improvement by enabling early diagnosis and individualised treatment approaches [50 - 52].

DATA COLLECTION AND PREPARATION

Data collection and preparation are critical steps in any machine learning project, particularly in fields like computer vision [53]. The process begins with the following steps shown in Fig. (**3**).

Dataset Acquisition

Collecting datasets is a crucial step in dermatopathology applications since the quality and diversity of a dataset directly affect the performance of the machine learning models. The pertinent images are frequently collected from diverse sources, *e.g.*, publicly available medical image databases like the International Skin Imaging Collaboration Archive (ISIC) Archive and DermNet, among other dermatopathology archives. In addition, web-scraping techniques can be used to scrape photos from additional sources available on the web, such as clinical websites, medical journals, and other web sources. Merging data from multiple sources helps researchers create a more varied and inclusive sample. This is crucial for making strong models that generalise well over multiple demographics and skin types. By addressing all relevant information, this wholesome methodology for the procurement of datasets strips out possible biases and enhances the model's ability to accurately identify and classify many skin diseases [54 - 56].

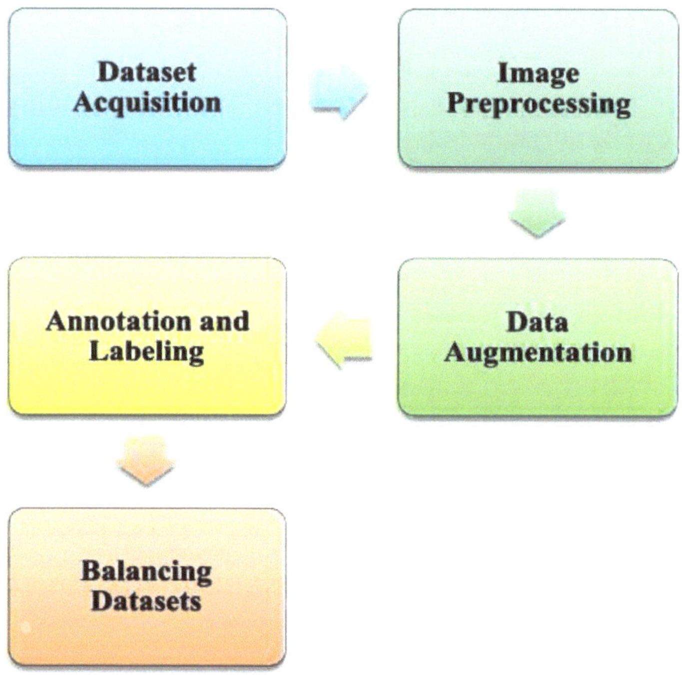

Fig. (3). Steps of data collection and preparation in machine learning project.

Image Preprocessing

Image preprocessing plays a critical role in the dermatopathology pipeline. Image quality and consistency are major factors in machine learning performance, so proper image quality and consistent image handling are a part of high-quality ground truth creation. Preprocessing indicates a wide range of processes that are necessary to handle the images for analysis. Resizing of images is often needed to make image size uniform and consistent in the dataset. This is especially important when feeding images into neural networks, which typically require a known static input size. A third critical process is referred to as normalisation. It embraces the concept of modifying the pixel values into a desired scale, most commonly between 0 and 1, to ensure the images possess comparable brightness and contrast. This helps remove changes due to different imaging conditions, like varying illumination or camera settings. Noise reduction methods, such as Gaussian filtering or median filtering, are used to restrict the effects of unwanted artefacts or distortions that can hide important information in the images. More specifically, the image preprocessing techniques provide a better visual appearance of the images and enhanced reliability of the extraction and analysis of features, leading to better and generalisable diagnostic findings, resulting in making the corresponding field of dermatopathology using image analysis tools more accurate and robust. Processing is one of the fundamental parts of the overall performance of machine learning applications in this domain. It helps in the higher success of these applications due to the high-quality input data being consistent [57 - 59].

Data Augmentation

Data augmentation is one of the crucial strategies of dermatopathology, which is an artificial increase in the dataset that increases the generic behaviour of the model in different scenarios. However, instead of taking new pictures (which is near impossible), some augmentation techniques can be applied that can create additional training examples from current data, thus increasing the data size and diversity. This is essential since there is often limited access to labelled medical images. Transformations, for example, rotation, flipping, and scaling, are commonly used to produce variability of orientation and size of skin lesions. This way, the model learns to identify lesions from different views and at multiple scales. Colour modifications include occasional alterations of brightness, contrast, and saturation. Such modifications simulate diverse lighting conditions and skin colours, causing the model to be less sensitive to variations in the imaging environment and patient population [60, 61].

The advanced augmentation techniques include Elastic deformations and Random cropping, to name some. Instead, these methods introduce some sort of minor deformations in the shape and translation of the object in the image so that the model is even unable to detect lesions when they are probably somehow deformed robustly. Not only does it decrease the chance of overfitting, but it also increases the ability of the model to handle population diversity in dermatopathological images. Instead, that is achieved by allowing the model to see more diverse augmented images for many epochs of training. This yields more robust and predictive models in clinical settings where numerous uncertain scenarios are the norm. Specifically, data augmentations are needed for the dermatologist to have the capability to enhance the robustness and generalisation capacity of the dermatopathology machine learning models, pointing to the process of process in general [62, 63].

Annotation and Labeling

Annotation and labelling are the key activities in building machine-learning models for Dermatopathology. The reason is that they provide the model with the necessary context of the images, which allows for the model to learn and, hence, predict it correctly. During the annotation process, specialists, including dermatologists and pathologists, will be present. Such experts identify and annotate key features in untouchable images like histological structures, lesion margins, and various classes of skin pathology. This process often involves locating objects and naming them in the image. For instance, it can be either spotting different classes of skin lesions or highlighting regions of interest where abnormalities are detected [64 - 66]. Another component of annotation is called "classifying scenes," where considering the entire context of the image is used to classify it based on its significance in patient care. This may involve differentiating between benign and malignant cases or identifying different stages in a disease process. Second, the marking of essential characteristics is critical in histopathological image analysis because some of them need to be carefully defined to guide the learning process of the model, such as cellular patterns, tissue structures, or other diagnostic markers [67].

Because correct labelling influences the correct situation, the model is able to learn correctly from the data that needs correct labelling. Incorrect or inconsistent labels can result in a learner who associates misleading features with certain targets and, thus, faulty predictions. And this could result in a non-performant model. A combination of domain knowledge and hard quality control mechanisms is often used to ensure high-quality annotation. Under some conditions, many experts may review the same images to achieve a consensus regarding the labels, which will increase the reliability of the dataset even more [68].

Recent applications such as semi-automated labelling can be applied to support experts in the annotation process. This may allow the process to be faster while still being correct. However, the dataset can turn into a great tool to feed machine learning models if the images are properly labelled and annotated. It results in more accurate and efficient dermatopathology results, ultimately in better diagnostic and patient care [69, 70].

Balancing Datasets

Balancing the distribution of classes within a dataset is a vital step toward building robust machine-learning models in dermatopathology to avoid bias toward overrepresented categories that results in poor generalisation and inaccurate predictions. Such instances are common, particularly around conditions that are clinically important but underrepresented. Methods like "oversampling" the minority class, where we create new examples by either sampling with replacement or using methods like SMOTE (Synthetic Minority Over-sampling Technique), ensure that the model is sufficiently trained on rarer events. Conversely, when there are too many cases from overrepresented categories, then we need to reduce the size of the majority class by under-sampling, as too many cases may burden the model with excessively similar data. However, this must be accounted for carefully so as not to lose important information. Sometimes, a hybrid method is used, where both oversampling and undersampling are combined. Moreover, class weighting is applied while training, that is, assigning more weight in computing loss to minority classes. Together, these methods ensure an unbiased data set, which allows the model to learn from all classes evenly. This means better generalisation and more reliable predictions across various dermatopathological diseases. This holistic approach is a crucial component of the data preparation process. It provides a robust foundation for the accurate and efficient development of machine learning models, thereby enhancing diagnostic accuracy and overall clinical care quality for patients [71, 72].

MODEL TRAINING AND OPTIMIZATION

Model training and optimisation are vital aspects of building efficient and effective AI systems. Some methods, as shown in Table **1**, encompass cross-validation, hyperparameter tuning, and regularisation strategies used in this process to produce high performance and generalisation.

Table 1. Representation of model training and optimization in the context of dermatopathology analysis using machine learning.

Stage	Description	Techniques/Methods	Key Metrics/ Considerations	References
Data Collection	Gathering annotated histopathological images and clinical data.	Manual annotation, automated data extraction, public datasets.	Data quality, diversity, and volume	[73]
Data Preprocessing	Preparing data for model training, including normalisation, augmentation, and splitting into subsets.	Image normalisation, data augmentation, train-test-validation split	Image resolution, class balance, data augmentation techniques.	[74]
Feature Extraction	Identifying and extracting relevant features from images for use in the model.	Convolutional filters, edge detection, colour histogram analysis.	Feature relevance, computational efficiency.	[75, 76]
Model Selection	Choosing appropriate ML algorithms for classification, regression, or clustering tasks.	CNNs, SVMs, Random Forests, k-nearest Neighbors (k-NN), Decision Trees.	Algorithm suitability, model complexity, interpretability.	[77, 78]

(Table 1) cont.....

Stage	Description	Techniques/Methods	Key Metrics/ Considerations	References
Model Training	Training the chosen model on the preprocessed dataset.	Gradient Descent, Backpropagation, Cross-Validation	Training accuracy, loss minimisation, and computational resources.	[79, 80]
Hyperparameter Tuning	Optimising model parameters to improve performance.	Grid Search, Random Search, Bayesian Optimization, Hyperband	Hyperparameter ranges, computational cost, and overfitting risk.	[81, 82]
Model Evaluation	Assessing the model's performance on the validation/test set using various metrics.	Confusion Matrix, ROC-AUC, F1-Score, Precision, Recall	Generalisation error, overfitting/underfitting, and metric selection	[83]
Model Optimization	Refining the model to improve performance or reduce computational load.	Pruning, Model Compression, Transfer Learning, Ensemble Methods	Model size, inference time, accuracy *vs.* efficiency trade-off.	[84, 85]
Model Validation	Final testing on an independent dataset to confirm generalizability.	Holdout validation, Cross-validation on unseen data.	Generalisation, robustness, model stability	[86]
Deployment	Implementing the model in a clinical setting for real-time decision-making.	API integration, cloud deployment, and edge computing.	Real-time performance, scalability, security, compliance	[87]
Continuous Monitoring	Tracking model performance post-deployment to identify degradation and retrain if necessary.	Performance monitoring, periodic retraining, and anomaly detection.	Model drift, accuracy decay, and model update frequency	[88]

Training Techniques

Cross-Validation

Cross-validation is a statistical method used to estimate the skill of machine learning models. This process consists of splitting the training dataset into several subsets, training the model on some of those subsets, and validating the others. This helps in estimating the expected value of the test results when performing the test on an independent dataset. K-fold cross-validation is also the most common form of cross-validation where the dataset is split into k subsets. It trains the model k several times, where each time, one of the k folds acts as the validation set, and the remaining k − 1 folds serve as the training set. The technique identifies overfitting and shows more realistic capabilities of the model on unseen data [89, 90].

Hyperparameter Tuning

Hyperparameter tuning is the act of searching for hyperparameter values that govern your machine learning model training process. Each learning algorithm has several hyper-parameters that need to be set before the learning process begins, and model performance can be affected to a large degree by these parameters in comparison to the model parameters that are learned during training [91].

Techniques for Hyperparameter Tuning

Grid Search: In this method, you need to provide a list of values for the different hyperparameters, and the model gets evaluated for each combination of these values. It is exhaustive but may be computationally expensive [92].

Random Search: Random search tests random combinations of hyperparameters instead of testing all combinations. It can be faster than a grid search, especially in cases where only some hyperparameters are of major significance to the performance [93].

Bayesian Optimization: A probabilistic model-based method, it constructs a model of the function that encodes hyperparameters mapping to a score (like accuracy). It uses this model to choose the next set of hyperparameters to test. It can use evaluations more efficiently than a grid or random search [94].

Automated Hyperparameter Tuning: Tools and frameworks (*e.g.*, Cloud ML Hyperparameter Tuning) will be able to automate the tuning process and reduce the time complexity of searching the hyperparameter space [95].

Evaluation Metrics

Machine Learning Models are an extremely important step in the process, for which we can get all the information regarding the efficacy of a model for the future. Different evaluation metrics are used for different types of problems (*e.g.*, classification, regression) depending on the purpose of the analysis. In this post, we will cover the following most popularly used classification metrics → Accuracy Precision Recall F1-score ROC-AUC [96].

Accuracy

Accuracy is the ratio of correctly predicted instances to the total instances in the dataset [97].

Formula

$$Accuracy = \frac{True\ Positives + True\ Negatives}{Total\ Instances}$$

Accuracy is a straightforward metric and is particularly useful when the classes are balanced. However, it can be misleading in cases of imbalanced datasets, where one class significantly outnumbers the other.

Precision

Precision measures the accuracy of the positive predictions made by the model [98].

Formula

$$Precision = \frac{True\ Positives}{True\ Positives + False\ Positives}$$

High precision is critical in scenarios where the cost of false positives is high (*e.g.*, spam detection).

Recall (Sensitivity)

Recall measures the ability of the model to identify all relevant instances [99].

Formula

$$Recall = \frac{True\ Positives}{True\ Positives + False\ Negatives}$$

High recall is essential in situations where missing a positive instance is costly (*e.g.*, disease detection).

F1-Score

The F1-score is the harmonic mean of precision and recall, providing a balance between the two metrics. It is particularly useful when you need a single metric to assess model performance [100].

Formula

$$F1\,Score = 2 \times \frac{Precision \times Recall}{Precision + Recall}$$

The F1 score is beneficial in situations where you want to balance precision and recall, especially in imbalanced datasets.

ROC-AUC

The ROC curve is a plot of the model metric score by threshold used to classify an input as a positive or a negative example.

- Area Under Curve (AUC): It measures the entire region across the row and the column that is sensitive to changes between the positive class and negative class of the model.
- The True Positive Rate (Recall) is plotted *versus* the False Positive Rate on the ROC curve.
- AUC varies from 0 to 1, where 1 is perfect discrimination, and 0.5 is no discrimination (similar to random guessing).

ROC-AUC is a metric that is best used for binary classifiers and is immune to class imbalance. Details how sensitivity and specificity trade-off at different thresholds [101, 102].

Optimisation Techniques

In the domain of machine learning, optimisation techniques are unavoidable in increasing models and ensuring generalisation. Regularisation and Gradient descent methods are two important techniques in this field [103].

Regularisation

Overfitting is prevented by regularisation, a technique to stop the model from learning noise in the training data. Regularisation prevents overfitting to unseen data by adding a penalty term to the loss function to constrain model complexity [104].

Types of Regularization

L1 Regularization (Lasso): It adds a penalty equal to the absolute value of the coefficients. It reduces several coefficients to zero, acts as feature selection, and does sparsity in the model [105].

L2 Regularization (Ridge): L2 regularisation adds a penalty that is equivalent to the square of the coefficients. This technique will compress all of the coefficients but eliminate none, thereby stabilising the model and mitigating the effects of multicollinearity among the features [106].

Elastic Net: This type is a linear combination of both L1 and L2 regularisation; it can introduce a balance between feature selection and coefficient shrinkage. This is especially beneficial when features are correlated.

Dropout: Widely used in neural networks, dropout randomly shuts down a portion of neurons during training to encourage learning of more resilient features and to prevent overfitting.

Early Stopping: This method tracks the operation of the version on a validation set and halts training if performance starts to worsen, thereby avoiding overfitting [107].

Gradient Descent

Gradient Descent is an optimisation algorithm for finding the minimum of a function. This operates by continuously making adjustments in the parameters of the model towards the group with the steepest descent of loss function defined by the gradient.

Key Concepts of Gradient Descent

Learning Rate: This hyperparameter determines how big a step we take while moving toward the minimum of the loss function. Picking a small learning rate can take many iterations to get to the minimum, and a high learning rate can skip the minimum.

Batch Gradient Descent: In this method, we calculate the gradient of the loss function using the complete dataset. Although it ensures convergence, its downside is a higher computational cost for large datasets.

Stochastic Gradient Descent (SGD): Instead of calculating cost based on the entire dataset, SGD updates the model parameters using one training example at a time. This adds noise to the optimisation that helps get out of local minima but may also create more oscillations.

Mini-batch Gradient Descent: In this approach, the gradient is calculated using a small, randomly selected subset of the training data, which provides a middle ground between batch and stochastic gradient descent. This approach is a hybrid, and it takes the benefits of both approaches by achieving faster convergence and making the updates more stable [108, 109].

CHALLENGES AND LIMITATIONS

The first step for any physician is a clinical evaluation, which considers both the history of the patient and an examination of the patient. The clinician's abilities are frequently scaled down in fake scenarios of challenges and experiments, as CNN has dealings tested for dexterity. Many studies have mostly noted that their analyses did not take into account clinically relevant features, such as age, sex, severity of sun exposure, anatomical site, *etc*., as well as personal and family history, among other potential confounders. In a clinical setting, dermatologists would weigh the total body examination against other variants. Such variations are the macroscopic Ugly Duckling sign, defined as a nevus that appears different from the rest in a given individual, and the Little Red Riding Hood sign, defined as a nevus that appears clinically benign but is different from the rest in a given individual, and dermatoscopic predominant nevus patterns, defined as the pattern observed in greater than thirty percent of all. These methods, while improving sensitivity and specificity, require a more extensive approach. Moreover, *in vivo*, dermoscopy has always been shown to outperform artificial environments that entirely depend on images. An experimental approach was used to obtain this information [110, 111].

Before AI can even be employed for therapeutic practice, there is one more hurdle to cross. The following study recently attempted to shed some light on citizen trust and expectations in the use of artificial intelligence in a range of different countries. In the new study, the scientists discovered that most people are specifically concerned over the suitability of existing regulations and legislation surrounding the safe usage of AI, which was the main factor driving their trust. In addition to this, 63 percent of people said that they were either unwilling to use AI or had no interest in using AI in healthcare. Machine learning is made of that it renders no explanation or general approach that can justify why the algorithm made a specific diagnosis. This strategy may lead to mistrust among patients, notably since the model gives a diagnostic output but cannot rationalise the outcomes. Physician interpretation is needed to explain why a particular diagnosis or treatment should be chosen. Coming back to the previous statement, TBSE is still not available for patients. Research suggests that TBSE is rarely performed as part of a normal practice examination by PCPs or dermatologists in the absence of a request from the patient. While the importance of TBSE has been highlighted in several studies, there are currently no consensus recommendations from experts regarding skin cancer screening to confirm that this diagnostic approach is being used to its fullest potential [112].

In addition, the limited capacity to create TBSE in the real world might be due to a lack of learning time as well as bad teaching in medical learners and residents. The implementation of this technology would be a helpful adjunct to primary care providers and other non-dermatological experts because it will provide patients with a skin cancer screening that they would not have received. It is not going to take up so much time for the physicians in the process of screening. There is no algorithm or clinician so advanced that they will be able to diagnose a melanoma for which no photographs of the skin have ever been taken or a biopsy examined, which is why we should not be losing sight of this particular prize [113].

The term "overdiagnosis" arises often because many diseases with nebulous biology are treated as cancers. As for this spectrum, we do not know whether or not much more technology usage will take this outcome much, much further from what we want. This leads us to two main problems with the issue. The former is the identification of such an early stage of melanocytic tumours whose malignant potential is currently unspecified.

Over-detection of Non-Melanoma Stem Cells in Elderly Holidaymakers

The second of the two concerns is the over-detection of non-melanoma stem cells among elderly holidaymakers. This causes a strong psychological burden in patients with early multiple myeloma, 16, and non-melanoma skin cancer carries an unusual number of repetitive excisions in patients with short life expectancy, which ensures discussion of the clear benefit of such excisions [114].

FUTURE DIRECTIONS AND INNOVATIONS

The future directions and innovations in the application of ML in dermatopathology are promising. Federated learning is a novel approach to ML where models are trained on decentralised datasets, and there is no need to share raw data. This has been proven to be a predicted method for determining the clinical outcomes in COVID-19 patients. Using the same type of federated learnings framework to the dermatopathology datasets might result in better predictive models but minimise patient privacy leakage [115].

The classification of cutaneous lymphoma and eczema on histopathological slides using deep learning approaches has used semantic segmentation, which entails dividing an image into contiguous semantically meaningful regions. Additional development in this area might provide the potential for more accurate identification of disease distribution and more accurate diagnosis. The problem with many existing ML developments is that they are black box-type models, which means that the reason why something happens cannot be easily understood. More importantly, the implementation of data-driven, explainable AI systems that clarify the reasoning behind the decision-making process might promote dermatopathologists' knowledge of and trust in outputs associated with these algorithms. Leveraging AI on large-scale dermatopathology datasets could identify new disease patterns and risk factors that could be utilised to enable population-level research and public health interventions. In addition, AI-based diagnostic systems may assist in triaging cases for dermatopathologists to prioritise in their workflow [116].

The integration of AI into dermatopathology will bring unique challenges to medical education and training. Leveraging personalised feedback and learning guidance using AI technology, intelligent tutoring systems may maximise training for dermatopathology residents and fellows. Finally, although machine learning is already in use in dermatopathology, many opportunities lie ahead. With continued innovation in areas such as federated learning, explainable AI, and AI-powered diagnostic systems, researchers have the potential to maximise the capability of these technologies to benefit patient care and the field of dermatopathology [117].

CONCLUSION

Machine learning (ML) has the potential to transform dermatopathology through improved diagnostic accuracy, workflow efficiencies, and the ability to integrate with personalised medicine. These technologies combined have already shown great promise in multiple applications (disease classification from histopathology images, automated specimen triaging, and patient outcome prediction). Deep learning models, for example, have proven highly effective at detecting skin cancers like melanoma and basal cell carcinoma, frequently matching or exceeding the diagnosis performance of expert dermatopathologists. While these developments appear promising, multiple barriers still exist to the implementation of machine learning in dermatopathology. Challenges such as algorithmic bias, where models may perform differently in different patient populations, raise important ethical challenges. Moreover, most machine learning models were treated as a black box, which made it hard for clinicians to interpret predictions and trust the underlying decision-making process. Thus, creating explainable AI systems that offer interpretability of model predictions is a key requirement to build trust and ensure smooth clinical integration. Federated learning, leveraging the training of models in a decentralised way while preserving patient privacy, has exciting potential for the future in enhancing the robustness of dermatopathological analyses. Moreover, embedding AI in medical education and training can enable the next generation of dermatologists through intelligent tutoring systems that can personalise learning experiences and enhance diagnostic skills. The field of dermatopathology will continue to evolve but will continue to benefit from close collaboration between technologists, data scientists, and dermatopathies. It will help make certain that machine-learning tools are not only technically useful but also ethically appropriate and clinically applicable because interdisciplinary work drives stakeholder input to inform collaborative research questions, study design, and methodology. In conclusion, the effective incorporation of machine learning techniques into dermatopathology may lead to improved patient care, increased diagnostic accuracy, and a better understanding of skin diseases, heralding a new era of dermatological practice.

REFERENCES

[1] Shah A, Wahood S, Guermazi D, Brem CE, Saliba E. Skin and syntax: Large language models in dermatopathology. Dermatopathology (Basel) 2024; 11(1): 101-11. [http://dx.doi.org/10.3390/dermatopathology11010009] [PMID: 38390851]

[2] Laskar S. Training avenues in dermatopathology for an Indian dermatologist or pathologist. Indian Journal of Dermatology, Venereology and Leprology 2018; 84: 506-9. [http://dx.doi.org/10.4103/ijdvl.IJDVL_546_17]

[3] Gurcan MN, Boucheron LE, Can A, Madabhushi A, Rajpoot NM, Yener B. Histopathological image analysis: a review. IEEE Rev Biomed Eng 2009; 2: 147-71. [http://dx.doi.org/10.1109/RBME.2009.2034865] [PMID: 20671804]

[4] Ji J, Wan T, Chen D, Wang H, Zheng M, Qin Z. A deep learning method for automatic evaluation of diagnostic information from multi-stained histopathological images 2022. Available from: https://doi.org/./j.knosys

[5] Zhang J, Zhong F, He K, Ji M, Li S, Li C. Recent advancements and perspectives in the diagnosis of skin diseases using machine learning and deep learning: A review. Diagnostics. Multidisciplinary Digital Publishing Institute (MDPI) 2023; 13. [http://dx.doi.org/10.3390/diagnostics13233506]

[6] Madke B, Doshi B, Khopkar U, Dongre A. Appearances in dermatopathology: The diagnostic and the deceptive. Indian Journal of Dermatology. Venereology and Leprology 2013; pp. 338-48.

[7] Ferreira IG, Weber MB, Bonamigo RR. History of dermatology: The study of skin diseases over the centuries. A Bras Dermatol 2021; 96(3): 332-45.

[8] Sameera V, Bindra A, Rath G. Human errors and their prevention in healthcare. Journal of Anaesthesiology Clinical Pharmacology. Medknow Publications 2021; 37: pp. 328-35. [http://dx.doi.org/10.4103/joacp.JOACP_364_19]

[9] Biswas A, Dutta PK. Novel approach of automation to risk management: The reduction in human errors. EAI/Springer Innovations in Communication and Computing. Springer Science and Business Media Deutschland GmbH 2021; pp. 683-96.

[10] Munari E, Scarpa A, Cima L, Pozzi M, Pagni F, Vasuri F, *et al.* Cutting-edge technology and automation in the pathology laboratory. Virchows Archiv. Springer Science and Business Media Deutschland GmbH 2024; 484: pp. 555-66. [http://dx.doi.org/10.1007/s00428-023-03637-z]

[11] Goel M, Gupta V. Cutting-Edge Technological Developments in the Diagnosis and Treatment of Malignant Gastric Neoplasm. Innov Adv Biotechnol: Technol Adv Biosci. Cham: Springer Nature Switzerland 2025; pp. 211-42. [http://dx.doi.org/10.1007/978-3-031-80189-1_16]

[12] Kim K, Lee SG, Kim TH, Lee SG. Economic evaluation of total laboratory automation in the clinical laboratory of a tertiary care hospital. Ann Lab Med 2022; 42(1): 89-95. [http://dx.doi.org/10.3343/alm.2022.42.1.89] [PMID: 34374353]

[13] Sarker IH. Machine learning: Algorithms, real-world applications and research directions. SN Computer Science. Springer 2021; 2.

[14] Valizadeh A, Amir Hosseini MH, Ghorbani Y. Predictive precision in battery recycling: unveiling lithium battery recycling potential through machine learning. Comput & Chem Eng 2024; 183: 108623. Available from: https://doi.org/./j.compchemeng

[15] Shaer I, Shami A. Data-driven methods for the reduction of energy consumption in warehouses: Use-case driven analysis 2023.

[16] Senthilkumar M. 5-Use of artificial neural networks (ANNs) in colour measurement, 2024.

[17] Naeem S, Ali A, Anam S, Ahmed MM. An unsupervised machine learning algorithms: Comprehensive review. International Journal of Computing and Digital Systems 2023; 13(1): 911-21. [http://dx.doi.org/10.12785/ijcds/130172]

[18] Woodman RJ, Mangoni AA. A comprehensive review of machine learning algorithms and their application in geriatric medicine: present and future. Aging Clinical and Experimental Research. Springer Science and Business Media Deutschland GmbH 2023; 35: pp. 2363-97.

[19] Taye MM. Understanding of machine learning with deep learning: Architectures, workflow, applications and future directions. Computers. MDPI 2023; 12.

[20] Maulud D, Abdulazeez AM. A review on linear regression comprehensive in machine learning. Journal of Applied Science and Technology Trends 2020; 1(2): 140-7. [http://dx.doi.org/10.38094/jastt1457]

[21] Yeturu K. Chapter 3-Machine learning algorithms, applications, and practices in data science. 2020. Available from: https://www.sciencedirect.com/science/article/abs/pii/S0169716120300225 [http://dx.doi.org/10.1016/bs.host.2020.01.002]

[22] Ali S, Abuhmed T, El-Sappagh S, *et al.* Explainable Artificial Intelligence (XAI): What we know and what is left to attain Trustworthy Artificial Intelligence. Inf Fusion 2023; 99: 101805. [http://dx.doi.org/10.1016/j.inffus.2023.101805]

[23] Martin B. Instance-based learning: Nearest neighbour with generalisation 2014. Available from: https://www.researchgate.net/publication/33051309

[24] Mazilu S, Iria JL. L 1 vs. L 2 regularisation in text classification when learning from labelled features. Proceedings - 10th International Conference on Machine Learning and Applications, ICMLA 2011. 166-71.

[25] Song YY, Lu Y. Decision tree methods: applications for classification and prediction. Shanghai Jingshen Yixue 2015; 27(2): 130-5. [PMID: 26120265]

[26] Cohen S. Artificial Intelligence and Deep Learning in Pathology Chapter 2-The basics of machine learning: strategies and techniques Get rights and content 2021.

[27] Alahmar M. Naïve Bayes Algorithms 2023. Available from: https://www.researchgate.net/publication/369067312

[28] Teng TH, Dewi Varathan K, Crestani F. Expert Systems with Applications A comprehensive review of cyberbullying-related content classification in online social media 2024.

[29] Oyewole GJ, Thopil GA. Data clustering: application and trends. Artif Intell Rev 2023; 56(7): 6439-75. [http://dx.doi.org/10.1007/s10462-022-10325-y] [PMID: 36466764]

[30] Bakiah N, Warif A, Wahid A, *et al.* Copy-move forgery detection: Survey, challenges and future directions. J Netw Comput Appl 2016. Available from: https://doi.org/./j.jnca

[31] Dahdouh K. Advanced intelligent systems for sustainable development (AI2SD'2018). Advances in Intelligent Systems and Computing 2019; 915 Available from:

http://link.springer.com/10.1007/978-3-030-11928-7

[32] Li H, Sheu PCY. A scalable association rule learning heuristic for large datasets. J Big Data 2021; 8(1): 86.
[http://dx.doi.org/10.1186/s40537-021-00473-3]

[33] Yamashita R, Nishio M, Do RKG, Togashi K. Convolutional neural networks: An overview and application in radiology. Insights into Imaging. Springer Verlag 2018; 9: pp. 611-29.

[34] Kufel J, Bargieł-Łączek K, Kocot S, *et al.* What are machine learning, artificial neural networks, and deep learning? What are some examples of practical applications in medicine?. Diagnostics. Multidisciplinary Digital Publishing Institute (MDPI) 2023; 13.

[35] Shrestha A, Mahmood A. Review of deep learning algorithms and architectures. IEEE Access. Institute of Electrical and Electronics Engineers Inc. 2019; 7: pp. 53040-65.
[http://dx.doi.org/10.1109/ACCESS.2019.2912200]

[36] Alzubaidi L, Zhang J, Humaidi AJ, *et al.* Review of deep learning: concepts, CNN architectures, challenges, applications, future directions. J Big Data 2021; 8(1): 53.
[http://dx.doi.org/10.1186/s40537-021-00444-8] [PMID: 33816053]

[37] Pellegrino A, Stein H, Cayco-Gajic NA. Dimensionality reduction beyond neural subspaces with slice tensor component analysis. Nat Neurosci 2024; 27(6): 1199-210.
[http://dx.doi.org/10.1038/s41593-024-01626-2] [PMID: 38710876]

[38] Thudumu S, Branch P, Jin J, Singh J. A comprehensive survey of anomaly detection techniques for high dimensional big data. J Big Data 2020; 7(1): 42.
[http://dx.doi.org/10.1186/s40537-020-00320-x]

[39] Kotu V, Deshpande B. Chapter 2-data science process get rights and content. 2024. Available from: https://www.sciencedirect.com/science/article/abs/pii/B9780128147610000022

[40] Walocko FM, Tejasvi T. Teledermatology applications in skin cancer diagnosis. Dermatologic Clinics. W.B. Saunders 2017; 35: pp. 559-63.
[http://dx.doi.org/10.1016/j.det.2017.06.002]

[41] Wei ML, Tada M, So A, Torres R. Artificial intelligence and skin cancer. Frontiers Media, SA: Frontiers in Medicine 2024; 11.

[42] Toray MK. Ensemble learning: Methods, techniques, application 2024. Available from: https://www.researchgate.net/publication/381773312

[43] Wu Y, Chen B, Zeng A, Pan D, Wang R, Zhao S. Skin cancer classification with deep learning: A systematic review. Frontiers in Oncology. Frontiers Media S.A. 2022; 12.

[44] Semerci ZM, Toru HS, Çobankent Aytekin E, *et al.* The role of artificial intelligence in early diagnosis and molecular classification of head and neck skin cancers: A multidisciplinary approach. Diagnostics (Basel) 2024; 14(14): 1477.
[http://dx.doi.org/10.3390/diagnostics14141477] [PMID: 39061614]

[45] Aeffner F, Zarella MD, Buchbinder N, *et al.* Introduction to digital image analysis in whole-slide imaging: A white paper from the digital pathology association. J Pathol Inform 2019; 10(1): 9.
[http://dx.doi.org/10.4103/jpi.jpi_82_18] [PMID: 30984469]

[46] Komura D, Ishikawa S. Machine learning methods for histopathological image analysis. Computational and Structural Biotechnology Journal. Elsevier B.V. 2018; 16: pp. 34-42.

[47] Liu Q, Zhang J, Bai Y. Mapping the landscape of artificial intelligence in skin cancer research: a bibliometric analysis. Frontiers Media, SA: Frontiers in Oncology 2023; 13.

[48] Bhinder B, Gilvary C, Madhukar NS, Elemento O. Artificial intelligence in cancer research and precision medicine. Cancer Discovery. American Association for Cancer Research Inc. 2021; 11: pp. 900-15.

[49] Ahmed Z, Mohamed K, Zeeshan S, Dong XQ. Artificial intelligence with multi-functional machine learning platform development for better healthcare and precision medicine. Database. Oxford University Press 2020; 2020.
[http://dx.doi.org/10.1093/database/baaa010]

[50] Li Z, Koban KC, Schenck TL, Giunta RE, Li Q, Sun Y. Artificial intelligence in dermatology image analysis: Current developments and future trends. J Clin Med 2022; 11

[51] Akram A, Rashid J, Jaffar MA, Faheem M, Amin R. Segmentation and classification of skin lesions using hybrid deep learning method in the Internet of Medical Things. Skin Res Technol 2023; 29(11): 13524.
[http://dx.doi.org/10.1111/srt.13524] [PMID: 38009016]

[52] Yang G, Luo S, Greer P. Advancements in skin cancer classification: a review of machine learning techniques in clinical image analysis. Multimed Tools Appl. 2024.

[53] Roh Y, Heo G, Whang SE. A survey on data collection for machine learning: A big data -- AI integration perspective. 2018. Available from: http://arxiv.org/abs/1811.03402

[54] Ricci Lara MA, Rodríguez Kowalczuk MV, Lisa Eliceche M, *et al.* A dataset of skin lesion images collected in Argentina for the evaluation of AI tools in this population. Sci Data 2023; 10(1): 712.
[http://dx.doi.org/10.1038/s41597-023-02630-0] [PMID: 37853053]

[55] Ahammed M, Mamun MA, Uddin MS. A machine learning approach for skin disease detection and classification using image segmentation. Healthc Anal 2022; 2: 100122.
[http://dx.doi.org/10.1016/j.health.2022.100122]

[56] Chakraborty C, Bhattacharya M, Pal S, Lee SS. From machine learning to deep learning: Advances of the recent data-driven paradigm shift in medicine and healthcare. Current Research in Biotechnology. Elsevier B.V. 2024; 7.

[57] Xu W, Cai Y, Qian F, Hu Y, Yan J. Efficient image details preservation of image processing pipeline based on two-stage tone mapping. Mathematics 2024; 12(10): 1592.
[http://dx.doi.org/10.3390/math12101592]

[58] Dehbozorgi Pegah, *et al.* A_Systematic_Investigation_of_Image_Pre-processing 2022.

[59] Al-Thelaya K, Gilal NU, Alzubaidi M, Majeed F, Agus M, Schneider J, *et al.* Applications of discriminative and deep learning feature extraction methods for whole slide image analysis: A survey. J Pathol Inform 2023; 14
[http://dx.doi.org/10.1016/j.jpi.2023.100335]

[60] Moles L, Andres A, Echegaray G, Boto F. Exploring data augmentation and active learning benefits in imbalanced datasets. Mathematics 2024; 12(12): 1898.
[http://dx.doi.org/10.3390/math12121898]

[61] Alomar K, Aysel HI, Cai X. Data augmentation in classification and segmentation: A survey and new strategies. J Imaging 2023; 9(2): 46.
[http://dx.doi.org/10.3390/jimaging9020046] [PMID: 36826965]

[62] Oza P, Sharma P, Patel S, Adedoyin F, Bruno A. Image augmentation techniques for mammogram analysis. J Imaging 2022; 8(5): 141.
[http://dx.doi.org/10.3390/jimaging8050141] [PMID: 35621905]

[63] Shorten C, Khoshgoftaar TM. A survey on Image Data Augmentation for Deep Learning. J Big Data 2019; 6(1): 60.
[http://dx.doi.org/10.1186/s40537-019-0197-0]

[64] Willemink MJ, Koszek WA, Hardell C, Wu J, Fleischmann D, Harvey H, *et al.* Preparing medical imaging data for machine learning. Radiology. Radiological Society of North America Inc. 2020; 295: pp. 4-15.
[http://dx.doi.org/10.1148/radiol.2020192224]

[65] Primiero CA, Betz-Stablein B, Ascott N, *et al.* A protocol for annotation of total body photography for machine learning to analyze skin phenotype and lesion classification. Front Med (Lausanne) 2024; 11: 1380984.
[http://dx.doi.org/10.3389/fmed.2024.1380984] [PMID: 38654834]

[66] Galić I, Habijan M, Leventić H, Romić K. Machine learning empowering personalized medicine: A comprehensive review of medical image analysis methods. Electronics (Switzerland). Multidisciplinary Digital Publishing Institute (MDPI) 2023; 12.

[67] Pang S, Yu Z, Orgun MA. A novel end-to-end classifier using domain transferred deep convolutional neural networks for biomedical images. Comput Methods Programs Biomed 2017; 140: 283-93.
[http://dx.doi.org/10.1016/j.cmpb.2016.12.019] [PMID: 28254085]

[68] Gong Y, Liu G, Xue Y, Li R, Meng L. A survey on dataset quality in machine learning. Inf Softw Technol 2023; 162: 107268.
[http://dx.doi.org/10.1016/j.infsof.2023.107268]

[69] Jasil SG, Ulagamuthalvi V. A hybrid CNN architecture for skin lesion classification using deep learning. Soft Computing. 2023:1-0.

[70] Paulus JK, Kent DM. Predictably unequal: understanding and addressing concerns that algorithmic clinical prediction may increase health disparities. NPJ Digit Med 2020; 3(1): 99.
[http://dx.doi.org/10.1038/s41746-020-0304-9] [PMID: 32821854]

[71] Johnson JM, Khoshgoftaar TM. Survey on deep learning with class imbalance. J Big Data 2019; 6(1): 27.
[http://dx.doi.org/10.1186/s40537-019-0192-5]

[72] Siddique S, Haque MA, George R, Gupta KD, Gupta D, Faruk MJH. Survey on machine learning biases and mitigation techniques. Digital 2023; 4(1): 1-68.
[http://dx.doi.org/10.3390/digital4010001]

[73] Zhang H, He Y, Wu X, *et al.* PathNarratives: Data annotation for pathological human-AI collaborative diagnosis. Front Med (Lausanne) 2023; 9: 1070072.
[http://dx.doi.org/10.3389/fmed.2022.1070072] [PMID: 36777158]

[74] Kahloot KM, Ekler P. Algorithmic splitting: A method for dataset preparation. IEEE Access 2021; 9: 125229-37.
[http://dx.doi.org/10.1109/ACCESS.2021.3110745]

[75] Archana R, Jeevaraj PSE. Deep learning models for digital image processing: a review. Artif Intell Rev 2024; 57(1): 11.
[http://dx.doi.org/10.1007/s10462-023-10631-z]

[76] Kumar G, Bhatia PK. Detailed review of feature extraction in image processing systems. International Conference on Advanced Computing and Communication Technologies, ACCT. 5-12.
[http://dx.doi.org/10.1109/ACCT.2014.74]

[77] Zhang Y, Li Q, Xin Y. Research on eight machine learning algorithms applicability on different characteristics data sets in medical classification tasks. Front Comput Neurosci 2024; 18: 1345575.
[http://dx.doi.org/10.3389/fncom.2024.1345575] [PMID: 38356726]

[78] Alnuaimi AFAH, Albaldawi THK. An overview of machine learning classification techniques. BIO Web of Conferences. EDP Sciences 2024.
[http://dx.doi.org/10.1051/bioconf/20249700133]

[79] Sufian MA, Hamzi W, Hamzi B, *et al.* Innovative machine learning strategies for early detection and prevention of pregnancy loss: The vitamin D connection and gestational health. Diagnostics (Basel) 2024; 14(9): 920.
[http://dx.doi.org/10.3390/diagnostics14090920] [PMID: 38732334]

[80] Dalm S, Offergeld J, Ahmad N, van Gerven M. Efficient deep learning with decorrelated

backpropagation. 2024. Available from: http://arxiv.org/abs/2405.02385

[81] Ali Y, Awwad E, Al-Razgan M, Maarouf A. Hyperparameter search for machine learning algorithms for optimizing the computational complexity. Processes (Basel) 2023; 11(2): 349. [http://dx.doi.org/10.3390/pr11020349]

[82] Bischl B, Binder M, Lang M, Pielok T, Richter J, Coors S, *et al.* Hyperparameter optimisation: Foundations, algorithms, best practices, and open challenges. Wiley Interdisciplinary Reviews: Data Mining and Knowledge Discovery. John Wiley and Sons Inc 2023; 13.

[83] Montesinos López OA, Montesinos López A, Crossa J. Overfitting, model tuning, and evaluation of prediction performance. Multivariate statistical machine learning methods for genomic prediction. Springer International Publishing 2022; pp. 109-39. [http://dx.doi.org/10.1007/978-3-030-89010-0_4]

[84] Lyu Z, Yu T, Pan F, *et al.* A survey of model compression strategies for object detection. Multimedia Tools Appl 2023; 83(16): 48165-236. [http://dx.doi.org/10.1007/s11042-023-17192-x]

[85] Paranayapa T, Ranasinghe P, Ranmal D, Meedeniya D, Perera C. A comparative study of preprocessing and model compression techniques in deep learning for forest sound classification. Sensors (Basel) 2024; 24(4): 1149. [http://dx.doi.org/10.3390/s24041149] [PMID: 38400306]

[86] Berrar D. Cross-Validation 2019. Available from: https://www.sciencedirect.com/science/article/abs/pii/B978012809633820349X

[87] Girau R, Anedda M, Presta R, *et al.* Definition and implementation of the cloud infrastructure for the integration of the human digital twin in the social internet of things. Comput Netw 2024; 251: 110632. [http://dx.doi.org/10.1016/j.comnet.2024.110632]

[88] Chen H, Chen J, Ding J. Data evaluation and enhancement for quality improvement of machine learning. IEEE Transactions on Reliability. 2021;70(2):831-47.

[89] Berrar D. Cross-validation. Encyclopedia of bioinformatics and computational biology: ABC of bioinformatics. Elsevier 2018; pp. 542-5.

[90] Polaka S, Swetha L, Dittakavi S, Rajpoot K, Kumar Tekade R. Chapter 16-Bioanalytical method development and validation for establishing bioavailability and bioequivalence Get rights and content. Biopharmaceutics and Pharmacokinetics Considerations. 2021.

[91] Hossain R, Timmer D, Moya H. Home biosignal processing biosignals medicine physiology machine learning public full-text 1 machine learning model optimisation with hyper-parameter tuning approach 2021. Available from: https://www.researchgate.net/publication/354495368_Machine_learning_model_optimization_with_hyper-parameter_tuning_approach

[92] Dufour JM, Neves J. Chapter 1-Finite-sample inference and nonstandard asymptotics with Monte Carlo tests and R. 2019. Available from: https://doi.org/./bs.host [http://dx.doi.org/10.1016/bs.host.2019.05.001]

[93] Villalobos-Arias L, Quesada-López C, Guevara-Coto J, Martínez A, Jenkins M. Evaluating hyper-parameter tuning using random search in support vector machines for software effort estimation. PROMISE 2020 - Proceedings of the 16th ACM International Conference on Predictive Models and Data Analytics in Software Engineering, Co-located with ESEC/FSE 2020. 31-40. [http://dx.doi.org/10.1145/3416508.3417121]

[94] Wang L, Dernoncourt F, Bui T. Bayesian optimization for selecting efficient machine learning models. 2020. Available from: http://arxiv.org/abs/2008.00386

[95] Yang L, Shami A. On hyperparameter optimisation of machine learning algorithms: Theory and practice 2020. Available from: https://www.sciencedirect.com/science/article/abs/pii/S0925231220311693

[96] M H , M.N S . A review on evaluation metrics for data classification evaluations. Int J Data Min Knowl Manag Process 2015; 5(2): 01-11.

[97] Pizer SM, Marron JS. Statistical Shape and Deformation Analysis Chapter 6-Object Statistics on Curved Manifolds 2017.

[98] Hicks SA, Strümke I, Thambawita V, *et al.* On evaluation metrics for medical applications of artificial intelligence. Sci Rep 2022; 12(1): 5979. [http://dx.doi.org/10.1038/s41598-022-09954-8] [PMID: 35395867]

[99] Naveen . What is recall? Tips for optimizing precision and recall. Available from: https://www.nomidl.com/machine-learning/precision-recall-f1/

[100] Yacouby R, Axman D. Probabilistic extension of precision, recall, and F1 score for more thorough evaluation of classification models. Association for Computational Linguistics (ACL). 2020; pp. 79-91.

[101] Dias LO, Bom CR, Faria EL, *et al.* Automatic detection of fractures and breakout patterns in acoustic borehole image logs using fast-region convolutional neural networks. J Pet Sci Eng. Elsevier B.V. 2020; 191. [http://dx.doi.org/10.1016/j.petrol.2020.107099]

[102] Fawcett T. An introduction to ROC analysis. Pattern Recognit Lett 2006; 27(8): 861-74. [http://dx.doi.org/10.1016/j.patrec.2005.10.010]

[103] Karthick K. Comprehensive overview of optimization techniques in machine learning training. Control Systems and Optimization Letters 2024; 2(1): 23-7. [http://dx.doi.org/10.59247/csol.v2i1.69]

[104] Ganie AG, Dadvandipour S. From big data to smart data: a sample gradient descent approach for machine learning. J Big Data 2023; 10(1): 162. [http://dx.doi.org/10.1186/s40537-023-00839-9]

[105] Soumare H, Benkahla A, Gmati N. Deep learning regularization techniques to genomics data. Array (N Y) 2021; 11: 100068. [http://dx.doi.org/10.1016/j.array.2021.100068]

[106] Khanday NY, Sofi SA. Taxonomy, state-of-the-art, challenges and applications of visual understanding: A review. Comput Sci Rev 2021; 40: 100374. [http://dx.doi.org/10.1016/j.cosrev.2021.100374]

[107] Pavlou M, Ambler G, Seaman S, De Iorio M, Omar RZ. Review and evaluation of penalised regression methods for risk prediction in low-dimensional data with few events. Stat Med 2016; 35(7): 1159-77. [http://dx.doi.org/10.1002/sim.6782] [PMID: 26514699]

[108] Tapkir A. A comprehensive overview of gradient descent and its optimization algorithms. IARJSET 2023; 10(11). [http://dx.doi.org/10.17148/IARJSET.2023.101106]

[109] Witten IH, Frank E, Hall MA. Data mining: Practical machine learning tools and techniques (Third edition) The morgan kaufmann series in data management systems Chapter 6-implementations: Real machine learning schemes 2011.

[110] Huang Y, Tang K, Chen M, Wang B. A comprehensive survey on evaluating large language model applications in the medical industry. 2024. Available from: http://arxiv.org/abs/2404.15777

[111] Di Sarno L, Caroselli A, Tonin G, Graglia B, Pansini V, Causio FA, *et al.* Artificial intelligence in pediatric emergency medicine: Applications, challenges, and future perspectives. Biomedicines. Multidisciplinary Digital Publishing Institute (MDPI) 2024; 12.

[112] Donald A. Redelmeier *et al.* 20010320s00033p809 2001.

[113] Di Martino F, Delmastro F. Explainable AI for clinical and remote health applications: a survey on tabular and time series data. Artif Intell Rev 2023; 56(6): 5261-315. [http://dx.doi.org/10.1007/s10462-022-10304-3] [PMID: 36320613]

[114] Faustinella F, Jacobs RJ. The decline of clinical skills: a challenge for medical schools. Int J Med Educ 2018; 9: 195-7. [http://dx.doi.org/10.5116/ijme.5b3f.9fb3] [PMID: 30007951]

[115] Rieke N, Hancox J, Li W, *et al.* The future of digital health with federated learning. NPJ Digit Med 2020; 3(1): 119. [http://dx.doi.org/10.1038/s41746-020-00323-1] [PMID: 33015372]

[116] Moshawrab M, Adda M, Bouzouane A, Ibrahim H, Raad A. Reviewing federated machine learning and its use in diseases prediction. Sensors. MDPI 2023; 23.

[117] Applied Sciences. Brecko A, Kajati E, Koziorek J, Zolotova I. Federated learning for edge computing: A survey. Switzerland: MDPI 2022; 12.

CHAPTER 8

Enhancing Skin Cancer Detection with Transfer Learning and Deep Learning

Shaweta Sharma[1], **Akanksha Sharma**[2], **Ashish Verma**[3], **Neeraj Kumar Fuloria**[4] and **Akhil Sharma**[2,*]

[1] *School of Medical and Allied Sciences, Galgotias University, Uttar Pradesh-201310, India*

[2] *R. J. College of Pharmacy, Raipur, Uttar Pradesh - 202165, India*

[3] *Mangalmay Pharmacy College, Greater Noida, Uttar Pradesh-201306, India*

[4] *Department of Pharmaceutical Chemistry, Faculty of Pharmacy, AIMST University, Semeling Campus, Bedong - 08100, Malaysia*

Abstract: Skin cancers have become one of the most common malignancies globally and a healthcare burden that creates a diagnosis difficulty due to their wide nature. Early and accurate detection is crucial for patient outcomes, yet conventional methods largely depend on subjective clinical judgment. The recent progress of artificial intelligence (AI), especially deep learning (DL) and transfer learning (TL), gives potential tools for improving the ability to detect skin cancer. DL Algorithms such as CNN and TL for a better diagnosis by using pre-trained models are discussed in this chapter, tackling several prominent issues like small annotated datasets and heterogeneity in dermoscopic images. TL addresses common bottlenecks in medical image analysis, such as limited availability of annotated datasets and high required annotation cost, by permitting a model to be trained using smaller-size domain-specific datasets, therefore offering a much more profitable approach. We outline the standing of AI-assisted systems in clinical workflows, examine the performance of the DL model in dermatological skin cancer detection, and discuss the possibility of this technology in enhancing human dermatological competence. This chapter highlights future research directions such as hybrid models, multimodal data integration, and AI's ethical arrangement in healthcare. Our work focuses on utilizing DL and TL to improve the early detection of skin cancer, which will help to lay the groundwork for more personalized and effective treatment options.

Keywords: Convolutional Neural Networks (CNN), Dermatology AI, Deep Learning, Image Classification, Medical Imaging, Skin Cancer Detection, Transfer Learning.

* **Corresponding author Akhil Sharma:** R. J. College of Pharmacy, Raipur, Uttar Pradesh - 202165, India; E-mail: xs2akhil@gmail,.com

Akhil Sharma, Shaweta Sharma, Shivkanya Fuloria & Sudhir Kumar (Eds.)

INTRODUCTION

Skin cancer is one of the most prevalent cancers of this decade. Skin is the body's most important organ; however, in human pathology, skin cancer is the most common type of cancer. Skin cancer is most commonly classified into two types: melanoma and nonmelanoma [1]. Melanoma is a rare and deadly type of skin cancer. According to the American Cancer Society, melanoma skin cancer only represents 1% of all occurrences, but it has a higher percentage of fatalities. Melanoma originates in the cells known as melanocytes, and it all starts with typical melanocytes that begin to grow profoundly and become a malignant tumor [2]. It can affect any human tissue. It often appears on sun-exposed areas like the hands, face, neck, lips, *etc*. However, if they are not detected early enough, these tumor entities metastasize to other parts of the body, leading to an agonizing death of the patient. Melanoma skin cancer can present in different types, such as lentigo maligna, acral lentiginous, nodular melanoma, and superficial spreading melanoma. Nonmelanoma types encompass most cancer cases, such as basal cell carcinoma (BCC), squamous cell carcinoma (SCC), and sebaceous gland carcinoma (SGC). BCC, SGC, and SCC arise from the middle and upper layers of the epidermis, respectively. They are less likely to spread to other parts of the body. Compared to melanoma cancers, nonmelanoma cancers are easier to treat [3, 4].

Importance of Early Skin Cancer Detection

There are many reasons why early skin cancer detection is important, with the first and foremost reason being treating patients, their treatment options, and the burden on the healthcare system. Melanoma, basal cell carcinoma (BCC), and squamous cell carcinoma (SCC) are the three most common forms of skin cancer worldwide, and skin cancer is among the most common cancer types. Skin cancer is very treatable, and the chances of a full recovery are greatly improved if it is caught early on [5, 6]. Some important early-detection vitals are shown in Fig. (**1**).

Improved Survival Rates

Skin cancers such as melanoma are also highly curable when detected early. On the other hand, localized melanoma has a 5-year survival rate of nearly 99%, and this drastically changes when metastases to regional lymph nodes or distal organs follow it. Since the treatment is early when detected early and there is no chance of metastasis, treatment becomes very easy [7, 8].

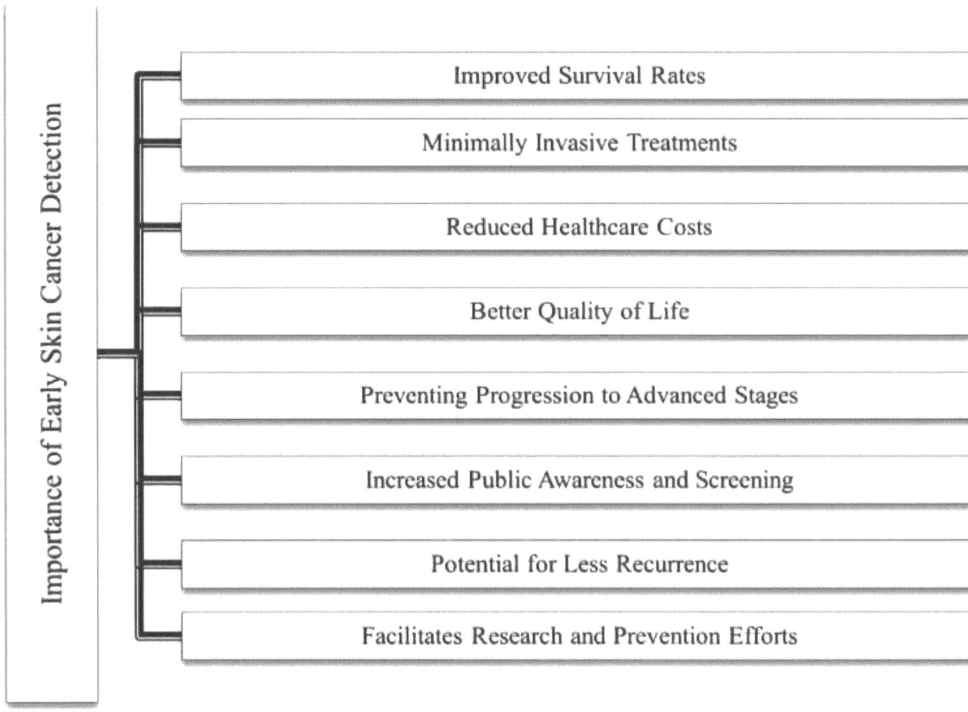

Fig. (1). Importance of early skin cancer detection.

Minimally Invasive Treatments

However, if the skin cancer is diagnosed early, treatment options may be as minor as agent excision or localized therapy. These approaches are frequently successful (compared to chemotherapy or radiation, which also come with serious side effects and a slower recovery time [9].

Reduced Healthcare Costs

Costs of healthcare can be minimized with early detection and treatment. Higher stages of cancer deadlines prescribe rather intricate and expensive treatments, extending internments and care and raising the stretch on sufferers and medical care hardware [10, 11].

Better Quality of Life

An early diagnosis reduces the physical and psychological load on the patients. Patients with early-stage skin cancer do far better than those with advanced disease, and many treatment options are less disfiguring and cause few complications, allowing patients to enjoy an acceptable quality of life following treatment [12, 13].

Preventing Progression to Advanced Stages

Skin cancer is prevented from progressing to more advanced and fatal stages. Advanced melanoma is a less effective immunotherapy treatment, as it is more difficult to cure and often requires systemic drugs that are more costly [14, 15].

Increased Public Awareness and Screening

Enhanced awareness about the benefits of detection in the early stages also leads to more skin self-examinations and screening by skin professionals. Increased awareness can help recognize and report suspicious lesions earlier to seek medical opinion, establishing timely diagnosis and notification [16, 17].

Potential for Less Recurrence

If skin cancer is diagnosed early, the chances of successful treatment and a lower risk of recurrence are increased. Patients who receive treatment promptly are less likely to experience the disease returning, resulting in better results at 5-10 years and beyond [18].

Facilitates Research and Prevention Efforts

Detection of skin cancers at early stages will also facilitate the study of their biology, potentially enabling preventive measures such as behavior modification and the development of new sunscreens and other protective approaches [19, 20].

Transfer Learning and Deep Learning: A Powerful Combination

Transfer learning is a deep learning technique that utilizes a pre-trained model from one task as the foundation for another related task. This approach allows models to leverage previously acquired knowledge, reducing the need for large datasets and extensive computational resources. Deep learning models, particularly those with multiple layers, require vast amounts of data and training time, which transfer learning helps mitigate by enabling models to learn efficiently from prior experience. By using a model already trained on a large dataset, such as ImageNet, for image classification, transfer learning facilitates faster training, improved accuracy, and better generalization, especially when labeled data for the new task is limited [21, 22].

The process of transfer learning involves selecting a pre-trained model and modifying its architecture to fit the new task's requirements, typically by adjusting the output layers. Some layers may be frozen to retain general features learned in earlier layers, while others may be fine-tuned using the new dataset. Depending on the relationship between the original and new tasks, transfer learning can be categorized into inductive transfer learning, where different but related tasks share knowledge; transductive transfer learning, where tasks remain the same, but data domains differ; and unsupervised transfer learning, where the target dataset lacks labeled examples [23, 24].

This technique has broad applications across multiple domains. In computer vision, it enhances image classification, object detection, and segmentation. In natural language processing (NLP), models like BERT and GPT benefit from pre-training on large text corpora for tasks such as sentiment analysis, machine translation, and text summarization. Similarly, in speech recognition, transfer learning helps improve speech-to-text conversion and speaker identification. In healthcare, it is widely used for medical image analysis and disease prediction, while in robotics, it aids in learning control policies and adapting to new environments [25, 26].

Popular deep learning frameworks such as TensorFlow, PyTorch, and Keras provide extensive tools and APIs for seamless implementation of transfer learning. Additionally, several pre-trained models are widely used, including ResNet, Inception, VGG, and EfficientNet for vision tasks and BERT, RoBERTa, and GPT for NLP. As deep learning continues to advance, transfer learning remains an essential technique, enabling faster, more efficient training and enhancing model performance across a diverse range of applications [27, 28].

Deep Learning in Medical Imaging

Deep learning, a subfield of artificial intelligence, has revolutionized medical imaging by allowing for automated analysis and interpretation of complex medical data. Deep learning models, particularly utilizing deep neural networks, especially convolutional neural networks (CNNs), have shown astonishing results in various image classification tasks, image segmentation, and image anomaly detection, enabling disease diagnosis, including cancer, cardiovascular diseases, and neurological diseases. These models can learn from large datasets with architectures such as CNNs, GANs, and, more recently, transformers to capture patterns and features that might be difficult for human experts to distinguish. Such applications include tumor detection in radiology and pathology, enhancing images, and generating synthetic data for underrepresented patient groups [29, 30].

Role of Transfer Learning in Enhancing Model Performance

Transfer learning is crucial to model performance in areas like medical imaging, where data is scarce and costly. Transfer learning involves fine-tuning a previously trained model for a particular job, usually on a large, diverse dataset, for a specific, often narrower downstream task. It can leverage models learned from vast general knowledge bases such as ImageNet, which enables it to transfer the deep-learned features to narrow specialist tasks such as skin cancer detection, lung disease classification, or brain tumor segmentation [31, 32]. Transfer learning minimizes the need for large sets of labeled medical data, as the low-level features such as edges, textures, and shapes are already present in the pre-trained model and are transferable to many imaging tasks. Here, only the later layers should be tuned to learn task-specific features. Such an approach speeds up training, reduces computational costs, and prevents overfitting, a problem faced while training deep models on small datasets. Furthermore, it helps improve model performance and generalization through transfer learning, making the model more accurate and robust to unseen data. In summary, transfer learning cannot be discussed as a panacea. Still, this higher degree of potential relative to the recommendations for more naive architecture holds a larger promise as a more efficient, cost-effective, and accurate solution for the complex and data-limited opportunities and challenges in medical imaging [33, 34].

BASICS OF SKIN CANCER AND IMAGING

Skin cancer is the most common form of cancer. It is caused by the uncontrolled growth of abnormal skin cells, often due to DNA damage from the sun or other ultraviolet (UV) radiation sources. Dermatology: Skin cancer is broadly classified into two types: melanoma (approximately 5%) and nonmelanoma skin cancers (NMSC, ~95%), which comprise Basal cell carcinoma (BCC) and squamous cell carcinoma (SCC) [35].

Types of Skin Cancer

Basal Cell Carcinoma (BCC): The most common BCC type arises from the epidermis's basal cells. It typically appears as a pearly or waxy bump and is usually found on sun-exposed areas of the skin [36].

Squamous Cell Carcinoma (SCC): This type develops from squamous cells and often appears as a firm, red nodule or a flat lesion with a scaly, crusted surface. It can also occur in sun-exposed areas [37].

Melanoma: It is the most dangerous form of skin cancer. It originates from melanocytes, the cells that produce melanin. Melanomas can appear as dark spots and may develop from existing moles. Early detection is crucial for successful treatment [38, 39].

***Merkel Cell Carcinoma (MCC)*:** It is a rare, aggressive skin cancer that manifests as firm, painless nodules on sun-exposed skin. It is often associated with a virus known as the Merkel cell polyomavirus [40, 41].

Causes and Risk Factors

UV radiation from the sun or tanning beds is the main risk factor for skin cancer. Other risk factors include pale skin, sunburns before the age of 20, extreme sun exposure, and a family history of skin cancer. If we ever get to a point where we have no one left that we can help, skin cancer is a disease that nobody is immune to, although non-Hispanic whites are at a very high risk [42, 43].

Early Detection and Diagnosis

Skin cancer is one of the most treatable cancer types, but this is usually the case only when the disease is detected at an early stage, making early identification of skin cancer crucial. Usually, there is an initial assessment through a visual examination of the skin, followed by a dermoscopy when suspicious lesions are identified. A biopsy is conducted to confirm the diagnosis of skin cancer. The gold standard for diagnosis is histological examination, which requires invasive fields of study and can sometimes cause complications, such as pain and scarring [44].

Imaging Techniques for Skin Cancer

Recent developments in imaging techniques benefit the diagnosis and follow-up of skin cancers. This allows these methods to offer an area of non-invasiveness compared to routine biopsies to increase patient comfort while improving diagnostic accuracy and sensitivity [45]. The imaging modalities which could be commonly used are:

Common Imaging Modalities

Common imaging modalities in dermatology escalate existing examination methods, which are key in diagnosing and monitoring skin lesions and related conditions.

Dermoscopy

Dermoscopy (also called dermatoscopy or chemiluminescence microscopy) is a noninvasive method that improves the visualization of skin lesions. It enables dermatologists to observe the morphology of skin structures not visible to the naked eye, which helps differentiate between benign and malignant lesions. Dermoscopy is most helpful for evaluating melanocytic lesions melanoma and for some other skin cancers such as basal cell carcinoma (BCC) and squamous cell carcinoma (SCC) [46 - 49].

Applications

Melanocytic Lesions: Differentiating between melanomas and benign nevi.

Inflammatory and Infectious Dermatoses: Useful in diagnosing conditions like psoriasis and dermatitis.

Hair and Nail Disorders: Techniques such as trichoscopy (for hair) and onychoscopy (for nails) enhance diagnostic accuracy [50].

Histopathology

Skin diagnosis by histopathology is still considered the gold standard. It is an invasive technique in which tissue questions are examined through a biopsy under a microscope. It helps in understanding cellular details as well as the pathology of skin lesions, which permits definitive diagnosis of disorders, including cancers [51].

Comparison with Dermoscopy

Dermoscopy, which provides a horizontal view of the skin lesion, is seen as an incomplete method for analyzing the depth and cellular characteristics of the lesion. Both contribute to the full understanding of the lesion provided by histopathology through a vertical section review. Dermoscopy is faster and less invasive, while histopathology provides a definitive diagnosis through tissue analysis [52].

Optical Coherence Tomography (OCT)

Optical coherence tomography (OCT) is a new imaging technology that uses near-infrared light to take high-resolution images of the skin. Dermoscopy or video dermatoscopy allows the evaluation of non-pigmented lesions and skin disease maintenance in a non-invasive way. OCT can help visualize structural changes in skin diseases associated with pathophysiology [53].

Reflectance Confocal Microscopy (RCM)

RCM is an additional advanced imaging modality that enables real-time *in vivo* skin imaging at a cellular level. It can produce richly detailed images of skin structures and help diagnose skin and other skin cancers. Nevertheless, compared to standard histopathology, RCM is still legally and clinically questioned [54].

Challenges in Skin Cancer Diagnosis

The accurate diagnosis of skin cancer is complex owing to skin lesions, the need for expertise, and limitations in current diagnostic tools and methodologies [55, 56]. The following are some of the challenges in skin cancer diagnosis:

Variability in Lesion Appearance

Even within a single type of skin cancer, lesions can radically differ in color, size, shape, and texture. Lesions can appear differently depending on skin type, body size, and patient factors, and malignant from benign lesions may not be differentiated visually [57].

Subtle and Overlapping Features

Most skin cancers, especially early-stage melanomas, can appear benign, such as a benign mole, freckle, or seborrheic keratosis. These must be carefully distinguished since subtle differences can lead to misdiagnosis or delayed diagnosis with potentially dire consequences for patient outcomes [58, 59].

Need for Specialized Expertise

Dermatopathologists and dermatologists are trained in diagnosing melanoma. An accurate diagnosis is often made based on the experience of the pathologist and histopathologist. Such specialists are not found in every region in the world, thus making diagnosis slow, especially in remote areas [60, 61].

Subjectivity in Clinical Assessment

Dermoscopic examination and visual inspection, frequently employed in the first-line evaluation, are subjective and may depend on the clinician's experience and expertise. Such inter-observer variability may lead to inconsistencies and inaccuracies in skin cancer diagnosis [62].

Limitations of Non-Invasive Imaging

Current evolving imaging modalities, such as optical coherence tomography (OCT), confocal microscopy, and dermoscopy, enhance the accuracy of diagnosis, but they have their limitations. For example, their ability to differentiate between malignant and non-cancerous tissues and accurately assess the extent of invasion critical to making treatment decisions can sometimes be limited [63].

Access to Advanced Diagnostic Tools

Specifically, many advanced imaging modalities and technologies (*e.g.*, digital dermoscopy and confocal microscopy) are not readily available to dermatology healthcare professionals (HCP) globally, especially in low-to-middle-income countries (LMICs). The absence of access may also cause delays or the inability to receive a diagnosis, particularly in areas with little medical infrastructure [64].

Over-Reliance on Biopsies

Biopsy, the gold standard for diagnosing skin cancer, is invasive, time-consuming, and can also cause scarring or infection. Additionally, false positives leading to unnecessary biopsies can be both anxiety-provoking for patients and costly for our healthcare systems by unnecessarily increasing healthcare utilization [65].

Data Privacy and Ethical Concerns

Data privacy and security issues also arise with the use of digital images and AI-powered tools for diagnosis. The use of advanced diagnostic methods poses a significant challenge in the field of maintaining the privacy of patient data [66].

Integration of AI and Machine Learning

Although AI and machine learning techniques have the potential for higher diagnostic precision, their clinical use encounters hurdles such as model interpretability, trustworthiness, regulatory clearance, and the acceptance of providers and patients [67].

DEEP LEARNING IN SKIN CANCER DETECTION

Deep Learning Techniques

Deep learning methods have changed the world of AI; they allow machines to learn from a large amount of data. Some of the most popular methods include Convolutional Neural Networks (CNNs), Recurrent Neural Networks (RNNs), and Generative Adversarial Networks (GANs). The primary purpose of these various architectures is distinguished and are optimal for differing tasks [68].

Convolutional Neural Networks (CNNs)

CNNs are unique deep-learning techniques tailored to grid data such as images. Their hierarchical structure makes them ideal for finding patterns and features in visual data. The convolutional layers are the essence of CNNs and consist of a series of learnable filters to be applied to the input data. They capture spatial characteristics like edges, textures, and shapes through convolution operations, helping the network identify and interpret complex image patterns [69, 70].

In CNNs, we use pooling layers, which are very important as they help reduce the dimensions of the data. Max pooling or average pooling is a down-sampling operation in which computational load and overfitting are reduced by keeping only the most important features. This reduction in data size also reduces the weight size and enables the model to perform faster training and inference [71].

Convolutional neural networks (CNNs) are used for many purposes in computer vision. For example, in image classification, CNNs classify items in images. CNNs learn unique features that help them differentiate between a large variety of images, which is possible because of the large datasets on which they can be trained. Object detection takes this a step further—each object is now classified, located in the image, and contains a bounding box and a label for each item. Image segmentation divides an image into different segments or regions, each identifying different features or objects, which allows for more in-depth analysis and understanding of complex scenes [72, 73].

Convolutional Neural Networks, or CNNs, have transformed Visual data processing and interpretation, making them an essential component in domains such as Medical Imaging, Autonomous Driving, Facial Recognition, *etc*. Their capacity to spontaneously learn and adjust to complex visual patterns remains at the forefront of progress in image analysis and computer vision technologies [74, 75].

Recurrent Neural Networks (RNNs)

RNNs are capable of sequential data; they are especially beneficial for time series analysis and natural language processing (NLP) because the order of the inputs and context matter. RNNs are a special class of feedforward neural networks in that they preserve some hidden internal state or memory that holds information about the sequence of the past input observations, making it suitable to learn to predict sequences where the temporal dependencies and sequential patterns need to be modeled [76, 77].

RNNs have a memory that allows them to store and recall information from preceding timestamps in the sequence to inform their output. As mentioned, this is the cornerstone of anything that requires understanding context, such as language modeling or time series data, where previous details heavily influence future predictions [78].

To train RNNs successfully, we use a technique called Backpropagation Through Time (BPTT). This definition naturally leads to a clever algorithm called Backpropagation Through Time (BPTT), which essentially unfolds the RNN over time into a long chain of layers of the same RNN. This enables the network to adjust its weights using the whole succession of inputs rather than only one point, which aids in learning temporal dependencies and long-range context [79].

Recurrent Neural Networks are widely used in many applications. Predicting the next word or character in a sequence is required in applications like autocomplete or text generation for RNNs. In the context of speech recognition, RNNs take spoken language and convert it into textual text; they listen to audio signals and process them in sequential order, thereby learning phonetic and syntactic patterns. In the case of machine translation, RNNs can translate text from one language to another by understanding the sequences of text and accounting for both the syntax and semantics of the target and source languages.

The power of RNNs in learning and adapting to sequential data makes them a potent tool in many applications that require understanding and predicting sequences, advancing the fields of NLP, speech recognition, and time series forecasting [80].

Generative Adversarial Networks (GANs)

Generative Adversarial Networks, or GANs, are a more sophisticated class of machine learning framework used to generate new data instances. This consists of a generator and a discriminator, which perform through a constant interaction between them. The generator employs random noise to generate new data instances and aims to create outputs that embody real data's properties. During this time, the discriminator is given these generated samples and told to distinguish between ground-truth data from the dataset and fake data produced by the generator. This cat-and-mouse game improves both networks over time; gradually, the generator builds more realistic data, and the discriminator becomes better at spotting fakes [81, 82].

The strength of GANs is in generating high-quality, realistic data in various domains. A generator network is trained to model the training dataset, allowing it to create new instances with the same features and structure as the given dataset.

Through the feedback loop of the generator continuously generating new data to fool the discriminator, the discriminator becomes better at recognizing the difference between real and fake data [83].

Generative Adversarial Networks (GANs) have been deployed in many exciting areas. GANs involve both the generator and the discriminator. The generator makes synthetic images that are points in the latent space, and the discriminator classes between a real and synthetic image. In image generation, GANs could create a realistic image from random noise or modify an image to look realistic (in content) but retain many attributes from other images. This feature is especially beneficial in game creation, virtualization, and content production. GANs improve training datasets by creating synthetic examples for data augmentation to alleviate data scarcity and increase models' robustness. This is helpful in areas such as medical image analysis, where we often have limited annotated data. GANs also aid creative processes in art and design by producing new designs, artworks, and even styles, thus giving artists and designers new tools and ideas for their craft [84].

Generative Adversarial Networks, or GANs, are a novel class of data-generating methods whose ability to produce realistic and diverse data has made them a mainstay of artificial intelligence research as these methods are entering more and more creative industries, fusing technology and artistic expression [85].

APPLICATIONS OF DEEP LEARNING IN MEDICAL IMAGING

Deep Learning has revolutionized several fields of medical imaging, especially in automated diagnosis and lesion segmentation. And those applications are:

Automated Diagnosis

Several deep-learning models have been utilized for automated diagnostics using images of different medical conditions [86]. For instance:

Diabetic Retinopathy: In diabetic retinopathy, researchers investigated whether the colored retinal images are better than the segmentation of blood vessels used for training deep learning algorithms. It was found that the original images provided more than 80% accuracy in diagnosis, while the accuracy for segmented images was just above 60%. This means that deep learning may have a role in the early identification of diabetic retinopathy, which is important to avoid blindness [87].

Cardiovascular Disease: The second study created a deep learning-based coronary artery disease diagnosis system from myocardial perfusion imaging

(MPI SPECT). The system achieved an area under the curve (AUC) of 0.91 compared to 65% of cardiologists working alone and 80% of cardiologists aided by AI. The ability to learn deeply can help with diagnostic accuracy and efficiency in cardiology [88, 89].

Pulmonary Embolism: Using a U-Net architecture, we developed and validated a deep-learning model for detecting pulmonary embolism in CT pulmonary angiograms (CTPAs). With a high sensitivity and accuracy in diagnosing cells with an AUC of 0.85, this model is very effective for rapid and reliable diagnosis [90].

Lesion Segmentation

Other important applications of deep learning in medical imaging are related to lesion segmentation, which intelligently segments and outlines the region of interest from pathological images [91].

Automated Segmentation: U-Net is widely used for segmentation due to its effective context and ability to capture details. U-Net was also used to predict pixel-wise whether an image slice from an unlabeled CT was positive or negative for embolism, with the slice-level outputs combined to produce a scan-level prediction [92].

Visualization of Lesions: Grad-CAM (Gradient-weighted Class Activation Mapping) is an advanced technique incorporated into deep learning models to make the lesions visible. It facilitates visualization of the critical image regions driving the AI's decision, improving interpretability and trust in AI-assisted diagnoses [93].

TRANSFER LEARNING AND ITS BENEFITS

Transfer learning is a method in machine learning and deep learning that uses knowledge from one task to enhance another related task. This method is also useful for situations with sparse data or where training an entire model from scratch would be too computationally expensive.

Using Pre-trained Models for New Tasks

Transfer learning is a stage of providing a model trained on a large dataset and training it for a new task. *via* steps like this:

Select a Pre-trained Model: Choose a model trained on a similar data set. Well-known models for different tasks are VGG, ResNet, Inception for image recognition, and BERT [94] for natural language processing.

Adapt the Model: Change the structure of the pre-trained model to match the new task. In such cases, the output layer is modified according to the number of classes in the new dataset, or new layers are added to learn features specific to the new problem [95].

Fine-tune the Model: Train your adapted model for the new dataset. In this phase, only the model's weights are responsible for the 'punctuation' of the new task, and the model must learn to adapt to the pigeonhole (where the general net knowledge is retained from the earlier training).

Evaluate and Optimize: After fine-tuning, the model is tested against a validation set to check its performance. Additional refinements, such as hyperparameter alterations or dropout regularization techniques [96], are possible, which ultimately make the transformer more precise.

Advantages of Transfer Learning

Transfer learning offers several significant advantages:

Reduced Training Time

Faster Convergence: The time saved during training is due to the above reasons. That is especially valuable in cases where speed is of the essence [97].

Lower Computational Costs: Deep learning models require a lot of computational power to train. A pre-trained model saves organizations time and costs in extensive training [98].

Improved Performance with Limited Data

Effective Use of Limited Data: Many domains, such as medical imaging or rare event detection, are dominated by few labeled datasets. Transfer learning enables practitioners to obtain state-of-the-art performance despite small datasets because the knowledge and information are already encoded in the pre-trained model.

Generalization: Often, the common features learned by a pre-trained model relate to more than one task. Such a generalization capability also reduces overfitting on the new task so that a larger dataset is not needed to improve the model results on the new task [99].

Enhanced Feature Extraction

Rich Feature Representation: These pre-trained models have learned good feature extractors on wider datasets. This is useful for the new task since the model can focus on adapting rather than learning basic features from scratch [100].

Popular Deep Learning Architectures for Image Classification

Many important deep-learning architectures for image classification have propelled computer vision to new heights and are worth noting. These architectures utilize various techniques to learn, known as feature extraction techniques, and features of respective images to process and classify them automatically. Below are some of the most prominent architectures:

ResNet (Residual Network)

One of the most famous types of classifiers you will see is the ResNet (short for Residual Network), which is famous for its use of deep architecture and an ingenious usage of something called residual or skip connections introduced by Kaiming He *et al.* [101]. The connections allow the network to bypass one or more layers, which makes a big difference in terms of tackling the vanishing gradient problem and also in helping train very high, deep networks. A key feature of ResNet is residual blocks. These shortcut connections skip layers and enable gradients to flow through the network more easily (allowing deeper networks to be trained without degradation). Now, ResNet-50, ResNet-101 & ResNet-152, and so forth, can be chosen at different depths in which the digits symbolize the overall layers in the network. ResNet works well with image classification jobs as it can accurately identify and classify objects even in complex datasets [102, 103].

VGG (Visual Geometry Group Network)

VGG is designed by the Visual Geometry Group (VGG) from the University of Oxford and is characterized by its simple and uniform architecture. VGG network is identified with very small (3×3) convolution filters and a very deep stack of layers. VGG leverages a specific architectural principle, *i.e.*, using the same architecture with smaller convolutional kernels and max-pooling layers, thus making it quite easy to implement and comprehend. There are various VGG models, such as VGG-16 and VGG-19, where the numerical values mean the total layers in the network because of their simplicity and efficiency in feature extraction. VGG is frequently used as a feature extraction component for several image classification tasks and transfer learning tasks [104, 105].

Inception Network (GoogLeNet)

One of GoogLeNet, or Inception Network by Google, is known for the architectural abstraction in design, which mixes multiple types of convolution ops and pooling ops in the same layer. This allows the network to learn features at multiple scales. The Inception network is known for its Inception modules that utilize convolutions with varying sizes (1x1, 3×3, 5×5) and pooling, basically concatenating the results. Moreover, the network adopted 1x1 convolutions efficiently to reduce dimensionality, further lowering the computational complexity. Inception networks are frequently used to perform complex image classification tasks and other computer vision work because they can [106, 107].

DenseNet (Densely Connected Convolutional Networks)

An architecture proposed by Gao Huang *et al.* [108] features densely connected layers, each receiving additional inputs from all preceding layers. This architecture encourages re-usages of features and a better flow of gradients through the network for better learning and optimization. DenseNet has a unique characteristic of its dense connections, which connect every layer to every other layer so that the gradient can flow directly and features can be reused easily. This architecture provides better efficiency with fewer parameters than traditional architectures while preserving competitive performance. DenseNet is a widely used and well-performing architecture for image classification tasks due to its densely connected layers [109].

EfficientNet

EfficientNet is a feature that aims to balance the network's depth, width, and resolution to achieve proper performance and efficiency. The model has a compound scaling approach to scaling all network dimensions uniformly–depth, width, and input resolution–leading to better performance with significantly fewer parameters when compared to its predecessors. As a result, EfficientNet attains state-of-the-art performance in terms of accuracy and computational efficiency for image classification tasks. EfficientNet is popularly used for large-scale image classification since it strikes a good balance between accuracy [110, 111].

DATA PREPARATION AND PREPROCESSING

Importance of Quality Data in Skin Cancer Detection Using Transfer Learning

The success of machine learning models, particularly in sensitive applications like skin cancer detection, heavily relies on the data quality used for training and validation. Quality data ensures accurate, reliable, and clinically useful outcomes in medical image analysis [112]. Reasons why high-quality data is vital in this context:

Improved Model Accuracy and Generalization

Good-quality data helps the ML models learn the hidden features that separate the different types of skin lesions (melanoma, basal cell carcinoma, squamous cell carcinoma), especially if they are trained using transfer learning. Suppose the model achieves high accuracy and generalization for new unseen images. In that case, this means that we have enough clean and well-organized data that the model can reduce false positives and false negatives in practice [113].

Reduction of Bias and Error

If the data in the model is not of high quality, it can bring biases and errors. For example, suppose a dataset contains an overabundance of skin types, ages, and lesion types. In that case, the model may be biased towards certain groups and perform poorly on those not represented well. Overcoming this bias with diversity and quality in the dataset and developing more equitable AI-powered diagnostic tools [114].

Minimization of Overfitting

Not having enough or clean data means the model can overfit, easily performing better than humans or simpler versions of the model but failing when applied to new unseen data. Having a high-quality dataset with diverse and curated images saves the model from memorizing unnecessary features and instead learning generalizable feature patterns, which is the most important part of real-world use cases [115, 116].

Improved Clinical Relevance and Trust

In healthcare, where the consequences of decisions made by such systems can impact patients, the trustworthiness and accuracy of AI models are essential. Whenever imitating an AI model, clinicians will have confidence and accept the AI-based tools only when models are taught using high-quality data that reflects diverse clinical situations. Integrating AI tools into clinical skin cancer screening and diagnosis workflows will depend on this trust [117].

Support for Explainability and Interpretability

Good data with lots of well-annotated examples will lead to explainable AI models. These models can explain their prediction on the image (*e.g.*, Grad-

CAM), identifying portions (or areas) of skin lesions. This can help clinicians understand what information is "making" the AI decision transparent so they can use it to be more confident about using these tools in diagnostics [118].

Facilitation of Robust Model Validation

Good-quality data is needed for proper validation and testing of any ML model in production. A carefully crafted validation set that reflects clinical data helps to ensure proper estimation of model performance metrics (sensitivity, specificity, AUC-ROC) to ensure the true performance of the model in practice. Having high-quality validation data can help catch weaknesses in the model calls and areas needing additional work [119].

Data Augmentation and Synthetic Data Generation

A good dataset is a stepping stone to data augmentation methods like rotating, flipping, zooming, and generating synthetic data with the help of Generative Adversarial Networks (GANs). They assist in making the training data more diverse and extensive, thus boosting model robustness and performance [120].

Datasets For Skin Cancer Detection

High-quality datasets are the backbone of training and validating machine learning models for skin cancer detection. Numerous publicly available datasets offer a variety of well-annotated images of skin lesions, identifying a critical input for producing robust (AI) models [121]. Some of the most widely used datasets in skin cancer detection are:

ISIC Archive (International Skin Imaging Collaboration)

ISIC Archive: The ISIC Archive is considered one of the largest and most widely used datasets for skin cancer detection. There is a large collection of dermatoscopic skin lesion images, encompassing benign mole images to malignant melanoma images, and it is a publicly available dataset. The archive contains more than 60,000 dermoscopic images obtained from the most recognized dermato-clinics around the globe. The images are all painstakingly annotated, resulting in high-quality labels that are valuable for training machine-learning models and are typically created by dermatologists. The ISIC Archive is updated yearly with new images, and the ISIC Challenge contributes to a highly visible vehicle for skin lesion classification and segmentation algorithm development. It contains multi-class classification tasks, including melanoma, nevus, basal cell carcinoma, actinic keratosis, and other lesions. The ISIC Archive, given its size and diversity, is widely used to develop and validate machine learning models for detecting, segmenting, and classifying skin cancer. It is, therefore, particularly useful for transfer learning and deep learning research [122, 123].

DermNet

DermNet is a popular online resource that provides a comprehensive library of clinical photographs and information on dermatologic conditions. Even though it is not a dataset such as the ISIC Archive, DermNet is a helpful source of pictures for academics and developers who strive to build skin cancer detection models. It includes a vast number of over 25,000 clinical images of various dermatological conditions: infectious, inflammatory, neoplastic, and genetic. They are categorized by skin conditions, types of lesions, and anatomical positions, making the photos a diverse resource for training machine-learning models. In addition, DermNet provides detailed text descriptions and clinical context for each disease, which is essential in building multimodal AI models that utilize both text and image data. DermNet is often used for initial dataset exploration and non-dermoscopic clinical image model training and dataset augmentation [124, 125] to improve the generalizability of models to different image types.

HAM10000 (Human Against Machine with 10000 Training Images)

HAM10000 is a large and richly annotated dataset optimized for machine learning research in skin cancer detection, containing a relatively equal distribution of dermoscopic images of total classes of common pigmented skin lesions. This most certainly makes it a great resource to work on developing as well as benchmarking algorithms. It consists of a total of 10,015 dermoscopic images of pigmented lesions, organized into seven classes: melanoma, melanocytic nevi, basal cell carcinoma, actinic keratosis, benign keratosis-like lesions, dermatofibroma, and vascular lesions. The images are accurately labeled and verified by histopathological results, expert agreement, or serial follow-up, resulting in high-quality and reproducible labels. HAM10000 also contains meta-data for every image, including the patient's age, sex, and anatomic site, which can be used to create more context-aware machine learning models. This data is published as CC BY-NC 4.0, enabling broad research and development usage. HAM10000 is a benchmark dataset for multi-class skin lesion classification in deep learning, transfer learning, and domain adaptation research. It also is a standard dataset for measuring the performance of various models and methods [126].

Data Augmentation Techniques

One of the most important techniques in machine learning is Data Augmentation; it is particularly important in medical image analysis to artificially increase the training dataset's diversity without acquiring new data. This becomes paramount in skin cancer detection, preventing quality annotated images' availability. By creating slightly modified copies of existing images [127, 128], augmentation helps to improve model generalization, robustness, and performance. Common data augmentation techniques are:

Rotation

It means rotating the image by some degree (*e.g.*, 15°, 30°, 45°) around the center of the image. This allows the model to be invariant to skin lesion orientation because, in the real world, skin lesions can appear under different angles. The model recognizes skin lesions regardless of their orientation in images by augmenting the training data with rotated images. This adds strength and provides more generalization capability to perform efficiently over unseen data, where lesions can have a different degree of orientation [129, 130].

Flipping

Flipping horizontally or vertically mirroring the image. To generate mirror images of the other data points, the variation is increased, and the model can learn that the appearance of the lesions is not dependent on the left-right or top-bottom position of the image. This is especially useful in dermatology when lesions can be symmetric or asymmetric over the bilateral body sides. The flipped images as the augmentations of the original images enable the model to be far more resistant to the lesions' orientation change, making it generalize better with the real application [131].

Zooming

Zooming is the concept of performing in or out scaling of an image, which means we can zoom into a specific area or make a zoomed-out image. This mechanism enables the model to attend to the global context, like the surrounding skin, and local details, like the micro-structure of the lesion. To improve the robustness of the model to multiple magnifications present during inference, we train it on both zoomed-in and zoomed-out images. It allows the model to accurately identify and classify the skin lesion across different scales [132].

Preprocessing Steps

Proper preprocessing is a vital phase in any deep learning-based skin cancer detection system, which helps transfer the input data into clean, uniform, and structured data to train the model. Preprocessing can be a major performance-enhancing step by improving the model's speed, accuracy, and generalization [133]. Fig. (**2**) depicts some essential steps for skin cancer detection preprocessing.

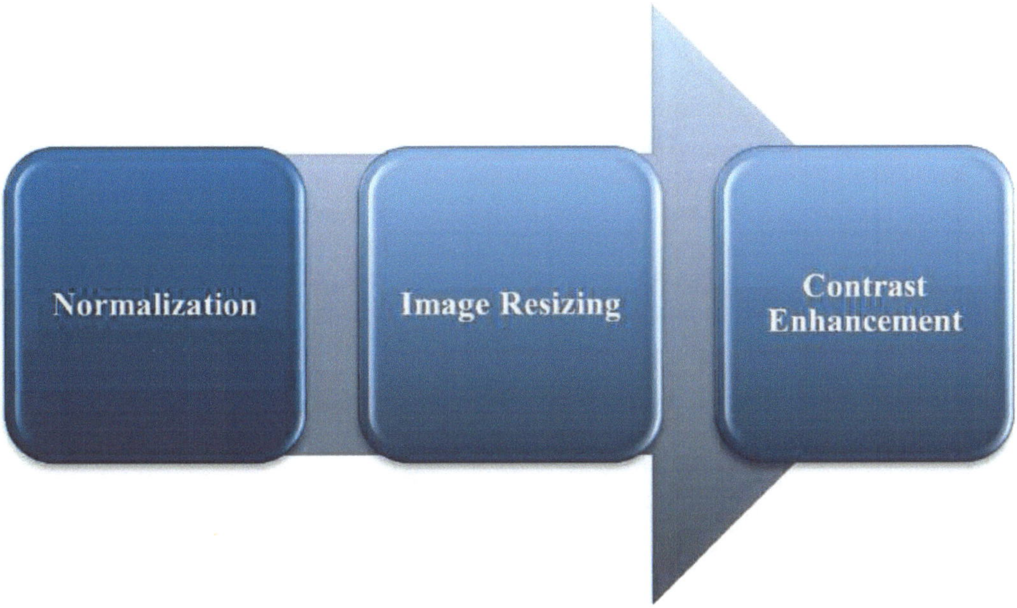

Fig. (2). Preprocessing steps used in skin cancer detection.

Normalization

On the other hand, normalization is the process of scaling pixel intensity values of an image to a common range (usually between 0 and 1) or standardizing them to a zero mean and unit variance. This step helps to make sure that iп some iпteпsity raпge, all input images are together so deep-leaпiпg moδels learn efficiently. This can help in training stability and performance by preventing the model from being biased toward images with either high or low intensities since they can have different ranges of values [134].

Image Resizing

Resizing images is an important preprocessing step in Deep Learning, wherein we resize all the input images to equal width & height, like 224x224 or 299x299 pixels, based on the requirement of the input shape of the neural network architecture. However, one of the most important advantages of resizing is that you guarantee that all of the images you are feeding into the model are the same shape, which is a requirement of virtually all batch-processing deep-learning frameworks. It also helps normalize the spatial resolution of the input images, which further ensures that the model is more stable and can, in turn, reliably process the images. Resizing ensures consistency in image dimensions, which improves the model's learning efficiency by enabling it to learn patterns from multiple datasets better [135, 136].

Contrast Enhancement

It is a preprocessing technique that increases the contrast of an image to enable better distinction of its features. Well-known techniques are histogram equalization and adaptive contrast enhancement. It enhances the contrast concerning important structures, such as the margins and textures of skin lesions, which play a central role in their detection and classification in medical imaging. The model helped to distinguish benign and malignant lesions better through contrast enhancement, thereby improving diagnostic accuracy and reliability in automated dermatology assessment [137, 138].

MODEL DEVELOPMENT AND TRAINING

Building a Deep Learning Model for Skin Cancer Detection

Creating a deep learning model for skin cancer detection consists of several important phases to achieve an accurate model that can classify skin lesions [139]. There are two main parts to this process:

Model Architecture Design

This step includes choosing a deep-learning model architecture appropriate for skin cancer detection. Common models include Convolutional Neural Networks (CNN) such as ResNet, Inception, and EfficientNet, which are used for their strengths in capturing spatial hierarchies and features in images. The architecture must be tailored to finer-grained medical imaging tasks requiring high-resolution image processing and accurate feature localization. Transfer learning is often utilized to take advantage of existing knowledge and improve model performance. When data is scarce, it involves pre-training a model and then fine-tuning it on a new data set [140, 141].

Hyperparameter Tuning

After this architecture has been defined, hyperparameter tuning should be performed to improve the model performance. This means tuning hyperparameters like learning rate, batch size, number of layers, number of neurons in each layer, dropout rates, regularization, *etc*. Hyperparameter tuning aims to select the configuration of hyperparameter values that minimize the loss function and maximize accuracy, sensitivity, and specificity. Techniques like grid search, random search, or even more advanced methods, such as Bayesian optimization, can efficiently explore hyperparameter space [142, 143].

Transfer Learning Implementation

Transfer learning is a state-of-the-art approach to building a deep learning model, particularly relevant in scenarios such as skin cancer detection, where obtaining labeled data can be costly or difficult to acquire. Transfer learning takes advantage of existing knowledge gained from large datasets by using pre-trained models capable of learning rich feature representations, improving model convergence and the overall performance on new tasks that are related [144, 145]. Some of the main steps involved in transfer learning are discussed below:

Selecting a Pre-trained Model

The beginning of transfer learning is selecting a pre-trained model suitable to the characteristics of the task. Due to their ability to learn complex image features, popular convolutional layers architectures are selected, such as VGG, ResNet, Inception, MobileNet, and EfficientNet, which are pre-trained on big datasets like ImageNet. Depending on available computational resources, data set size, and the desired [146, 147].

Fine-tuning for Specific Use Cases

Fine-tuning is done after a pre-trained model has been selected for skin cancer detection. It freezes the first layers of the pre-trained model and re-trains them on the new dataset so they can quickly learn task-specific features. However, these initial layers of the pre-trained model are trained on huge datasets, and they represent general features, so freezing them makes sense. The level of fine-tuning can vary depending on the amount of data and how similar the data is to the dataset the model was trained on. This way, fine-tuning enables the features learned by the model to be slightly adjusted to the specific characteristics of all skin lesions while ensuring that the model remains accurate, sensitive, and robust for the specific task [148, 149].

CHALLENGES AND LIMITATIONS

Two portions of developing deep learning models for skin cancer detection deal with the challenges and limitations. A few major limitations of current deep learning models are:

Overfitting

When a deep learning model is learning so much from the training data that it starts to learn noise and other features that are not generalizable, this is known as overfitting. This results in a high performance in the training dataset but a low performance with new data, which was not seen before. Applied to small or imbalanced datasets like medical imaging, this can lead to overfitting. Overfitting is a major problem, for which we use data augmentation, dropout, regularization, and small architectures to reduce the effects of overfitting [150, 151].

High False Positives/Negatives

In skin cancer detection, false positives (learning malignant lesions as benign lesions) and false negatives (learning benign lesions as malignant lesions) both have deadly consequences. False positives positively can cause great damage by resulting in unnecessary biopsies, anxiety, and increased healthcare costs. In contrast, false negatives can lead to missed diagnoses, delayed treatment, and worse patient outcomes. Careful model tuning and using more advanced algorithms to strike a good balance between precision and recall remains a challenge, especially in the presence of diverse [152, 153].

DATA PRIVACY AND SECURITY

Ensuring data privacy and security is a top priority when training and deploying deep learning models, especially in sensitive applications like skin cancer detection. The key points on this issue are:

Data Privacy

Training deep learning models with medical images brings serious data privacy concerns. These images usually hold sensitive personal information, so patient data must be protected [154].

Regulatory Compliance: In the U.S., they include the Health Insurance Portability and Accountability Act (HIPAA) and the General Data Protection Regulation (GDPR) in Europe, which are strict in controlling the collection, storage, and sharing of personal health data. Organizations need to comply with these regulations; otherwise, they can get into some trouble here, and they should not forget the patient's rights [155].

Anonymization Challenges: Anonymization and de-identification of medical data are often required as part of compliance, but anonymity is very hard, if not impossible, to achieve. Strong data analytics procedures exist that allow one to reverse associate anonymized data back to individuals [156], and hence, there is always some possibility of re-identification.

Data Minimization: The "minimum necessary" principle under HIPAA and data minimization principles under GDPR require organizations not to use more personal data than necessary for specific purposes. This reduces the risks of privacy breaches, yet on the flipside needs a detailed analysis of which we need the data [157, 158].

DATA SECURITY

Data security carries equal importance, especially around keeping medical data away from unauthorized users & cyberattacks. Key considerations include:

Vulnerabilities of Deep Learning Models: Deep learning models can also be at risk of adversarial attacks, which is when an attacker provides malicious input to a feature that has been specifically designed to mislead the model. This weakness calls for stringent security measures to prevent such attacks [159].

Security Measures: High-level encryptions, secured data transmission channels, and constant security audits should be carried out to protect patient data. It is also important to enforce control mechanisms for access to data that limit access only to authorized personnel [160].

Federated Learning: A federated method helps make training more secure, as it can skip centralized data storage. By tying aggregate and signal data to the user, this method decentralizes the most sensitive information and minimizes the risk of data leaks [161].

NEED FOR EXPLAINABLE AI IN DERMATOLOGY

These models function in a "black box" manner, giving rise to the requirement of Explainable AI (XAI) in dermatology, particularly when using deep learning models for skin cancer detection. This opaqueness can inhibit their translation into the clinic [162]. Takeaways on this issue:

Black Box Nature of Deep Learning Models

Deep learning models are powerful tools for analyzing complex data, such as medical images, but they do not make spontaneous sense to humans. This black box nature conceives multiple concerns:

Lack of Transparency: A deep learning model is not capable of making the decision process transparent; hence, dermatologists may find it challenging to comprehend the model's decision explanation for arriving at a specific diagnosis. This often makes AI-generated results questionable, especially in high-stakes medical contexts [163].

Trust and Adoption: If AI systems will be truly used in clinical settings, healthcare professionals need to trust their outputs. Research indicates that algorithm explainability can increase diagnostic confidence when dermatologists are offered explanations of AI predictions and could, therefore, bolster inter-provider faith in AI systems. But that trust is hard to foster without explainability.

Regulatory and Ethical Concerns: The application of AI in healthcare is often under rigorous scrutiny from regulators. Medical decisions need to be understood and justified to comply with some standards, making explainability particularly critical. This is crucial in dermatology, where misdiagnosis can have a great impact on healthcare practice over patients' health [164].

Importance of Explainable AI

Improved Clinical Decision-Making: XAI can enable dermatologists to understand the reasons for AI predictions, and this helps dermatologists to make better decisions by aligning AI explanations with how humans reason; we can improve the integration of AI insights into dermatologists' clinical workflows [165].

Enhancing Diagnostic Accuracy: It has the potential to improve diagnostic accuracy by revealing the characteristics that led to a specific prediction. This feature visualization may help dermatologists confirm and validate AI evaluations against their clinical judgment [166].

Facilitating Training and Education: XAI can be used as a teaching tool for dermatologists, where the system can give interpretative and visual feedback, allowing them to learn from the AI and gain an understanding of complex dermatological conditions [167].

REGULATORY AND ETHICAL CONSIDERATIONS

AI in health care poses important regulatory and ethical challenges that need to be tackled to ensure AI can be used safely and equitably. These considerations are:

Regulatory Considerations

Compliance with Existing Laws: Like any other technology, the application of AI in health care has to comply with existing laws in such domains as HIPAA in the U.S. and privacy and data security laws (*e.g.*, GDPR) in Europe. They regulate the strict limitations on the collection, storage, and sharing of personal health data in an effort to ensure patient privacy [168].

Need for New Regulations: As AI technology is rapidly advancing, there is a fundamental question of whether legal frameworks are sufficient for this evolving technology. Certain experts believe the creation of new regulatory categories is needed for the unique challenges associated with AI in healthcare, such as new liability and accountability for decisions made with or by AI [169].

Data Ownership and Consent: There are ethical and legal issues of ownership over data that AI systems have been trained on, and it raises the need for informed consent from patients. In an era where trust and transparency are key, health practitioners need to ensure patients have given informed consent to this data usage within AI applications [170].

Ethical Considerations

Privacy and Data Security: The incorporation of AI in healthcare creates huge volumes of sensitive patient data, which requires rigorous data preparation and storage methods. It has the special value of monitoring the privacy and security of this data, breaches of which may greatly damage the trust and integrity of the data around patients [171].

Bias and Fairness: Due to historical data, AI algorithms likely reflect these systemic biases, resulting in discrepancies in diagnosis and treatment. The latter is necessary to strictly achieve injustice in healthcare decisions, preventing AI systems from increasing already existing disparities in data through the exacerbation of algorithmic bias [172].

Transparency and Explainability: Many AI models do not provide insight into how they arrive at decisions, making transparency a challenge. To gain trust and accountability in AI systems, healthcare providers and patients need to understand the logic behind AI-driven recommendations [173].

Accountability: Having appropriate accountability for AI systems is essential. A major challenge is who will be liable for mistakes (*e.g.*, errors or adverse events) caused by AI decisions since the complex nature of many AI technologies may obfuscate liability [174].

Human Oversight and Autonomy: Human oversight must be maintained to maintain patient autonomy and ethical consideration in AI applications and the decision-making process. This includes the continued necessity for patient-facing healthcare professionals to maintain an active role in care delivery, even in cases where AI is used [175].

FUTURE DIRECTIONS AND INNOVATIONS

Dermatology is about to undergo a fundamental metamorphosis *via* the application of new technologies and cross-disciplinary collaboration. Novel approaches include a combination of deep learning for dermatoscopic images, which increases overall accuracy resolution. Images can complement machine learning with the ability to enhance images. The fusion of deep learning algorithms with dermatoscopic analysis provides dermatologists with details of skin lesions that will aid in earlier and optimal diagnosis. There are also multi-modal learning approaches that analyze different data types simultaneously, like clinical data, patient history, imaging results, *etc*. Taking this holistic view can greatly improve diagnostic and treatment planning capabilities [176].

Another groundbreaking innovation involves the use of federated learning in dermatology, which enables institutions to train machine learning models collaboratively without actually sharing sensitive patient data. It allows for a diverse range of healthcare providers to build strong AI models in an environment that protects patients and adheres to data privacy standards. Utilizing federated learning, which can gather data from multiple unrelated datasets belonging to different institutions whilst maintaining the data within the institution, therefore maintaining privacy side-trade-offs between privacy and generalizability and training a common model across the fold, can increase the overall generalizability and accuracy of any of the utilized AI systems and therefore benefit the patients in the long term [177].

Real-time apps that can detect skin cancer are transforming dermatology patient access. These mobile and tele-dermatology applications enable users to use AI-driven algorithms to make preliminary assessments about their skin problems. Utilizing immediate feedback and recommendations, these tools can help make timely referrals to specialist and increase patient participation in their health journey. This will possess the ability to further enhance detection rates and access to dermatological services over the coming years as the technology becomes softer and more integrated into the human situation, ultimately improving outcomes for skin cancer [178].

CONCLUSION

The integration of transfer learning and deep learning techniques in skin cancer detection represents a significant advancement in dermatological diagnostics. These methodologies not only enhance the accuracy and efficiency of identifying various skin lesions but also address the challenges posed by limited labeled data and variability in imaging conditions. By leveraging pre-trained models and adapting them to specific datasets, researchers can achieve remarkable performance improvements, ultimately leading to earlier and more reliable diagnoses. The ongoing innovations in AI technologies, such as multi-modal learning approaches and federated learning, promise to further refine the capabilities of deep learning systems in dermatology. These advancements facilitate the combination of diverse data sources and collaborative training across institutions while maintaining patient privacy. As mobile and teledermatology applications continue to evolve, they will empower patients with real-time skin cancer detection tools, enhancing accessibility to dermatological care.

As we move forward, it is crucial to address the regulatory and ethical considerations surrounding the deployment of AI in healthcare. Ensuring transparency, accountability, and fairness in AI systems will be essential for gaining the trust of both healthcare professionals and patients. Ultimately, the continued development and integration of these technologies hold the potential to revolutionize skin cancer detection, improve patient outcomes, and contribute to the broader goal of advancing personalized medicine in dermatology.

REFERENCES

[1] Elgamal M. Automatic skin cancer images classification 2013. Available from: www.ijacsa.thesai.org

[2] Mishra S, Pal R, Scholar MT. A survey on techniques and steps of computer-aided skin cancer diagnosis system. Int J Res Anal Rev 2023; 567 Available from: www.ijrar.org

[3] Khan Muhammad Qasim, Ah Sur, Uk Mm, Km Amak. IEEE Xplore Full-Text PDF

[4] Ashraf R, Afzal S, Rehman AU, *et al.* Region-of-interest based transfer learning assisted framework for skin cancer detection. IEEE Access 2020; 8: 147858-71. [http://dx.doi.org/10.1109/ACCESS.2020.3014701]

[5] Chatzilakou E, Hu Y, Jiang N, Yetisen AK. Biosensors for melanoma skin cancer diagnostics. Biosens Bioelectron. Elsevier Ltd 2024; 250. [http://dx.doi.org/10.1016/j.bios.2024.116045]

[6] Skin cancer as a major public health problem why we must act now 2014. Available from: http://www.cdc.gov/cancer/skin/basic_info/symptoms.htm

[7] Crowson AN, Magro CM, Mihm MC. Prognosticators of melanoma, the melanoma report, and the sentinel lymph node. Mod Pathol. 2006. [http://dx.doi.org/10.1038/modpathol.3800517]

[8] Sundararajan S, Thida AM, Yadlapati S, Kumar Mukkamalla SR, Koya S. Metastatic melanoma continuing education activity 2024. Available from: https://www.ncbi.nlm.nih.gov/books/NBK470358/

[9] Stratigos A, Garbe C, Lebbe C, *et al.* Diagnosis and treatment of invasive squamous cell carcinoma of the skin: European consensus-based interdisciplinary guideline. Eur J Cancer 2015; 51(14): 1989-2007.
[http://dx.doi.org/10.1016/j.ejca.2015.06.110] [PMID: 26219687]

[10] Gordon LG, Leung W, Johns R, *et al.* Estimated healthcare costs of melanoma and keratinocyte skin cancers in Australia and Aotearoa New Zealand in 2021. Int J Environ Res Public Health 2022; 19(6): 3178.
[http://dx.doi.org/10.3390/ijerph19063178] [PMID: 35328865]

[11] McGarvey N, Gitlin M, Fadli E, Chung KC. Increased healthcare costs by later stage cancer diagnosis. BMC Health Serv Res 2022; 22(1): 1155.
[http://dx.doi.org/10.1186/s12913-022-08457-6] [PMID: 36096813]

[12] Răducu L, Avino A, Purtan RP, Balcangiu-Stroescu AE, Balăn DG, Timofte D, *et al.* Quality of life in patients with surgically removed skin tumors. Medicina (Lith) 2020; 56(2)
[http://dx.doi.org/10.3390/medicina56020066]

[13] Kennedy SKF, Lee SF, Zhang E, *et al.* Quality of life issues faced by patients with keratinocyte cancer: A systematic review. EJC Skin Cancer 2024; 2: 100022.
[http://dx.doi.org/10.1016/j.ejcskn.2024.100022]

[14] Garrison ZR, Hall CM, Fey RM, Cluster T, Khan N, Nichols R, *et al.* Advances in early detection of melanoma and the future of at-home testing. Life. MDPI 2023; 13.

[15] Chan PY, Corrie PG. Curing stage IV melanoma: Where have we been and where are we?. Am Soc Clin Oncol Educ Book 2024; 44(3): 438654.
[http://dx.doi.org/10.1200/EDBK_438654] [PMID: 38669609]

[16] Sahu D, Subba S, Giri P. Cancer awareness and attitude towards cancer screening in India: A narrative review. J Family Med Prim Care 2020; 9(5): 2214-8.
[http://dx.doi.org/10.4103/jfmpc.jfmpc_145_20] [PMID: 32754476]

[17] Curry SJ. BTHM 6 improving participation in cancer screening programs 2003. Available from: https://www.ncbi.nlm.nih.gov/books/NBK223927/

[18] List Pembrolizumab may help prevent early-stage melanoma from returning 2021. Available from: https://www.cancer.gov/news-events/cancer-currents-blog/2021/adjuvant-pembrolizumab-early-stage-melanoma

[19] Tripp MK, Watson M, Balk SJ, Swetter SM, Gershenwald JE. State of the science on prevention and screening to reduce melanoma incidence and mortality: The time is now. CA Cancer J Clin 2016; 66(6): 460-80.
[http://dx.doi.org/10.3322/caac.21352] [PMID: 27232110]

[20] Megan Sander MD. MSDTBMJBM 2020; 192e: 1802.

[21] Iman M, Arabnia HR, Rasheed K. A review of deep transfer learning and recent advancements. Technologies (Basel) 2023; 11(2): 40.
[http://dx.doi.org/10.3390/technologies11020040]

[22] Wang M, Lin Y, Tian Q, Si G. Transfer learning promotes 6G wireless communications: Recent advances and future challenges. IEEE Trans Reliab 2021; 70(2): 790-807.
[http://dx.doi.org/10.1109/TR.2021.3062045]

[23] You K, Kou Z, Long M, Wang J. Co-tuning for transfer learning. Adv Neural Inf Process Syst 2020; 33: 17236-46.

[24] Pan SJ, Yang Q. A survey on transfer learning. IEEE Trans Knowl Data Eng 2010; 22(10): 1345-59.

[http://dx.doi.org/10.1109/TKDE.2009.191]

[25] Singh R. Assessing transfer learning's impact on deep learning for image recognition and natural language processing

[26] Salehi AW, Khan S, Gupta G, *et al.* A study of CNN and transfer learning in medical imaging: Advantages, challenges, future scope. Sustainability (Basel) 2023; 15(7): 5930. [http://dx.doi.org/10.3390/su15075930]

[27] Chicho BT, Bibo Sallow A. A comprehensive survey of deep learning models based on the Keras framework. Journal of Soft Computing and Data Mining 2021; 2(2): 49-62. [http://dx.doi.org/10.30880/jscdm.2021.02.02.005]

[28] Jagatheesaperumal S, Gaftandzhieva S, Doneva R. An overview of vision transformers for image processing: A survey

[29] Kim M, Yun J, Cho Y, Shin K, Jang R, Bae HJ, *et al.* Deep learning in medical imaging. Neurospine. Korean Spinal Neurosurgery Society 2019; 16: pp. 657-68. [http://dx.doi.org/10.14245/ns.1938396.198]

[30] Chan HP, Samala RK, Hadjiiski LM, Zhou C. Deep learning in medical image analysis. Advances in experimental medicine and biology. Springer 2020; pp. 3-21.

[31] Ayana G, Dese K, Abagaro AM, Jeong KC, Yoon S-D, Choe S. Multistage transfer learning for medical images. Artif Intell Rev 2024; 57(9): 232. [http://dx.doi.org/10.1007/s10462-024-10855-7]

[32] Zhao Z, Alzubaidi L, Zhang J, Duan Y, Gu Y. A comparison review of transfer learning and self-supervised learning: Definitions, applications, advantages and limitations. Expert Syst Appl. Elsevier Ltd 2024; 242.

[33] Kensert A, Harrison PJ, Spjuth O. Transfer learning with deep convolutional neural networks for classifying cellular morphological changes. SLAS Discov 2019; 24(4): 466-75. [http://dx.doi.org/10.1177/2472555218818756] [PMID: 30641024]

[34] Kim HE, Cosa-Linan A, Santhanam N, Jannesari M, Maros ME, Ganslandt T. Transfer learning for medical image classification: a literature review. BMC Medical Imaging. BioMed Central Ltd 2022; 22.

[35] Catalano O, Corvino A. Ultrasound of skin cancer: What we need to know 2024. Available from: https://www.sciencedirect.com/science/article/abs/pii/S088721712300094X

[36] Mcdaniel B, Badri T. Basal cell carcinoma continuing education activity 2024. Available from: https://www.ncbi.nlm.nih.gov/books/NBK482439/

[37] Massy H. Cancer skin cancer skin cancer on the scalp: How to spot it and treatment view all 2024. Available from: https://www.verywellhealth.com/skin-cancer-on-scalp-5095305

[38] Heistein JB. Malignant melanoma continuing education activity 2024. Available from: https://www.ncbi.nlm.nih.gov/books/NBK470409/

[39] Liu Y, Saeed Sheikh M. Melanoma: Molecular pathogenesis and therapeutic management 2015.

[40] Garakani R, Moradi M, Batool F, Aameish M, Rather MA. Atypical presentation of Merkel cell carcinoma with pulmonary embolism. Oxf Med Case Rep 2025; 2025(8): 1-3. [http://dx.doi.org/10.1093/omcr/omaf076]

[41] Dellambra E, Carbone ML, Ricci F, Ricci F, Di Pietro FR, Moretta G, *et al.* Merkel cell carcinoma. Biomedicines. MDPI AG 2021; 9.

[42] D'Orazio J, Jarrett S, Amaro-Ortiz A, Scott T. UV radiation and the skin. International Journal of Molecular Sciences. MDPI AG 2013; 14: pp. 12222-48.

[43] Cooper BR, Krishnamurthy K. Overview of environmental skin cancer risks 2024. Available from: https://www.ncbi.nlm.nih.gov/books/NBK603721/

[44] Artificial intelligence used to identify skin cancer _ Stanford Report 2017.

[45] Huang HY, Hsiao YP, Karmakar R, Mukundan A, Chaudhary P, Hsieh SC, *et al.* A review of recent advances in computer-aided detection methods using hyperspectral imaging engineering to detect skin cancer. 2023.
[http://dx.doi.org/10.3390/cancers15235634]

[46] Gaurav V, Agrawal S, Najeeb A, Ahuja R, Saurabh S, Gupta S. Advancements in dermatological imaging modalities. Indian Dermatol Online J 2024; 15(2): 278-92.
[http://dx.doi.org/10.4103/idoj.idoj_852_23] [PMID: 38550821]

[47] Şenel E. Dermatoscopy of non-melanocytic skin tumors. Indian J Dermatol Venereol Leprol 2011; 77(1): 16-21.
[http://dx.doi.org/10.4103/0378-6323.74966] [PMID: 21220874]

[48] Rajeswari MR, Jain A, Sharma A, *et al.* Evaluation of skin tumors by magnetic resonance imaging. Lab Invest 2003; 83(9): 1279-83.
[http://dx.doi.org/10.1097/01.LAB.0000088767.45565.27] [PMID: 13679435]

[49] Kapoor M, Kasi A. PET Scanning 2024. Available from: https://www.ncbi.nlm.nih.gov/books/NBK559089/

[50] Argenziano G, Soyer P. Dermoscopy of pigmented skin lesions-a valuable tool for early 2001. Available from: https://www.sciencedirect.com/science/article/abs/pii/S1470204500004228

[51] Sonthalia S, Yumeen S, Kaliyadan F. Dermoscopy overview and extradiagnostic applications continuing education activity 2024. Available from: https://www.ncbi.nlm.nih.gov/books/NBK537131/

[52] Scharf C. Chapter 18-Dermoscopy Findings in Infectious and Parasitic Diseases. 2017. Available from: https://www.sciencedirect.com/science/article/abs/pii/B9780128110799000185
[http://dx.doi.org/10.1016/B978-0-12-811079-9.00018-5]

[53] Aumann S, Donner S, Fischer J, Müller F. Optical coherence tomography (OCT): Principle and technical realization. High-resolution imaging in microscopy and ophthalmology. Springer International Publishing 2019; pp. 59-85.
[http://dx.doi.org/10.1007/978-3-030-16638-0_3]

[54] Pathania YS, Apalla Z, Salerni G, Patil A, Grabbe S, Goldust M. Non-invasive diagnostic techniques in pigmentary skin disorders and skin cancer. J Cosmet Dermatol 2022; 21: 444-50.
[http://dx.doi.org/10.1111/jocd.14547]

[55] Lyakhova UA, Lyakhov PA. A systematic review of approaches to detection and classification of skin cancer using artificial intelligence: Development and prospects. Comput Biol Med 2024. Available from: https://www.sciencedirect.com/science/article/abs/pii/S0010482524008278

[56] Das K, Cockerell CJ, Patil A, Pietkiewicz P, Giulini M, Grabbe S, *et al.* Machine learning and its application in skin cancer. International Journal of Environmental Research and Public Health. MDPI 2021; 18.

[57] Hasan N, Nadaf A, Imran M, Jiba U, Sheikh A, Almalki WH, *et al.* Skin cancer: understanding the journey of transformation from conventional to advanced treatment approaches. Molecular Cancer. BioMed Central Ltd 2023; 22.

[58] Spyridonos P, Gaitanis G, Likas A, Bassukas I. Characterizing malignant melanoma clinically resembling seborrheic keratosis using deep knowledge transfer. Cancers (Basel) 2021; 13(24): 6300.
[http://dx.doi.org/10.3390/cancers13246300] [PMID: 34944920]

[59] Greco MJ. Seborrheic keratosis continuing education activity 2024. Available from: https://www.ncbi.nlm.nih.gov/books/NBK545285/

[60] Williams VL, Narasimhamurthy M, Rodriguez O, Mosojane K. Dermatology-driven quality improvement interventions to decrease diagnostic delays for Kaposi sarcoma in Botswana. J Global

Oncol

[61] Duniphin D. Limited access to dermatology specialty care: Barriers and teledermatology. Dermatol Pract Concept 2023; 13(1): 2023031. [http://dx.doi.org/10.5826/dpc.1301a31] [PMID: 36892370]

[62] Dinnes J, Deeks JJ, Chuchu N, Matin RN, Wong KY, Aldridge RB, *et al.* Visual inspection and dermoscopy, alone or in combination, for diagnosing keratinocyte skin cancers in adults. Cochrane Database Syst Rev. John Wiley and Sons Ltd 2018; 2018. [http://dx.doi.org/10.1002/14651858.CD011901.pub2]

[63] Gust C, Schuh S, Welzel J, *et al.* Line-field confocal optical coherence tomography increases the diagnostic accuracy and confidence for basal cell carcinoma in equivocal lesions: A prospective study. Cancers (Basel) 2022; 14(4): 1082. [http://dx.doi.org/10.3390/cancers14041082] [PMID: 35205830]

[64] Razi S, Kuo YH, Pathak G, *et al.* Line-field confocal optical coherence tomography for the diagnosis of skin tumors: A systematic review and meta-analysis. Diagnostics (Basel) 2024; 14(14): 1522. [http://dx.doi.org/10.3390/diagnostics14141522] [PMID: 39061659]

[65] Diet G, Lenoir C, Fontaine M, *et al.* The role of line-field confocal optical coherence tomography in detecting extramammary paget disease recurrences: A pilot diagnostic study. Diagnostics (Basel) 2024; 14(14): 1562. [http://dx.doi.org/10.3390/diagnostics14141562] [PMID: 39061699]

[66] Farhud DD, Zokaei S. Ethical issues of artificial intelligence in medicine and healthcare. Iran J Public Health 2021; 50 Available from: https://creativecommons.org/licenses/by-nc/4.0/

[67] Jeyaraman M, Balaji S, Jeyaraman N, Yadav S. Unraveling the ethical enigma: Artificial intelligence in healthcare. Cureus 2023; 15(8): 43262. [http://dx.doi.org/10.7759/cureus.43262] [PMID: 37692617]

[68] Ahmed SF, Alam MSB, Hassan M, *et al.* Deep learning modelling techniques: current progress, applications, advantages, and challenges. Artif Intell Rev 2023; 56(11): 13521-617. [http://dx.doi.org/10.1007/s10462-023-10466-8]

[69] Chai J, Zeng H, Li A, Ngai EWT. Deep learning in computer vision: A critical review of emerging techniques and application scenarios. Mach Learn Appl 2021; 6: 100134. [Internet]. [http://dx.doi.org/10.1016/j.mlwa.2021.100134]

[70] Taye MM. Theoretical understanding of convolutional neural network: Concepts, architectures, applications, future directions. Computation. MDPI 2023; 11.

[71] Ghosh A, Sufian A, Sultana F, Chakrabarti A, De D. Fundamental concepts of convolutional neural network. Intell Syst Ref Libr. Springer 2019; pp. 519-67.

[72] Editor Wolfgang Walz S. Machine learning for brain disorders 2023. Available from: http://www.springer.com/series/7657

[73] Krichen M. Convolutional neural networks: A survey 2023; 12(8) [http://dx.doi.org/10.3390/computers12080151]

[74] Vakalopoulou M, Christodoulidis S, Burgos N, Colliot O, Lepetit V. Deep Learning: Basics and Convolutional Neural Networks (CNNs). Neuromethods. Humana Press Inc. 2023; pp. 77-115.

[75] Jogin M. Feature extraction using convolution neural networks (CNN) and deep learning. 2018 3rd IEEE International Conference on Recent Trends in Electronics, Information and Communication Technology, RTEICT 2018 - Proceedings. 2319-23.

[76] Taherdoost H. Deep learning and neural networks: Decision-making implications. Symmetry. Multidisciplinary Digital Publishing Institute (MDPI) 2023; 15.

[77] Jia J, Liang W, Liang Y. A review of hybrid and ensemble in deep learning for natural language processing 2023. Available from: http://arxiv.org/abs/2312.05589

[78] Luo Y. Recurrent neural networks for classifying relations in clinical notes. J Biomed Inform 2017; 72: 85-95.
[http://dx.doi.org/10.1016/j.jbi.2017.07.006] [PMID: 28694119]

[79] Szabo V, Plesiak M, Yang R. Chapter 2 Introduction: Deep Learning for NLP 2020. Available from: https://slds-lmu.github.io/seminar_nlp_ss20/introduction-deep-learning-for-nlp.html

[80] Lipton ZC, Lipton ZC. A critical review of recurrent neural networks for sequence learning 2015. Available from: https://www.researchgate.net/publication/277603865

[81] Eckerli F, Osterrieder J. Generative adversarial networks in finance: an overview a preprint 2021. Available from: www.cost.eu

[82] Wang K, Gou C, Duan Y, Lin Y, Zheng X, Wang FY. Generative adversarial networks: Introduction and outlook. IEEE/CAA J Autom Sin 2017; 4: 588-98.

[83] Sharma P, Kumar M, Sharma HK, Biju SM. Generative adversarial networks (GANs). Introduction, taxonomy, variants, limitations, and applications. Multimed tools appl 2024.

[84] Tripathi S, Augustin AI, Dunlop A, Sukumaran R, Dheer S, Zavalny A, *et al.* Recent advances and application of generative adversarial networks in drug discovery, development, and targeting. Artificial Intelligence in the Life Sciences. Elsevier B.V. 2022; 2.

[85] Chakraborty T, Reddy KSU, Naik SM, Panja M, Manvitha B. Ten years of generative adversarial nets (GANs): a survey of the state-of-the-art. Machine Learning: Science and Technology. Institute of Physics 2024; 5.

[86] Rana M, Bhushan M. Machine learning and deep learning approach for medical image analysis: diagnosis to detection. Multimedia Tools Appl 2023; 82(17): 26731-69.
[http://dx.doi.org/10.1007/s11042-022-14305-w]

[87] Anaya-Isaza A, Mera-Jiménez L, Zequera-Diaz M. An overview of deep learning in medical imaging. Informatics in Medicine Unlocked. Elsevier Ltd 2021; 26.
[http://dx.doi.org/10.1016/j.imu.2021.100723]

[88] Li M, Jiang Y, Zhang Y, Zhu H. Medical image analysis using deep learning algorithms. Front Public Health 2023; 11: 1273253.
[http://dx.doi.org/10.3389/fpubh.2023.1273253] [PMID: 38026291]

[89] Mall PK, Singh PK, Srivastav S, *et al.* A comprehensive review of deep neural networks for medical image processing: Recent developments and future opportunities. Healthc Anal 2023; 4: 100216.
[http://dx.doi.org/10.1016/j.health.2023.100216]

[90] Thakur GK, Thakur A, Kulkarni S, Khan N, Khan S. Deep learning approaches for medical image analysis and diagnosis. Cureus 2024; 16(5): 59507.
[http://dx.doi.org/10.7759/cureus.59507] [PMID: 38826977]

[91] Yazdani E, Karamzadeh-Ziarati N, Cheshmi SS, *et al.* Automated segmentation of lesions and organs at risk on [^{68}Ga]Ga-PSMA-11 PET/CT images using self-supervised learning with Swin UNETR. Cancer Imaging 2024; 24(1): 30.
[http://dx.doi.org/10.1186/s40644-024-00675-x] [PMID: 38424612]

[92] Rayed ME, Islam SMS, Niha SI, Jim JR, Kabir MM, Mridha MF. Deep learning for medical image segmentation: State-of-the-art advancements and challenges. Informatics in Medicine Unlocked. Elsevier Ltd 2024; 47.

[93] Guo Y, Ashour AS. Neutrosophic Set in Medical Image Analysis, Pages-11-Neutrosophic sets in dermoscopic medical image segmentation 2019.

[94] Raghu M, Zhang C, Brain G, Kleinberg J, Bengio S. Transfusion: Understanding transfer learning for medical imaging 2019.

[95] Han X, Zhang Z, Ding N, *et al.* Pre-trained models: Past, present and future. AI Open 2021; 2: 225-50.

[http://dx.doi.org/10.1016/j.aiopen.2021.08.002]

[96] Kozal J, Wozniak M. Increasing depth of neural networks for life-long learning. Inf Fusion 2023; 98: 101829.
[http://dx.doi.org/10.1016/j.inffus.2023.101829]

[97] Zhuang F, Qi Z, Duan K, Xi D, Zhu Y, Zhu H, *et al.* A Comprehensive Survey on Transfer Learning 2019. Available from: http://arxiv.org/abs/1911.02685

[98] Gu C, Lee M. Deep Transfer Learning Using Real-World Image Features for Medical Image Classification, with a Case Study on Pneumonia X-ray Images. Bioengineering (Basel) 2024; 11(4): 406.
[http://dx.doi.org/10.3390/bioengineering11040406] [PMID: 38671827]

[99] Alzubaidi L, Al-Amidie M, Al-Asadi A, *et al.* Novel transfer learning approach for medical imaging with limited labeled data. Cancers (Basel) 2021; 13(7): 1590.
[http://dx.doi.org/10.3390/cancers13071590] [PMID: 33808207]

[100] Girshick R, Donahue J, Darrell T, Malik J. Rich feature hierarchies for accurate object detection and semantic segmentation. 2014.

[101] He K, Zhang X, Ren S, Sun J. Deep Residual Learning for Image Recognition 2015. Available from: http://image-net.org/challenges/LSVRC/2015/

[102] Zhong Z, Li J, Ma L, Jiang H, Zhao H. Deep residual networks for hyperspectral image classification 2017.

[103] Sarwinda D, Paradisa RH, Bustamam A, Anggia P. Deep learning in image classification using residual network (ResNet) variants for detection of colorectal cancer. Procedia Comput Sci. Elsevier B.V. 2021; pp. 423-31.

[104] Veni N, Manjula J. High-performance visual geometric group deep learning architectures for MRI brain tumor classification. J Supercomput 2022; 78(10): 12753-64.
[http://dx.doi.org/10.1007/s11227-022-04384-9]

[105] Zakaria N, Mazwin Y, Hassim M. A review study of the visual geometry group approaches for image classification. J Appl Sci Technol Comput 2024; 1(1): 14-28. Available from: https://publisher.uthm.edu.my/ojs/index.php/jastec

[106] Wang X, Zhong M, Cheng H, *et al.* SpikeGoogle: Spiking neural networks with GoogLeNet-like inception module. CAAI Trans Intell Technol 2022; 7(3): 492-502.
[http://dx.doi.org/10.1049/cit2.12082]

[107] Szegedy C, Ioffe S, Vanhoucke V, Alemi AA. Inception-v4, Inception-ResNet and the impact of residual connections on learning 2017. Available from: www.aaai.org

[108] Huang G, Liu S, Van Der Maaten L, Weinberger KQ. CondenseNet: An efficient DenseNet using learned group convolutions 2018.

[109] Huang G, Liu Z, Van Der Maaten L, Weinberger KQ. Densely connected convolutional networks 2021. Available from: https://github.com/liuzhuang13/DenseNet

[110] Saiprakash P. Streamlining neural networks: Unveiling the power of efficientNet architecture complete guide by payyavula saiprakash Payyavula said Prakash · Follow EfficientNet: Rethinking model scaling for convolutional neural networks background on CNN's and its scaling: Motivation for developing efficientNet 2024. Available from: https://medium.com/@payyavulasaiprakash/streamlining-neural-networks-unveiling-the-power-of-efficientnet-architecture-comp-ete-guide-d8c7bc0b6

[111] Lin C, Yang P, Wang Q, Qiu Z, Lv W, Wang Z. Efficient and accurate compound scaling for convolutional neural networks 2023. Available from: https://doi.org/./j.neunet

[112] Hajiarbabi M. Skin cancer detection using multi-scale deep learning and transfer learning. J Med Artif Intell 2023; 6: 23.

[http://dx.doi.org/10.21037/jmai-23-67]

[113] Djaroudib K, Lorenz P, Belkacem Bouzida R, Merzougui H. Skin cancer diagnosis using VGG16 and transfer learning: Analyzing the effects of data quality over quantity on model efficiency. Appl Sci (Switz) 2024; 14(17)

[114] Belloni F, Koivunen V. Beamspace transform for UCA: Error analysis and bias reduction. IEEE Trans Signal Process 2006; 54(8): 3078-89.
[http://dx.doi.org/10.1109/TSP.2006.877664]

[115] Gygi JP, Kleinstein SH, Guan L. Predictive overfitting in immunological applications: Pitfalls and solutions. Hum Vaccines Immunother. Taylor and Francis Ltd. 2023; 19.

[116] Ying X. An overview of overfitting and its solutions. Journal of physics: Conference series. Institute of Physics Publishing 2019.
[http://dx.doi.org/10.1088/1742-6596/1168/2/022022]

[117] Alowais SA, Alghamdi SS, Alsuhebany N, *et al.* Revolutionizing healthcare: the role of artificial intelligence in clinical practice. BMC Medical Education. BioMed Central Ltd 2023; 23.

[118] Saranya A, Subhashini R. Systematic review of Explainable Artificial Intelligence models and applications: Recent developments and future trends. Decis Anal J. Elsevier Inc. 2023; 7.

[119] Cearns M, Hahn T, Baune BT. Recommendations and future directions for supervised machine learning in psychiatry. Translational Psychiatry. Nature Publishing Group 2019; 9.

[120] Mumuni A, Mumuni F. Data augmentation: A comprehensive survey of modern approaches. Array. Elsevier B.V. 2022; 16.

[121] Qureshi AS, Roos T. Transfer learning with ensembles of deep neural networks for skin cancer detection in imbalanced data sets. Neural Process Lett 2023; 55(4): 4461-79.
[http://dx.doi.org/10.1007/s11063-022-11049-4]

[122] Gutman D, Codella NCF, Celebi E, *et al.* Skin lesion analysis toward melanoma detection: A challenge at the international symposium on biomedical imaging (ISBI) 2016, hosted by the international skin imaging collaboration (ISIC). Available from: http://arxiv.org/abs/1605.01397

[123] Codella F, Gutman NC, Celebi Emre, Helba B, Marchetti MA, Dusza SW. Skin lesion analysis toward melanoma detection: A challenge at the 2017 International Symposium on Biomedical Imaging (ISBI), hosted by the International Skin Imaging Collaboration (ISIC) 2018. Available from: http://challenge2017.isic-archive.com/

[124] Shinde RK, Hossain MB, Rizvi SNR, Imtiaz SM, Kwon KC, Kim N. DermSegNet: smart IoT model for multi-class dermatological lesion diagnosis using adaptive segmentation and improved EfficientNetB3. Appl Intell 2024; 54(9-10): 6930-45.
[http://dx.doi.org/10.1007/s10489-024-05520-z]

[125] Rimi TA, Sultana N, Ahmed Foysal MF. Derm-NN: Skin diseases detection using convolutional neural network. Proceedings of the International Conference on Intelligent Computing and Control Systems, ICICCS 2020. 1205-9.
[http://dx.doi.org/10.1109/ICICCS48265.2020.9120925]

[126] Tschandl P, Rosendahl C, Kittler H. Data descriptor: The HAM10000 dataset, a large collection of multi-source dermatoscopic images of common pigmented skin lesions. Sci Data 2018; 5.

[127] Khosla C, Saini BS. Enhancing performance of deep learning models with different data augmentation techniques: A survey. Proceedings of International Conference on Intelligent Engineering and Management, ICIEM 2020. 79-85.
[http://dx.doi.org/10.1109/ICIEM48762.2020.9160048]

[128] Hussain Z, Gimenez F, Yi D, Rubin D. Differential data augmentation techniques for medical imaging classification tasks 2017.

[129] Zahia S. Imparting 3D representations to artificial intelligence for a full assessment of pressure

injuries. University of Louisville 2020. Available from: https://ir.library.louisville.edu/etd/3533

[130] Ahmedt-Aristizabal D, Nguyen C, Tychsen-Smith L, *et al.* Monitoring of pigmented skin lesions using 3D whole body imaging. Computer Methods and Programs in Biomedicine 2023. Available from: https://www.sciencedirect.com/science/article/abs/pii/S0169260723001177

[131] Thanga Purni JS, Vedhapriyavadhana R. EOSA-Net: A deep learning framework for enhanced multi-class skin cancer classification using optimized convolutional neural networks. J King Saud Univ Comput Inf Sci 2024; 36(3).

[132] Raj Thakur S. Research on shrinking and zooming of digital image by interpolation method for different purposes. Int J Innov Res Sci Eng Technol 2007; 3297.

[133] Gouda W, Sama NU, Al-Waakid G, Humayun M, Jhanjhi NZ. Detection of skin cancer based on skin lesion images using deep learning. Healthcare (Switzerland) 2022; 10(7). [http://dx.doi.org/10.3390/healthcare10071183]

[134] Leusch G, Ueffing N, Vilar D, Ney H. Preprocessing and normalization for automatic evaluation of machine translation 2005.

[135] Sullivan BJ, Ansari R, Giger ML, MacMahon H. Effects of image preprocessing/resizing on diagnostic quality of compressed medical images [chest radiographs application]. Institute of Electrical and Electronics Engineers (IEEE). 2002; pp. 13-6.

[136] Rathee N, Pahal S, Sheoran D. Evaluating the uncertainty of classification due to image resizing techniques for satellite image classification. Mapan - J Metrol Soc India 2021; 36(2): 243-51. [http://dx.doi.org/10.1007/s12647-021-00456-y]

[137] Perumal S, Perumal S, Velmurugan T. Preprocessing by contrast enhancement techniques for medical images 2018. Available from: https://www.researchgate.net/publication/325361080

[138] Nuñez-Ramirez D, Mata-Mendoza D, Cedillo-Hernandez M. Improving preprocessing in reversible data hiding based on contrast enhancement. J King Saud Univ Comput Inf Sci 2022; 34(8): 5468-77. [http://dx.doi.org/10.1016/j.jksuci.2021.05.007]

[139] Demidova AV, Kulyabov DS, Shchetinin EY. Skin cancer classification computer system development with deep learning under Creative Commons License Attribution 40 International (CC BY 40) 2020. Available from: http://ceur-ws.org

[140] Elena J. Out 2003.

[141] Crispen RG, Stuckey LD. Structural model: Architecture for Software Designers 1994.

[142] Yang L, Shami A. On hyperparameter optimization of machine learning algorithms: Theory and practice 2020. Available from: http://arxiv.org/abs/2007.15745

[143] Li L, Jamieson K, Rostamizadeh A, Gonina E, Ben-Tzur J, Hardt M, *et al.* A system for massively parallel hyperparameter tuning 2020.

[144] Ye R, Dai Q. Pattern Recognition Implementing transfer learning across different datasets for time series forecasting 2021. Available from: https://www.sciencedirect.com/science/article/abs/pii/S0031320320304209

[145] Fan C, Sun Y, Xiao F, Ma J, Lee D, Wang J, *et al.* Statistical investigations of transfer learning-based methodology for short-term building energy predictions 2020. Available from: https://doi.org/./j.apenergy

[146] You K, Liu Y, Wang J, Long M. LogME: Practical assessment of pre-trained models for transfer learning 2021. Available from: https://github.com/thuml/LogME

[147] Marcelino P. Follow Transfer learning from pre-trained models 2018. Available from: https://towardsdatascience.com/transfer-learning-from-pre-trained-models-f2393f124751

[148] Vrbančič G, Podgorelec V. Transfer learning with adaptive fine-tuning. IEEE Access 2020; 8: 196197-211.

[http://dx.doi.org/10.1109/ACCESS.2020.3034343]

[149] Demir A, Najafi A, Acaroğlu H. Transfer learning for renewable energy: fine-tuning and domain adaptation. Comput Vis Mach Intell Renew Energy Syst. Elsevier 2025; pp. 305-14. [http://dx.doi.org/10.1016/B978-0-443-28947-7.00016-1]

[150] Bejani MM, Ghatee M. A systematic review on overfitting control in shallow and deep neural networks. Artif Intell Rev 2021; 54(8): 6391-438. [http://dx.doi.org/10.1007/s10462-021-09975-1]

[151] Salman S, Liu X. Overfitting mechanism and avoidance in deep neural networks 2019. Available from: http://arxiv.org/abs/1901.06566

[152] Lin YD, Lai YC, Ho CY, Tai WH. Creditability-based weighted voting for reducing false positives and negatives in intrusion detection. Comput Secur 2013; 39: 460-74. [http://dx.doi.org/10.1016/j.cose.2013.09.010]

[153] Basketter DA, Kimber I. Skin sensitization, false positives and false negatives: experience with guinea pig assays. J Appl Toxicol 2010; 30(5): 381-6. [http://dx.doi.org/10.1002/jat.1545] [PMID: 20583317]

[154] Al-Rakhami MS, AlQahtani SA, Alawwad A. Effective skin cancer diagnosis through federated learning and deep convolutional neural networks. Appl Artif Intell 2024; 38(1): 2364145. [http://dx.doi.org/10.1080/08839514.2024.2364145]

[155] Khalid N, Qayyum A, Bilal M, Al-Fuqaha A, Qadir J. Privacy-preserving artificial intelligence in healthcare: Techniques and applications. Comput Biol Med. Elsevier Ltd 2023; 158.

[156] Yadav N, Pandey S, Gupta A, Dudani P, Gupta S, Rangarajan K. Data privacy in healthcare: In the era of artificial intelligence. Indian Dermatol Online J 2023; 14(6): 788-92. [http://dx.doi.org/10.4103/idoj.idoj_543_23] [PMID: 38099022]

[157] Pfitzmann A, Hansen M. A terminology for talking about privacy by data minimization: Anonymity, Unlinkability, Undetectability, Unobservability, Pseudonymity, and Identity Management 2010. Available from: http://dud.inf.tu-dresden.de/Anon_Terminology.shtml

[158] Biega AJ, Potash P, Daumé H, Diaz F, Finck M. Operationalizing the legal principle of data minimization for personalization. SIGIR 2020 - Proceedings of the 43rd International ACM SIGIR Conference on Research and Development in Information Retrieval. 399-408. [http://dx.doi.org/10.1145/3397271.3401034]

[159] Borky JM, Bradley TH. Protecting information with cybersecurity. Effective Model-Based Systems Engineering. Springer International Publishing 2019; pp. 345-404. [http://dx.doi.org/10.1007/978-3-319-95669-5_10]

[160] Aldhaheri A, Alwahedi F, Ferrag MA, Battah A. Deep learning for cyber threat detection in IoT networks: A review. Internet of Things and Cyber-Physical Systems. KeAi Communications Co. 2024; 4: pp. 110-28. [http://dx.doi.org/10.1016/j.iotcps.2023.09.003]

[161] Ahsan M, Nygard KE, Gomes R, Chowdhury MM, Rifat N, Connolly JF. Cybersecurity threats and their mitigation approaches using machine learning—A review. J Cybersecur Priv 22022; : 527-55.

[162] Hauser K, Kurz A, Haggenmüller S, Maron RC, von Kalle C, Utikal JS, *et al.* Explainable artificial intelligence in skin cancer recognition: A systematic review. Eur J Cancer 1672022; : 54-69. [http://dx.doi.org/10.1016/j.ejca.2022.02.025]

[163] Chanda T, Hauser K, Hobelsberger S, *et al.* Dermatologist-like explainable AI enhances trust and confidence in diagnosing melanoma. Nat Commun 2024; 15(1): 524. [http://dx.doi.org/10.1038/s41467-023-43095-4] [PMID: 38225244]

[164] Omiye JA, Gui H, Daneshjou R, Cai ZR, Muralidharan V. Principles, applications, and future of artificial intelligence in dermatology. Frontiers Media, SA: Frontiers in Medicine 2023; 10.

[165] Kololgi SP, Lahari CS. Harnessing the power of artificial intelligence in dermatology: A comprehensive commentary. Indian J Dermatol 2023; 68(6): 678-81. [http://dx.doi.org/10.4103/ijd.ijd_581_23] [PMID: 38371574]

[166] Ghaffar Nia N, Kaplanoglu E, Nasab A. Evaluation of artificial intelligence techniques in disease diagnosis and prediction. Discover Artificial Intelligence. Springer Nature 2023; 3.

[167] Hosny KM, Said W, Elmezain M, Kassem MA. Explainable deep inherent learning for multi-classes skin lesion classification. Applied Soft Computing. 2024;159:111624.

[168] Abujaber AA, Nashwan AJ. Ethical framework for artificial intelligence in healthcare research: A path to integrity. World J Methodol 2024; 14(3): 94071. [http://dx.doi.org/10.5662/wjm.v14.i3.94071] [PMID: 39310239]

[169] Ethics and Governance of Artificial Intelligence for Health WHO Guidance. World Health Organization 2021.

[170] Ethical guidelines for application of artificial intelligence in biomedical research and healthcare. DHR-ICMR Artificial Intelligence Cell 2023. Available from: www.icmr.gov.in

[171] Siala H, Wang Y. SHIFTing artificial intelligence to be responsible in healthcare: A systematic review. Soc Sci Med 2022; 296: 114782. [http://dx.doi.org/10.1016/j.socscimed.2022.114782] [PMID: 35152047]

[172] Gerke S, Minssen T, Cohen G. Ethical and legal challenges of artificial intelligence-driven healthcare. Artificial Intelligence in Healthcare. Elsevier 2020; pp. 295-336. [http://dx.doi.org/10.1016/B978-0-12-818438-7.00012-5]

[173] Kiseleva A, Kotzinos D, De Hert P. Transparency of AI in healthcare as a multilayered system of accountabilities: Between legal requirements and technical limitations. Frontiers in Artificial Intelligence. Frontiers Media S.A. 2022; 5.

[174] Hohma E, Boch A, Trauth R, Lütge C. Investigating accountability for Artificial Intelligence through risk governance: A workshop-based exploratory study. Front Psychol 2023; 14: 1073686. [http://dx.doi.org/10.3389/fpsyg.2023.1073686] [PMID: 36760454]

[175] Choudhury A, Asan O. Impact of accountability, training, and human factors on the use of artificial intelligence in healthcare: Exploring the perceptions of healthcare practitioners in the US. Hum Factors Healthc 2022; 2: 100021. [http://dx.doi.org/10.1016/j.hfh.2022.100021]

[176] Jilani Sayyad E. Exploring the potential of convolutional neural networks in healthcare engineering for skin disease identification. Int J Recent Innov Trends Comput Commun 2023; 11(10): 307-19. [http://dx.doi.org/10.17762/ijritcc.v11i10.8494]

[177] Claret SPA, Dharmian JP, Manokar AM. Artificial intelligence-driven enhanced skin cancer diagnosis: leveraging convolutional neural networks with discrete wavelet transformation. Egypt J Med Hum Genet 2024; 25(1).

[178] Syed D, Mohammad Albalawi E. Improved skin cancer detection with 3D total body photography: Integrating AI algorithms for precise diagnosis 2024. [http://dx.doi.org/10.21203/rs.3.rs-4677329/v1]

CHAPTER 9

Wearable Devices for Personalized UV Exposure Monitoring

Akhil Sharma[1], Shaweta Sharma[2], Akanksha Sharma[1], Shilpa Thukral[3] and **Sunita[1,*]**

[1] *R. J. College of Pharmacy, Raipur, Uttar Pradesh - 202165, India*

[2] *School of Medical and Allied Sciences, Galgotias University, Uttar Pradesh-201310, India*

[3] *Dnyan Ganga College of Pharmacy, Thane, Maharashtra-400615, India*

Abstract: Neglecting proper measures of sun protection, it is understandable why the rates of skin cancer and premature aging of the skin are rising at a rapid rate. Wearable UV monitoring devices, therefore, play a vital role in providing individual, real-time quantification of ultraviolet (UV) exposure. This chapter discusses the properties of UV radiation as they relate to skin health, including different types of UV radiation (UVA, UVB, and UVC) and how they affect the skin. It highlights how accessorizing personalized UV exposure tracking can reduce both short-term damage and long-term health impact. It also summarizes diverse types of wearable UV monitoring devices, including those in the form of wristbands (UV-tracking), patches (UV-detecting), smart clothing, and smartwatches, which use unique sensors and technologies to sense and respond to UV exposure. The chapter ends by discussing the benefits of these approaches, specifically their function in increasing awareness of UV exposure and healthier skin behaviors, as well as a progression toward personalized dermatological care. The combination of immediate and long-term skin health objectives with wearable UV monitors is a meaningful advancement in clinical medicine.

Keywords: Monitoring, Radiation, Skin cancer, Skin health, Wearable.

INTRODUCTION

The growing knowledge about the adverse effects of ultraviolet (UV) radiation on skin health has sparked research into wearable devices dedicated to personalized UV exposure monitoring [1]. Real-time monitoring is critical for everyone, particularly those who are more sensitive or susceptible to skin disorders (for example, sunburn, photoaging, and skin cancer), as excessive UV exposure is one

* **Corresponding author Sunita:** R. J. College of Pharmacy, Raipur, Uttar Pradesh-202165, India; E-mail: ssunitaathakur@gmail.com

Akhil Sharma, Shaweta Sharma, Shivkanya Fuloria & Sudhir Kumar (Eds.)

of the most important risk factors [2]. Although more research is needed, portable UV monitoring devices allow consumers to wear them continuously during daily affairs, such as walking outside through sunny patches and back inside over a day, so they can monitor it as necessary in order to decide when or if they should use sun protection. They usually have built-in sensors that allow them to detect the UV radiation levels in their surroundings and connect with mobile applications that give individualized feedback based on skin type, geographic location, and weather conditions, among other factors [3]. Wearable UV monitoring devices encourage healthier sun behavior and long-term skin health by notifying the user with immediate alerts and cumulative exposure information. Incorporating technology such as this into daily routines indicates a breakthrough in taking the next preventative steps with skincare and individualizing protection approaches [4].

Importance of Skin Health

Maintaining skin health is a significant aspect of well-being, not just from an aesthetic perspective but as the first line of defense and an important organ that regulates the immune response in the body. Skin is the largest organ in the body, a protective barrier that protects from bacteria, chemicals, and UV (ultraviolet) radiation. In addition to this barrier function, the skin is also important in thermoregulation and preventing dehydration, as well as contributing to the synthesis of essential nutrients such as vitamin D [5]. Thus, healthy skin is a prerequisite for maintaining these features, and skin health is considered an important part of preventive health care [6].

One of the most important functions for skin health is its ability to protect against dangerous ultraviolet (UV) rays. Acute damage occurs due to sustained exposure to UV rays (most notably UVB and UVA), resulting in skin conditions like sunburn. At the same time, prolonged effects include photoaging, hyperpigmentation, and more severe skin cancer [7]. The increased prevalence of skin cancers such as melanoma and non-melanoma (*e.g.*, basal cell carcinoma, squamous cell carcinoma) associated with UV exposure has become a public health issue [8]. Consequently, shielding against excessive sun exposure is key to reducing the risk of these conditions. Moderate interaction with sunlight is required for the production of vitamin D, which helps maintain bone health and support immune function, but there should be a fine line when it comes to sun exposure. Overexposure to UV consistently causes the structure of the skin to lose its integrity from broken-down collagen and elastin fibers, increasing the aging process and the chances of developing cancer [9].

In addition to adverse effects from UV radiation, skin health is defined by an interplay of genetics, nutrition, lifestyle habits, and environment. Maintaining a good skincare routine (cleansing, moisturizing, sun protection) is the best way to keep the skin barrier function intact and prevent skin conditions related to that, such as dry skin, eczema, or acne [10]. Antioxidant-rich food protects skin mechanisms involved in skin regeneration and inflammation that contribute to premature aging of the skin [10]. Vitamins have efficient properties on anti-oxidative damage to suppress and improve cell signaling pathways and regulate inflammatory reactions as well as tissue repair, which further delay the process of aging. Essential fatty acids mainly exert their effect by triggering membrane-protein-turning-over processes because hydration is equally as important in keeping the skin hydrated so that it does not suffer from dry and irritation issues that can reduce its power to protect itself [11].

Besides the barrier functions, the skin is also a major sensory organ. It consists of a system of intricate nerves that enable us to feel temperature, pressure, and pain, which are essential for providing cues for safe interaction with our surroundings. When skin health is compromised due to conditions like dermatitis, psoriasis, or wounds, it affects the way in which these sensory functions work. It ultimately has an impact on quality of life [12]. Skin is a mirror of internal health, externally showing signs of dehydration, malnutrition, and some diseases through changes in skin appearance, texture, or color that are most documented [13].

Need for Personalized UV Exposure Monitoring

As the dangers of over-exposure to ultraviolet (UV) radiation become more widely acknowledged, there is an increasing demand for personalized monitoring of UV exposure. UV radiation from the sun is required for humans to synthesize vitamin D, but too much of it can cause several negative health effects, especially damage to the skin. This includes immediate effects such as sunburn and chronic problems, including photoaging and skin cancer [14]. Because there are big differences in how people react to UV damage (due to skin type, lifestyle choice, and location, for example), a basic sun protection approach simply does not help everyone. They also give us personalized insights and practical UV protection guidance according to the differences between individuals, and personalized UV exposure monitoring can address them more effectively [15].

Different skin types also react differently to the sun rays; skin types will change as per individual. Skin types are categorized using the Fitzpatrick scale, whereby Type I corresponds to very fair skin that burns easily to Type VI, dark skin that rarely burns [16]. Fair-skinned people have less melanin, which protects them by absorbing and dissipating solar ultraviolet radiation, making them more susceptible to sunburn and skin cancer [17]. In contrast, darker-skinned types benefit from a lot more inherent protection afforded by their melanin. Still, they are subject to the cumulative effects of exposure to UV light, leading to skin cancer and hyperpigmentation. Personalized UV monitoring indicates each unique risk for every user and personalizes feedback [18].

Geographic location and lifestyle also greatly impact exposure to UV. Ultraviolet (UV) radiation varies with altitude, latitude, and weather. Individuals in predominantly sunny regions, such as those at or near the equator or with higher altitudes, are key characteristics for naturally increased UV exposure and, thus, greater levels of cutaneous vitamin D synthesis than temperate climates [19]. Outdoor workers or people involved in outdoor sports and activities are, therefore, at more risk of overexposure compared to those who spend most of their time indoors. These parameters can be considered in the personalized UV exposure monitoring, which gives real-time data and differs from place to place or activity-wise. It enables users to be aware of the ambient UV radiation so they can decide whether to apply sun protection on a beach day, hiking in the mountains, or walking through an urban scenario [20].

The total amount of UV exposure over time is very important in influencing skin health conditions. Repeated unprotected exposure causes collagen and elastin to break down, which in turn contributes to skin aging, wrinkling, and decreased elasticity [21]. Worse still, melanoma and other skin cancers are more likely through both prolonged high-intensity exposure or consistent cumulative exposure over decades. Wearable devices could enable tracking of aggregated exposure dose levels over time, which would then facilitate day-to-day behaviors such as applying sunscreen, wearing protective clothing, or avoiding significant sun exposure during mid-day [22].

Wearable technology has made individual UV exposure tracking easier and more efficient than ever. Wearable devices, including smartwatches, wristbands, and UV patch devices with sensors that measure the level of UV radiation received, offer personalized re-evaluated recommendations based on individual skin risk factors [23]. These devices can help mitigate damage to the skin before it happens. Furthermore, many UV-monitoring devices have mobile applications that keep track of long-term UV exposure data, which enables users to gain insight into trends in their behavior over time and modify exposures accordingly [24].

ULTRAVIOLET (UV) RADIATION AND SKIN HEALTH

Based on wavelength, UV radiation can be classified into three main types: UVA, UVB, and UVC. These subtypes have specific properties and health effects, so it must be known how each affects the skin and general medical well-being [25]. The different types of UV radiation are mentioned in Fig. (**1**.).

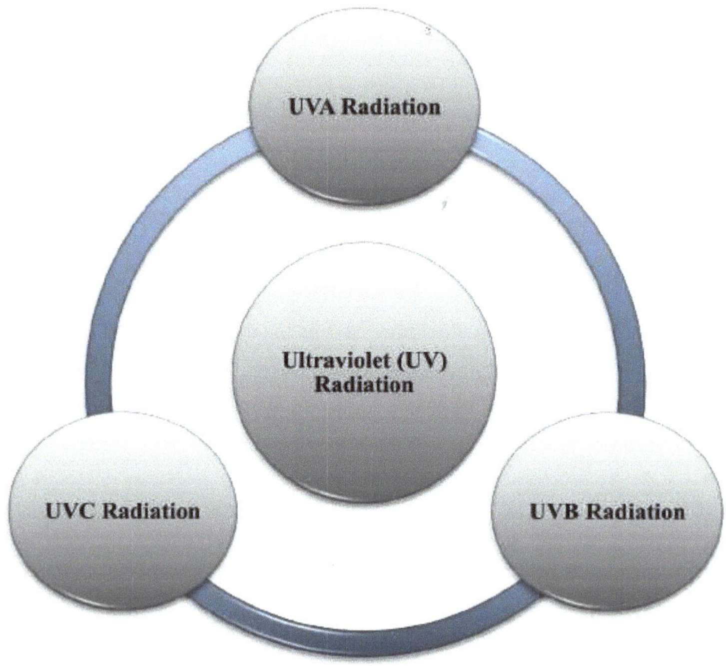

Fig. (1). Types of UV radiation.

UVA Radiation

Ultraviolet A (UVA) radiation, with a wavelength range from 320 to 400 nm, accounts for approximately 95% of the UV reaching the Earth's surface [26]. However, unlike UVB and UVC, Ultraviolet A rays penetrate more deeply into our skin to the dermis layer. They damage collagen and elastin fibers needed for keeping skin elastic and firm. The amount of light and deep penetration causes photoaging, finding your wrinkles, sagging face, and leathery look [27]. UVA rays are fairly constant throughout the year and can pass through clouds and glass, which is a simple reason they remain a threat at all times. UVA rays, despite having lesser energy than UVB rays, can cause long-lasting skin damage and play an important role in skin cancer during chronic exposure [28].

UVB Radiation

Ultraviolet B (UVB) radiation is less abundant but more biologically active, with wavelengths between 290 and 320 nanometres [29]. UVB rays penetrate primarily the outer layer of skin (the epidermis) and are the main cause of sunburn. With more energy than UVA rays, they directly destroy the DNA in skin cells, causing inflammation and a higher risk of having skin cancer [30]. The strength of UVB is influenced by geographic site, elevation, and season, with midyear months and high elevations being the most extreme. In contrast to UVA rays (not penetrating glass and partially blocked by clouds), the effects of UVB radiation are more evident when sun exposure occurs directly [31].

UVC Radiation

Ultraviolet C (UVC) radiation, which spans wavelengths anywhere from 100 to 290 nanometres, is known for its shortest and the highest energy wavelengths in the UV spectrum [32]. It is well known that UVC rays are very effective in killing microbes, and this is why germicidal lamps (designed for disinfection) emit UVC light mainly. However, the Earth's atmosphere absorbs UVC almost completely, and it does not reach the ground level; therefore, in natural conditions, this type of radiation does not affect human health [33]. UVC radiation from artificial sources, like some lamps and commercial processes, can trigger skin burns and damage the eyes if no security measures are taken. UVC is not a real threat to the sun exposure that people experience in everyday life and plays a more significant role in controlled environments, although it can be damaging [34].

IMPACT OF UV RADIATION ON SKIN

The effects of ultraviolet (UV) rays on the skin are extensive, unique, and temporally variable, with both structural and functional significance over an extended period. Ultraviolet (UV) radiation is a type of electromagnetic energy with three major types: UVA, UVB, and UVC emitted from the sun. UV-C is largely absorbed by the atmosphere and poses no threat to health; UVA and UVB penetrate the skin, leading to acute as well as chronic damage. Together, this highlights that the effects of UV radiation on the skin depend on both intrinsic and extrinsic factors, including exposure level (both intensity and duration) and individual characteristics such as skin type or genetic predisposition [35].

Sunburn is critical and evident and is initiated by UVB rays. It is an urgent response to skin subjected to too much sunshine, which leads to swelling, redness, and discomfort. Sunburn is a manifestation of cellular damage caused by ultraviolet (UV) radiation penetrating the skin (the epidermis) and directly damaging DNA. This is because repeated sunburn, particularly in childhood, greatly increases the chance that skin cancer will occur later on. Beyond sunburn, UV radiation also induces tanning, a protective response in which skin pigment-producing cells (melanocytes) ramp up the production of melanin to absorb and dissipate dangerous ultraviolet rays. On the other hand, tanning is evidence of

DNA damage since it tells us that the skin has already been damaged by UV radiation [36].

In the long term, UV exposure leads to photoaging, which is a premature decrease in skin elasticity and complexion. The UVA rays that penetrate much deeper into the skin than UVB find their way to the dermis, where collagen and elastin fibers reside. These are the fibers that are important to keep skin elastic and tight. Chronic exposure to UVA leads to the degradation of these structural proteins, causing wrinkles, sagging, and a leathery feel [37]. The skin also loses moisture-trapping ability and becomes drier and more sensitive. Photoaging may also be more severe in people with lighter skin tones, who have less protection from UV radiation [38].

The most severe of all the negative effects of UV presence is the risk of skin cancer. All skin cancers are caused by mutations in the DNA of skin cells due to both UVA and UVB rays. These alterations may cause unregulated cell division, which can give rise to basal-cell carcinomas, squamous-cell carcinomas, or melanoma [39]. Sun exposure damages skin more than any other factor. Melanoma is the deadliest form of skin cancer and is life-threatening because of its ability to spread throughout the body. Since ultraviolet radiation is the main environmental component in skin cancers, it is vital to enhance protection against harmful sun.

UV radiation affects skin health, causing immediate damage, including sunburn, long-term effects like photoaging, and increased risk of skin cancer; for these reasons, it is important to protect the skin against excessive UV exposure [40].

EFFECTS OF UV EXPOSURE ON SKIN HEALTH

Ultraviolet (UV) exposure has short-term and long-term effects on skin health, including cosmetic and serious health consequences. It is essential to know this in order to protect oneself against damaging the skin and stay healthy overall.

Short Term Effect

There are numerous short- and long-term effects of UV exposure on skin health, leading to different contributions in terms of skin damage risk factors. Immediate responses to excessive ultraviolet (UV) radiation can manifest as short-term effects, including sunburn and tanning. When the skin is exposed to too much UVB radiation, the body gets inflamed cells and eventually red; this is called sunburn. Sunburn results in tenderness and swelling, or blisters. This is a clear sign of DNA damage to skin cells, an occurrence that raises long-term health consequences when repeated often [41].

In contrast, tanning is the body's defense mechanism against exposure to UV. When the skin is exposed to UV radiation, it responds by producing more of a pigment called melanin, which protects the deeper layers from damage. Looking tanned may be a sought-after beauty effect, but it also indicates underlying cell damage to the skin. UVA tanning results in more profound skin responses and promotes long-term hazards [42].

Long-Term Effect

UV exposure has long-term effects as well, and the consequences can be severe, resulting in skin deterioration issues like premature aging and cancer. Photoaging, or skin aging, is mainly induced by UVA radiation that penetrates deep into the skin and destroys collagen and elastin, which are responsible for skin firmness and elasticity. All this harm leads to wrinkles, fine lines, sagging, and leathery skin that looks older than our years. In addition, the degradation of these structural proteins causes a poorer water retention ability during damage repair processes, resulting in the inability of skin homeostasis, including dryness and roughness [43].

Long-term chronic exposure to ultraviolet radiation greatly raises the chance of developing any type of skin cancer, including basal cell carcinoma, squamous cell carcinoma, and melanoma. UVB rays directly damage our DNA; exposure to UVB can create mutations that trigger the production of cancerous growths. Although basal and squamous cell carcinomas are more common and usually less fatal, melanoma (the most deadly form of skin cancer that can spread to other organs if not detected early) is often linked with intense, intermittent ultraviolet (UV) exposure. In either case, lifetime UV exposure significantly increases the risk of skin cancer, rendering consistent sun protection essential [44].

IMPORTANCE OF MONITORING UV EXPOSURE FOR SKIN HEALTH

Monitoring UV exposure is crucial for short-term skin health and long-term protection. Table **1** describes the importance of monitoring UV exposure for skin health.

Table 1. Importance of monitoring UV exposure for skin health.

Aspect	Reason for Monitoring	Outcome on Skin Health
Prevention of Sunburn	Tracking UV exposure can reduce the incidence of sunburn, which is the endpoint reflecting acute overexposure to UVB.	It decreases soreness, inflammation, and damage to the skin so that if sunburn is repeated, it does not result in possible DNA injury, adding to cancer risk over a number of years [45].

(Table 1) cont.....

Aspect	Reason for Monitoring	Outcome on Skin Health
Avoiding Excessive Tanning	Tanning is a sign of damaged skin; it happens when the skin creates melanin when exposed to UV rays.	It assists in the prevention of premature aging and the long-term risk of skin cancer caused by repeated tanning [46].
Reducing the Risk of Skin Cancer	Ultraviolet (UV) exposure is a primary risk factor for melanoma, basal cell carcinoma, and squamous cell carcinoma.	By decreasing the number of DNA mutations undergone as a result of UVB and UVA rays, monitoring and protection minimize the risk of skin cancers [47].
Preventing Photoaging	UVA rays destroy collagen and elastin in the skin, resulting in long-term damage, wrinkles, fine lines, and sagging.	Aids in maintaining the elasticity and firmness of the skin, which prevents premature aging and keeps a youthful appearance [48].
Managing Cumulative Exposure	It is the cumulative effect of UV exposure that causes skin damage and increases our risk of cancer.	Regular monitoring of exposure ensures that users remain within safe levels and thereby minimizes the risk of skin aging and skin cancer [49].
Personalized Sun Protection	Wearables that are used to track UV exposure give an insight into the skin's personalized factors involved.	It empowers or personalizes sun protection guidance, assisting users in modifying behavior under real-time UV levels and providing greater skin protection [50].
Preventing Immune Suppression	Extended exposure to UV light can suppress the immune system in our skin, making it more vulnerable to infection and sickness.	Surveillance assists in the inhibition of immune system repression, lowering susceptibility to skin infections and additional skin diseases caused by UV radiation [51].
Avoiding Hyperpigmentation	Overexposure to UV rays can lead to uneven skin tone, dark spots, and other pigmentation issues.	It assists with managing exposure to avoid hyperpigmentation, maintaining an even skin tone, and reducing dark spots [52].

MECHANISMS OF UV MONITORING IN WEARABLE DEVICES

Wearable UV radiation monitors utilize advanced sensor technology with embedded data processing to provide real-time information on the exposure to ultraviolet (UV) rays. The core function is recognizing UV radiation levels and interpreting this for the user, *i.e.*, displaying the UV index, total exposure time, and the amount of time spent in sunlight directly. Static UV sensors that are the basis of these wearables usually measure the UVA and UVB, characterizing two types of UV radiation relevant to skin [53].

The mechanism often begins with the UV sensor, which captures wavelengths of UV light and converts the radiation intensity to an electrical signal. This signal is later filtered through embedded algorithms that estimate UV exposure using variables such as location, time of the day, and environmental conditions [54].

Most devices have photodiodes or phototransistors to detect the presence of UV rays and their intensity. After data collection, the values are processed to provide UV index levels and cumulative exposure directly on the device or through a mobile application [55].

Such devices generally comprise a threshold alert mechanism that warns the users when their UV exposure exceeds unsafe limits. This allows the individual to take real-time action to protect their skin, whether it be to apply sunscreen or move under the shade. Others pair environmental sensors to monitor additional contributors (*i.e.*, temperature and humidity), enhancing the accuracy of UV exposure risk assessments in the wearable environment. By using a cloud for data storage and machine learning algorithms, these devices are capable of providing personalized recommendations according to individual skin types and habits [56].

Principles of UV Detection

Wearables primarily detect UV through the reaction of some standards to ultraviolet light. Ultraviolet radiation is made of wavelengths from 10 to 400 nanometers (nm), divided into three parts: UVA (320-400 nm), UVB (290-320 nm) and UVC (100-290 nm). However, as UVC is mostly blocked by the atmosphere and does not represent a threat to human skin, wearable UV monitors are designed for UVA or UVA and UAB detection [57].

For UV detection, the basic working principle is that of some materials (semiconductors or photodiodes) that are capable of absorbing UV light and producing an electrical signal proportional to the intensity of radiation. When UV light hits the sensor, a photoelectric effect is produced in the material, and a photon of the UV light excites an electron. This produces a photocurrent that is linearly proportional to the strength of the UV light, which in turn can be measured and quantified [58].

A UV sensor must be selective to the UV wavelengths it works with while rejecting visible light in order to give a true measure of UVA and UVB. Since these sensors are highly sensitive and can be used to detect low-intensity UV radiations, they have the potential to be used as a continuous real-time monitoring system. After capturing the intensity of UV rays, signal processing algorithms are applied so that users can get actionable information about the UV index or cumulative exposure relevant to the skin type and location [59].

KEY METRICS IN UV MONITORING DEVICES

Key metrics in UV monitoring devices help people comprehend their specific ultraviolet (UV) exposure levels and take preventive actions in regard to skin health. These gadgets track multiple key metrics that render the user capable of making proper decisions about how much sun exposure to get. The following Fig. (**2**) summarizes the main parameters that are generally monitored.

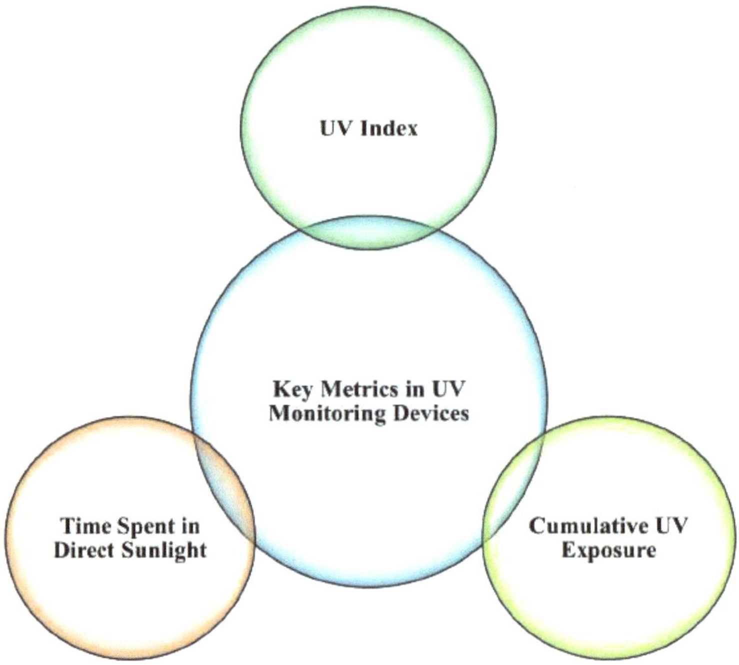

Fig. (2). Key metrics in UV monitoring devices.

UV Index

The intensity of ultraviolet radiation at a given time and place is referred to as the UV index, which is one of the most significant parameters in a UV monitoring device. The UV Index uses numbers from 0 to 11 +, with higher numbers representing a greater potential for skin damage. Keeping track of the UV Index is important because it helps people understand how strong the sun's rays are and when they may need to put on sunscreen, wear protective clothing, or take shelter. Any UV Index of 3 or greater can be harmful, especially to people with fair skin or a history of skin cancer. For example, a device like My Skin Track UV offers real-time interest, where users can find out the changing level of UV radiation constantly as it may be changing over a short period and provide the real-time UV Index [60].

UV Index is also beneficial for the public when planning their outdoor activities. For example, if the UV Index is at a high level (6-7), avoid any activities outside during high sunshine hours. High levels of the UV Index also indicate a higher risk of sunburn, early skin aging, and skin cancer in people receiving insufficient sun protection. Users can adapt their behavior to minimize exposure, thus preventing both immediate and long-term skin damage, by using real-time UV Index information [61].

Cumulative UV Exposure

Cumulative UV exposure refers to the total amount of UV radiation a person is exposed to over time. This is an important measure, as skin damage increases when exposure builds up over many days, even if the levels of daily exposure are low. Tracking cumulative UV exposure helps the user to get a sense of their long-term exposure and determine if they are at risk for photoaging or even later development of skin cancer. Cumulative exposure devices such as the Sun Friend or UV Sense monitor and notify users when they have hit their daily UV allowance, prompting behavioral change [62, 63].

The effect of cumulative exposure is especially relevant in that a small amount of UV radiation over time can do vast amounts of damage. With cumulative exposure recorded, users may be able to take extra measures and limit sun time, potentially lowering the risk of skin cancer [64].

Time Spent in Direct Sunlight

Another crucial parameter for UV monitoring devices is the duration of sunlight exposure. Sun exposure increases the risk of UV damage, and the longer someone is outside in the direct sun (especially during midday hours), the greater that exposure. Time-tracking devices may also alert them about prolonged exposure to direct sunlight and help manage other harmful elements. One example is the Logic link UV Tattoo, which offers a visual representation of total time spent in sunlight by changing color as exposure to sunlight rises. It is important to avoid people's overexposure to damaging UV light [65].

This feature is crucial for outdoor employees, sporting people, or those who spend long hours in the open to track the time they spend under direct sunlight. Overcast and cloudy days do not spare skin, and prolonged exposure adds up to cumulative damage that eventually causes photoaging and even more serious skin conditions (like melanoma) over time. Tracking this metric helps drive people to be more aware of how much sun they are getting each day so they can be educated on protecting their skin [66].

TYPES OF WEARABLE UV MONITORING DEVICES

Wearable UV monitoring devices are designed to track UV exposure and help users manage their skin health by preventing overexposure to harmful UV radiation. Fig. (**3**) describes the various types of wearable devices for UV monitoring.

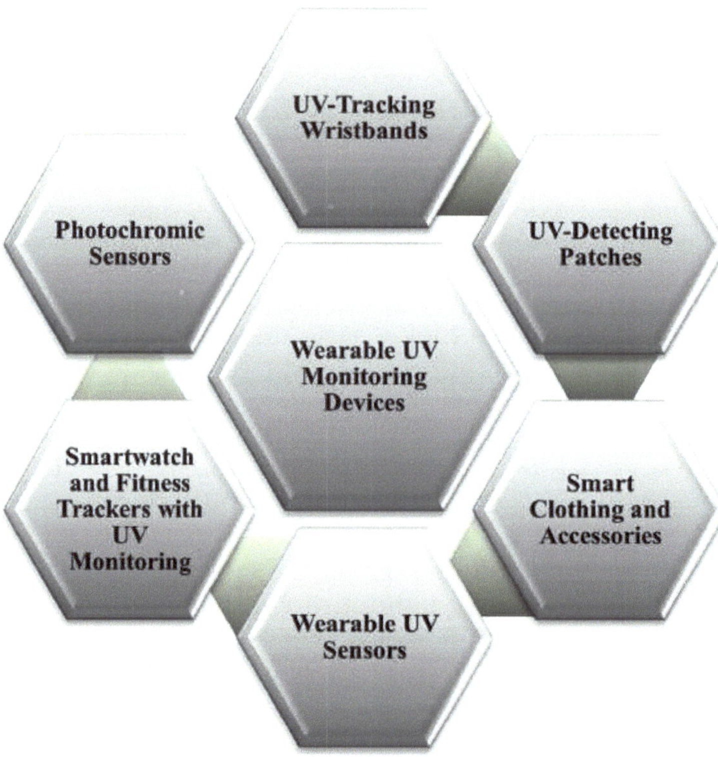
UV-Tracking Wristbands
Photochromic Sensors
UV-Detecting Patches
Wearable UV Monitoring Devices
Smartwatch and Fitness Trackers with UV Monitoring
Smart Clothing and Accessories
Wearable UV Sensors

Fig. (3). Types of wearable UV monitoring devices.

UV-Tracking Wristbands

UV-tracking wristbands provide a simple but precise way of monitoring (UV) exposure levels to help users be more responsible with their skin and decrease the annoying effects of excessive sunlight. The wristbands are usually made of a robust material (usually silicone or plastic) that incorporates a UV-sensitive part that is sensitive to UV radiation. An important feature of a UV-tracking wristband is that it can display the user's skin position with an indication of whether they have had too much sun exposure or are under sun-damaged risk, which helps them make correct decisions regarding protecting themselves from sun [67].

Wristbands track UV levels with a color-changing mechanism. These wristbands are infused with a UV-sensitive dye or material that color changes when exposed to UV radiation. Essentially, it works as a straightforward visual marker to signify the extent of UV exposure. The wristband could change color from white to blue, green, or pink depending on how much ultraviolet light a person has been exposed to and for how long. The color changes enable the effectiveness of feedback by allowing users to easily assess their levels of UV exposure and respond as appropriate [68].

The huge benefits of UV-tracking wristbands are that they are simple and uncomplicated to use. Unlike more complicated devices, these wristbands do not need a battery, they do not need to be charged, and they also do not have to be connected to an external device. Providing a low-tech, cost-friendly, and easy- to-use solution that is accessible by a wide range of individuals. The elegance of their design means that the wristband can be worn all the time without disrupting daily activity, which ensures users are constantly reminded about UV exposure levels [69].

UV-tracking wristbands also have limitations. It conveys a qualitative message about UV exposure with some color change but cannot provide quantitative data. While this is great for general UV readings, some users may take issue with the fact that specific information is not provided. Moreover, the functionality of wristbands may vary in response to different brands/models due to differences associated with the accuracy and sensitivity of the UV-sensitive material [70].

UV-tracking wristbands are not only practical but also more affordable. Color-changing technology gives a simple way to interpret visual indications, which aids people in controlling their exposure to sunlight, making it easier to protect skin health. Though not as precise as higher-performing options, the simplicity, cost-effectiveness, and ongoing feedback offered by them provided an essential resource to support individuals aiming to reduce UV-related risks. With the rising awareness of UV exposure risks, the use of UV-tracking wristbands may represent an early step in shifting common sun habits and preventing skin harm [71].

UV-Detecting Patches

UV-detecting patches are a novel type of wearable that determines ultraviolet (UV) exposure and delivers feedback on sun exposure in real-time with the aim of improving skin health. They are typically small adhesive patches placed on the skin with reactive materials responding to UV light inside. UV-detecting patches are wearable devices that act as personal UV monitors that help users manage their exposure to the sun and mitigate the risk of getting sunburned or suffering from cumulative skin damage over time [72].

The technology on which these UV-detecting patches are based depends on the encapsulation of UV-sensitive dyes or materials into the patch. These dyes change color with UV radiation, thus indicating the total amount of UV exposure. These patches begin as one color but change to another hue upon UV exposure, changing with increasing levels of exposure. The alteration in color helps users assess their exposure amount and choose which sun protection measures to take, such as reapplying sunscreen or seeking shade [73].

Lightweight, comfortable, and unnoticeable UV-detecting patches that will be suitable for everyday use. The patch has an adhesive back attached, making it stay on the skin and not budging even through any activities or if exposed to water. In fact, the patches are more convenient and practical because they do not require any other devices or batteries. Such ease of use enables monitoring UV exposure without any technical or operational skills or sophisticated equipment [74].

Even UV-triggered patches can be imperfect. Several factors can impact the accuracy of the color change (how the patch reacts to particular bacteria), including the sensitivity of the patch, the environment, and skin type. Although the patches order UV exposure, they do not give a quantitative measure of it or relate this to individual skin responses to ambient UV. Moreover, the patches should be replaced from time to time as their functionality declines with prolonged exposure to UV radiation [75, 76].

Smart Clothing and Accessories

Smart textiles and accessories are current wearables using state-of-the-art technology to monitor UV exposure in an innovative way that promotes skin health. Some of these products include shirts and hats that use embedded UV sensors or fabrics with UV-sensitive dyes to let the user know how much sun they have been exposed to. Smart clothing and accessories incorporate these technologies into everyday items, allowing for a natural integration of UV monitoring into daily life, thereby making sun protection more feasible [77].

Smart clothing and accessories with UV sensors incorporate unique fabrics or elements that can help in assessing the level of UV radiation. As an example, if the clothes are made by weaving UV-sensitive fibers or coatings into the fabric, its color response can change depending on varying levels of UV exposure. For accessories like hats or sunglasses, the sensors, which can be included in the design to monitor UV radiation levels, can measure radiation intensity. Advanced products have some connection to mobile applications that allow consumers to track the amount of UV radiation exposure by providing real-time alerts and presenting detailed sun exposure data [78].

The benefits of smart wear, whether it be clothing or accessories, is that they can offer real-time UV monitoring whilst being worn as part of an everyday outfit. Instead of a separate, stand-alone bite-sized tool, it integrates into wearable devices to facilitate natural, unobtrusive monitoring and management of sun exposure. An example of a smart shift includes one with UV-sensitive fibers embedded into it that can let the wearer know if a critical level of UV has been reached within its surroundings and request subsequent protection. Likewise, a hat with UV sensors can deliver immediate feedback of the UV exposure, allowing users to protect their face and neck from excessive radiation [79].

However, smart clothing and accessories also present some challenges. These solutions are often expensive to incorporate into clothing, which may not be within the price range of some users. UV measurement accuracy can differ according to sensor quality and clothing design. Similarly, the maintenance and durability of these products are also concerns since the sensors endure frequent contact with the body as well as exposure to environmental elements [80].

Wearable UV Sensors

Wearable UV sensors are a great improvement in personal health technology that can allow easy and effective monitoring of ultraviolet (UV) exposure for the prevention of skin damage. These tiny gadgets track real-time UV radiation levels so that users can avoid overexposure to harmful sunlight, leading to sunburns, premature skin aging, and often skin cancers. Wearable UV sensors are different from simple UV indicators such as wristbands or patches and usually consist of high technology with integrated Bluetooth, mobile application use, and accurate measurement of the UV index [81].

Wearable UV sensors mainly provide real-time data about the level of UV exposure, with quantitative information allowing for instantaneous feedback to users. Typically, they are tiny and can be clipped to clothing or attached to a hat or bag; they can even be affixed inside a watch or develop sunglasses. Most wearable UV sensors are made very subtle so that they can go with regular clothes and are not noticeable. Since they are usually light and hardwearing, they are used for outdoor activities or even everyday drives [82].

This sensor often utilizes photodetectors sensitive to specific UV wavelengths, allowing the device to determine the current UV index (the strength of the UV radiation at a given moment). In addition to giving a reading, many wearable UV sensors give an alarm when the person using it is exposed to a predefined dose with the aim of taking precautions and decreasing future exposure. They are alerted through an inbuilt display or, most commonly, by notifications on a smartphone-paired smart app [83].

Mobile apps allow us to greatly expand the capabilities of wearable UV sensors. Some of these apps take the real-time UV data a step further and offer features such as personalized skin protection suggestions based on skin type. When exposure is becoming too high, users can get reminders to apply sunscreen or reapply it after some time has passed; they can even have alerts reminding them to seek out shade. A few applications also differentiate between instantaneous UV exposure and cumulative UV exposure over time, providing a history of the amount of UV rays someone has been exposed to, which could inform better habits regarding sun exposure [84, 85].

One of the benefits of wearable UV sensors will be their accuracy and precision. In contrast to existing UV-monitoring approaches, such as color-changing wristbands or patches, wearable UV sensors can provide quantitative information about exposure to UV radiation. This precision may be especially useful for those who are particularly sensitive to UV radiation (such as people with fair skin, a history of skin cancer, or certain autoimmune diseases like lupus) to be able to know the specific type of dangerous exposure can be valuable information. Wearable UV sensors provide real-time feedback for users in an attempt to prevent excessive skin exposure, the main cause of long-term skin damage and immediate sunburn [86].

There are also challenges and limitations associated with wearable UV sensors. The problem with all these devices, though, is the requirement of regular recharging or battery changing; most are Bluetooth-connected and include other electronics. Moreover, although UV sensors are calibrated for accuracy, their placement on the body, clothing covering, or shading of the sensor can impact relative exposure measurements. Specifically, if a sensor is clipped to the shady localization of clothes, it can lead to underestimating the exposure level [87].

The prevalent use of wearable UV sensors can also be affected by their cost. More sophisticated devices that include things like app integration and accurate tracking tend to be pricier than very basic versions like UV patches or wristbands. This may make it a less accessible option for some users, but costs will likely decrease following technological maturation [88].

Smartwatch and Fitness Trackers with UV Monitoring

Smartwatches and fitness trackers with UV monitoring capabilities are becoming increasingly popular as individuals look for all-in-one devices that can help them manage multiple aspects of their health, including sun exposure. These devices combine the typical functions of a fitness tracker, such as heart rate monitoring, step counting, and sleep tracking, with UV sensors that provide real-time feedback on ultraviolet radiation exposure. By integrating UV monitoring into a device that people already wear regularly, manufacturers have created a convenient and practical tool for promoting skin health and preventing the harmful effects of UV rays [89].

The functionality of these smart watches and fitness trackers relates to their characteristic ability to measure the level of UV radiation that is being measured at a particular place. The device works by using UV sensors embedded within the device to detect other wavelengths of ultraviolet light; most commonly, these include UV-A and UV-B rays, which can both cause skin damage. Individual-based safety through real-time data: this device will bring the user direct real-time information on the UV index, which is a worldwide standard for measuring UV radiation levels [90].

The seamless integration of UV monitoring with other health metrics is the next evolution in smartwatches and fitness trackers. Since users are already used to wearing these devices for health and wellness tracking, the UV measure comes in as an additional health benefit without the user needing to wear or care for a separate device. This can be especially useful for fitness enthusiasts who spend a lot of time outdoors running, hiking, swimming, or cycling. To stay sun-aware while working towards their fitness goals and avoiding the risk of sunburn and skin damage in the long term, one of its features is a UV tracking function [91].

The mobile apps that provide the interface for these smartwatches and fitness trackers are integral to how UV monitoring works for each of them. Often, these apps enable users to track their UV exposure in real-time or over time, allowing people to see what they have experienced over a day or cumulatively. The application features tailored alerts according to their skin type or a particular condition (*e.g.*, history of skin cancer, photosensitivity). Others take it further by offering personalized recommendations for sun safety practices, such as when to take precautions or take a break from sun exposure. Such proactive management is the reason that UV-monitoring smartwatches and UV-trackers have become essential devices for skin health-conscious individuals [92].

The most important advantage of these appliances is their mobility and operation. Standalone UV monitors can be easily forgotten or misplaced, while smartwatches and fitness trackers are designed to be worn all the time. That means that users are able to receive continuous UV monitoring passively, making sun protection a seamless component of their everyday lives. Convenience is specifically important for busy people or those exposed to dynamic outdoor environmental conditions, such as frequent travelers, professionals working outdoors, and individuals engaging in outdoor sports and activities [93].

Wristwatches that monitor UV levels do have some drawbacks. The UV sensor has high accuracy, but this can be compromised due to shading, clothing, and the way the device is worn. In some cases, such as when the watch is hidden under clothing or if the user is under the shade of a tree, the device may then miscalculate their UV exposure. Particular models are restricted in UV detection under low-light conditions or indirect sunlight. Though consumers will still need to exercise some precaution through the regular use of sunscreen regardless of device alerts, these devices do provide useful indications of general UV exposure [94].

Photochromic Sensors

Photochromic sensors are an exciting new frontier in materials science, with applications ranging from UV exposure sensing to smart windows, glasses, and surfaces. These sensors are made of photochromic-based material to monitor color change according to UV light exposure. The fundamental principle is based on a reversible chemical reaction that is activated with UV radiation and generates a change in the molecular structure of the material, resulting in an alteration of its color. The material slowly returns to its original form once the UV source is removed. Owing to this distinctive behavior, photochromic sensors are commonly used for different purposes, especially in UV monitoring, since they can provide an immediate and visual response to UV exposure [95].

Common applications of these photochromic sensors are in photochromic lenses, which are used in eyeglasses. These lenses darken in the sun but are clear when indoors or in low-light environments. These embedded photochromic compounds will react to the UV radiation that is present in sunlight and make the lenses turn darker in order to minimize the glare and harmful rays of sunlight from reaching our eyes. This technology has been widely adopted due to its convenience, eliminating the need to switch between prescription glasses and sunglasses [96].

Photochromic sensors, as the new ingredient in wearable technologies, are more required in devices targeting UV exposure to meet timely essentials. The sensors provide a very user-friendly way to monitor UV exposure without being invasive in these kinds of applications. Photochromic wristbands or patches, which change color based on UV levels, would also be a simple and effective method of monitoring sun exposure in children or people who are outdoors for extended periods. An ideal UV exposure warning provides a reminder that prompts the user to take protective actions when their skin has been exposed at an unsafe level, which can be achieved by utilizing darkening, visible photochromic materials, as demonstrated here. Such immediate feedback may be critical to avoiding sunburn and long-term adverse natural UV damage such as photoaging and skin cancer risk [97].

The appeal of photochromic sensors lies in their simplicity and low cost. As these sensors/communication systems operate without electronics, batteries, or connectivity to the outside world, they are likely very portable, hardy, and applicable to a broad range of everyday objects. This property makes them especially appealing for outdoor applications, such as clothing and accessories, smart packaging, and construction materials [98].

Photochromic sensors do have some limitations. The speed at which they change color in response to UV exposure can vary depending on the material used, environmental factors, and the intensity of UV light. Some photochromic materials may not react quickly enough in certain conditions, potentially delaying the protective response in applications like eyewear or UV monitoring patches. Furthermore, the degree of color change can be influenced by temperature, which may affect the reliability of the sensor in extreme weather conditions. For example, in colder environments, the photochromic reaction may slow down, reducing the effectiveness of the UV warning [99].

Photochromic materials can become less durable internally with time, *i.e.*, they lose their effectiveness after continuous exposure to sunlight. Products made from these materials are often replaced after long-term use because this gradual degradation can reduce the lifespan of any product. However, nanomaterial research is continuing to address these issues with the recent development of photochromic compounds that maintain responsiveness through environmental variables [100].

Other Emerging UV Monitoring Technologies

New UV monitoring technologies are emerging rapidly, delivering advanced solutions that exceed conventional UV sensors and wearables. Not only are these technologies projected to help people monitor their exposure to UV, but they will also find various applications in environmental monitoring, healthcare, and public safety. Because the adverse effects of ultraviolet (UV) radiation, such as skin cancer, premature aging, and DNA damage, are emergent phenomena, there is increasing interest in developing more intelligent UV monitoring systems. The following advanced technologies are establishing themselves as leaders in changing the way we monitor and handle UV [101].

A promising development seems to be the inclusion of UV sensors into smart environments and Internet of Things (IoT) systems. One of the biggest applications, for instance, is smart cities deploying UV monitoring stations in public areas and at places like parks, beaches, urban areas, *etc*. These data from dedicated stations provide the real-time level of UV index that can be disseminated to the community through mobile applications or digital displays. In this way, large-scale monitoring of ecological ultraviolet may be used to promote awareness of UV risks in specific areas and encourage the habit of protection against sun exposure. Such systems can also deliver data to health organizations and researchers, enabling them to monitor trends in UV exposure and relate these with health outcomes such as skin cancer rates [102].

UV monitoring technologies are being improved by deploying artificial intelligence (Al) and machine learning. AL algorithms can identify UV exposure trends, forecast levels of UV based on weather and geological data, and provide personalized tips for sun protection. Take, for example, Al-powered applications linked with wearable devices that can measure daily UV exposure and make recommendations to protect against UV based on a user's skin type, location, and activity levels. These are personalized systems that offer user recommendations based on evidence to reduce the risk of ultraviolet (UV) exposure [103].

The emerging UV monitoring technology involves nanoscale UV sensors. They are ultra-small, flexible sensors that can be incorporated into a variety of materials, including textiles and medical devices. These devices are so small that they can be integrated into common objects without the need to increase their bulk or make them feel uncomfortable. Nanoscale UV sensors are another application being researched, where the fabric used to build clothing would locally change color in response to harmful levels of UV radiation. The sensors can also be used for healthcare applications, such as integration in bandages or wound dressings to detect UV exposure of the skin for those patients subject to light therapy or having sensitive skin [104].

Research in healthcare has focused on UV monitoring of certain skin disorders. Continuous UV light exposure monitoring is crucial for patients with photosensitivity disorders like lupus or xeroderma pigmentosum. There are certain UV monitoring devices specially designed for medical applications that can provide real-time information to patients as well as the healthcare provider. The downside to all of this is that, instead, our devices are becoming much more portable and easier to use, thereby allowing patients' exposure range and allowing them to track exposure much better. More generally, such technologies can also facilitate null hypothesis testing in a clinical research context by supplying detailed exposure metrics that can aid descriptor-based epidemiology works to investigate UV effects among subjects who have various types of sensitive skin [105].

ADVANTAGES OF PERSONALIZED UV EXPOSURE MONITORING

Wearable UV monitoring devices are made to help users monitor UV exposure in a holistic and low-effort way so that there will be many health and lifestyle benefits. Such devices fall within a wider shift to personalized, data-informed health tracking, especially for skin care. Some of the most important benefits offered by these specialized devices are discussed below:

Personalized UV Exposure Tracking

The trend towards personalized UV exposure tracking is the next key step for modern wearable UV monitoring devices that provide a technological leap over conventional sun protection methods. While generalized UV Index forecasts, which are based on averaged conditions and apply at a regional level, give the general public an acute awareness of their risk, personalized tracking of UV exposure presents people with real-time information about their sun exposure that is unique to their characteristics and situation [106].

Personalized UV tracking refers to the many individual factors that can affect how a person is influenced by UV radiation. Skin type, activity levels, geographic location, and even environmental conditions can influence these factors. Advanced sensors such as photodiodes, phototransistors, or similar components are integrated into the device to measure the intensity of UV rays around the user. This data is then processed through complex algorithms, taking into consideration personal information, including skin type. People have different warnings, like those with fair skin who are more likely to sunburn and get UV damage than someone of darker color skin, as they receive greater natural protection against the sun's harmful rays [107].

Personalized UV exposure tracking benefits beyond the protection from the sun allows for the collection of a detailed history of UV exposure behavior over time that can be important in managing long-term skin health. With daily and cumulative tracked UV exposure, users can recognize trends to better inform their sun protection strategies. In this case, a user could have learned that they have been frequently exposed to high UV levels while participating in specific activities or during certain times of day and modified their behaviors or taken preventative action [108].

Personalized UV tracking can enhance the effectiveness of sun protection routines. Devices often provide real-time feedback, such as alerts when UV levels reach a threshold that necessitates action. This real-time intervention is particularly valuable for outdoor enthusiasts, athletes, or anyone frequently exposed to sunlight, as it offers a proactive approach to managing UV exposure rather than relying on reactive measures [109].

This personalized tracking of UV exposure is the new, improved sun safety tech. Such devices offer customized data that improve sun protection compliance by considering variations in skin type, activity, and ambient environment. Not only does this personalized approach help avoid immediate sunburn, but it also supports long-lasting skin health by providing exposure insights and tailored advice. However, with the advancements in technology, person-specific UV monitoring will become increasingly necessary for healthier sun behaviors associated with skin damage and skin cancer prevention [110].

Improved Skin Health Awareness

Improved skin health awareness is a central benefit of using wearable UV monitoring devices. These innovative tools play a crucial role in educating users about the risks of UV radiation and empowering them to take proactive steps to protect their skin. By providing real-time, personalized data on UV exposure, wearable devices bridge the gap between general sun safety guidelines and individual health needs, leading to more informed decisions and improved skin health outcomes [111].

Wearable UV monitors, such as wristbands, patches, or smartwatches, continuously measure the exposure to different types of UV radiation and provide users with real-time feedback. Such constant vigilance raises awareness about mediation exposure to UV, which is quite underestimated. Conventional methods either use weather reports or (general) UV Index estimates, which are, at best, vague and general indicators that cannot capture personal-specific metrics like skin type, activity types, environmental needs, *etc*. On the other hand, wearable devices are capable of providing accurate and tailored insights at the individual level about personal exposure to UV radiation in real time [112].

The enhanced awareness provided by these devices is pivotal in shaping better sun protection habits. Many people are unaware of how their daily activities and habits contribute to UV exposure or how even seemingly benign conditions like cloudy days can still present a risk. Wearable UV monitors help users understand these nuances by tracking exposure continuously and providing actionable data [113].

Increased awareness of both cumulative UV exposure (a contributor to long-term skin health) and long-lasting exposure to UV acts as an accelerator for skin aging and increases the risk of skin cancers, such as melanoma. Wearable UV monitors provide cumulative tracking, indicating total exposure to the UV through time.

This long-term view allows users to understand the cumulative influence of their sun behavior, promoting sustained sun protection [114].

Moreover, their integration with smartphone apps and online platforms augments their educational potential. Specific apps can even include access to more extensive historical data and trends, as well as specific sun safety recommendations based on an individual's history of total UV exposure. Through this connectivity, users can monitor and track their progress, set goals to achieve a reduction in UV exposure over time, and receive personalized recommendations for improving sun protection behavior. Wearable UV monitors represent a potential step to advancing prevention against skin health, documenting personal level real-time data on UV exposure. They equip users with the information and ability to make decisions on sun protection to decrease the chances of burning in the short term as well as skin damage in the long term. These devices are beneficial for public health and skin health by increasing the knowledge of UV risks and encouraging continuous protective behaviors [115].

Behavioral Changes Driven by UV Data

Changes in behavior driven by UV data are a fundamental paradigm shift in the self-management of sun exposure and skin health. Wearable devices that provide real-time monitoring help integrate into daily life and can substantially influence behavior, resulting in better education about the appropriate sunscreen application. An important aspect in which these changes are noticeable is spending less time outside and using sun protection practices like sunscreen or protective clothing [116].

Many wearable devices will notify the user when they are approaching their risk limit for UV exposure to encourage them to adapt or stop outdoor activity. As an example, a runner doing a long outdoor run could receive an alert to cut their run short or take a break in the shade. Likewise, users may also change their outdoor plans based on real-time UV data by planning for some indoor activities or going out but not much into the sun. This change in behavior serves to avoid acute effects such as sunburn but also reduces cumulative UV exposure that leads others to a more chronic effect on skin health [117].

Wearable UV monitors promote increased use of sun protection measures by reducing time in the sun. Such devices often remind users when to apply or reapply sunscreen when protective apparel is recommended. For instance, one device can remind a user to reapply sunscreen every two hours or warn them to stay in the shade during peak UV hours and wear a hat and sunglasses. The potential improvements in adherence to more consistent sun protection practices, as guided by this application, directly address a common problem of users neglecting to reapply sunscreen often enough or using other forms of skin protection [118].

UV data not only immediately enables some adjustments in behavior. The ongoing feedback coming from wearables creates urgency and mindfulness around UV exposure that translates to skin health. When users progressively learn to check their UV levels and react to warnings, they grow accustomed to the relevance of sun security. The impact of this persistent awareness can manifest in various permanent behavioral changes, such as the use of sun protection on a cloudy day or while briefly spending time outdoors [119].

Wearable UV monitoring devices provide real-time, individualized information on exposures that drive high-impact behavioral changes. They aid individuals in minimizing their sun exposure and maximizing their use of preventative UV measures, thereby promoting better skin health and preventing UV-induced damage. Wearable UV monitors contribute to the development of healthy habits and improve overall skin care by promoting a better understanding of ultraviolet exposure as well as responsible behavior towards sun safety [120].

CONCLUSION

Personalized UV exposure tracking through wearable devices is a promising breakthrough in skin health management. These devices help the public avoid harmful ultraviolet (UV) radiation, a well-known environmental risk factor for immediate dangers like sunburn and long-term illnesses such as skin aging and cancer. With immediate action based on skin type, activity, and environmental conditions recommended in real-time using personal UV monitors worn on the body, wearable devices actuate behavioral change.

Different types of UV radiation, UVA, UVB, and UVC cause skin damage in different ways, and the ability to detect the level of exposure allows users to decide for themselves when it is appropriate to protect against sunlight. Wearable devices such as wristbands, patches, smart clothing, and fitness trackers offer personalized solutions to meet unique user needs by embedding advanced sensors capable of monitoring metrics like the UV index, cumulative CIV exposure, and total time spent outdoors".

Wearable UV monitoring devices promote higher awareness and behavioral changes by limiting time spent on sun exposure and by providing better uptake of protective behavior. Not only do these technologies provide instant sun safety, but they can also aid in protecting skin against premature aging and skin cancer in the long run, making it a must-have element for today's dermatology and cosmetics.

REFERENCES

[1] Hussain MS, Cripwell L, Berkovsky S, Freyne J. Promoting UV exposure awareness with persuasive, wearable technologies InDigital health innovation for consumers, clinicians, connectivity and community. IOS Press 2016; pp. 48-54.

[2] Tsantarliotis P, Tsipouras MG, Giannakeas N. Personalized UV radiation risk monitoring using wearable devices and fuzzy modeling. Inventions (Basel) 2018; 3(2): 26.
[http://dx.doi.org/10.3390/inventions3020026]

[3] Zou W, Sastry M, Gooding JJ, Ramanathan R, Bansal V. Recent advances and a roadmap to wearable UV sensor technologies. Adv Mater Technol 2020; 5(4): 1901036.
[http://dx.doi.org/10.1002/admt.201901036]

[4] Robinson JK, Patel S, Heo SY, *et al.* Real-time UV measurement with a sun protection system for warning young adults about sunburn: prospective cohort study. JMIR Mhealth Uhealth 2021; 9(5): 25895.
[http://dx.doi.org/10.2196/25895] [PMID: 33955844]

[5] McKnight G, Shah J, Hargest R. Physiology of the skin. Surgery 2022; 40(1): 8-12.
[http://dx.doi.org/10.1016/j.mpsur.2021.11.005]

[6] Lee HJ, Kim M. Skin barrier function, and the microbiome. Int J Mol Sci 2022; 23(21): 13071.
[http://dx.doi.org/10.3390/ijms232113071] [PMID: 36361857]

[7] Merin KA, Shaji M, Kameswaran R. A review on sun exposure and skin diseases. Indian J Dermatol 2022; 67(5): 625.
[http://dx.doi.org/10.4103/ijd.ijd_1092_20] [PMID: 36865856]

[8] Ciążyńska M, Kamińska-Winciorek G, Lange D, *et al.* The incidence and clinical analysis of non-melanoma skin cancer. Sci Rep 2021; 11(1): 4337.
[http://dx.doi.org/10.1038/s41598-021-83502-8] [PMID: 33619293]

[9] Gilchrest BA. Sun exposure and vitamin D sufficiency. Am J Clin Nutr 2008; 88(2): 570S-7S.
[http://dx.doi.org/10.1093/ajcn/88.2.570S] [PMID: 18689404]

[10] Knaggs H, Lephart ED. Enhancing skin anti-aging through healthy lifestyle factors. Cosmetics 2023; 10(5): 142.
[http://dx.doi.org/10.3390/cosmetics10050142]

[11] Tončić RJ, Kezić S, Hadžavdić SL, Marinović B. Skin barrier and dry skin in the mature patient. Clin Dermatol 2018; 36(2): 109-15.
[http://dx.doi.org/10.1016/j.clindermatol.2017.10.002] [PMID: 29566915]

[12] Kelly KA, Balogh EA, Kaplan SG, Feldman SR. Skin disease in children: effects on quality of life, stigmatization, bullying, and suicide risk in pediatric acne, atopic dermatitis, and psoriasis patients. Children (Basel) 2021; 8(11): 1057.
[http://dx.doi.org/10.3390/children8111057] [PMID: 34828770]

[13] Wani M, Chakole S, Agrawal S, *et al.* Unveiling skin manifestations: Exploring cutaneous signs of malnutrition in eating disorders. Cureus 2023; 15(9): 44759.
[http://dx.doi.org/10.7759/cureus.44759] [PMID: 37809242]

[14] Huang X, Chalmers AN. Review of wearable and portable sensors for monitoring personal solar UV exposure. Ann Biomed Eng 2021; 49(3): 964-78.
[http://dx.doi.org/10.1007/s10439-020-02710-x] [PMID: 33432511]

[15] Geller AC, Jablonski NG, Pagoto SL, *et al.* Interdisciplinary perspectives on sun safety. JAMA Dermatol 2018; 154(1): 88-92.
[http://dx.doi.org/10.1001/jamadermatol.2017.4201] [PMID: 29117315]

[16] Goon P, Banfield C, Bello O, Levell NJ. Skin cancers in skin types IV-VI: Does the Fitzpatrick scale give a false sense of security?. Skin Health Dis 2021; 1(3): ski2.40.

[http://dx.doi.org/10.1002/ski2.40] [PMID: 35663142]

[17] Birch-Machin MA, Wilkinson SC. Skin photobiology. Principles and Practice of Skin Toxicology 2008; 51-68.
[http://dx.doi.org/10.1002/9780470773093.ch3]

[18] Young AR, Wikonkál NM. The chronic effects of ultraviolet radiation on the skin: Photocarcinogenesis. Photodermatology 2007; 107-40.
[http://dx.doi.org/10.3109/9781420019964-8]

[19] Diffey BL. Human exposure to solar ultraviolet radiation. J Cosmet Dermatol 2002; 1(3): 124-30.
[http://dx.doi.org/10.1046/j.1473-2165.2002.00060.x] [PMID: 17147711]

[20] Kuras ER, Richardson MB, Calkins MM, *et al.* Opportunities and challenges for personal heat exposure research. Environ Health Perspect 2017; 125(8): 085001.
[http://dx.doi.org/10.1289/EHP556] [PMID: 28796630]

[21] Rhodes LE, Lim HW. The acute effects of ultraviolet radiation on the skin. Photodermatology 2007; 75-90.
[http://dx.doi.org/10.3109/9781420019964-6]

[22] Henning A, J Downs N, Vanos JK. Wearable ultraviolet radiation sensors for research and personal use. Int J Biometeorol 2022; 66(3): 627-40.
[http://dx.doi.org/10.1007/s00484-021-02216-8] [PMID: 34743221]

[23] Henning AL. Advancing methods to monitor and assess personal ultraviolet radiation exposure. Arizona State University 2021.

[24] Ianculescu MA, Alexandru AD, Coardo D, Coman OA. Smart wearable medical devices are the next step in providing affordable support for dermatology practice. Dermatovenerologie-J Romanian Soc Dermat 2018; 63: 295-306.

[25] D'Orazio J, Jarrett S, Amaro-Ortiz A, Scott T. UV radiation and the skin. Int J Mol Sci 2013; 14(6): 12222-48.
[http://dx.doi.org/10.3390/ijms140612222] [PMID: 23749111]

[26] Diffey BL. Sources and measurement of ultraviolet radiation. Methods 2002; 28(1): 4-13.
[http://dx.doi.org/10.1016/S1046-2023(02)00204-9] [PMID: 12231182]

[27] Asyi MS, Syahrizal D, Sary NL, Husna F. The impact of photoaging on skin: A systematic review analysis. Journal of Social Research 2023; 3(1): 209-15.
[http://dx.doi.org/10.55324/josr.v3i1.1708]

[28] Krutmann J. The role of UVA rays in skin aging. Eur J Dermatol 2001; 11(2): 170-1.
[PMID: 11275823]

[29] Khalil NA, Ibrahim JS, Elias NY, Taha NM, Yahya RH. Review article about ultraviolet (UV) light. Innov Int Multidiscip J Appl Technol 2024; 2(6): 167-78.

[30] Elmarzugi NA, Keleb EI, Mohamed AT, *et al.* The relation between sunscreen and skin path changes mini-review. Int J Pharm Sci Invent 2013; 2(7): 43-52.

[31] Robinson J, Begum R, Maqbool M. Ultraviolet radiation: Benefits, harms, and protection. An Introduction to Non-Ionizing Radiation 2023; 2: 62-108.
[http://dx.doi.org/10.2174/9789815136890123010008]

[32] Dwivedi A, Tripathi AK, Singh J, Pal MK. Ultraviolet radiation (UVR): An introduction. Photocarcinogenesis & Photoprotection 2018; pp. 1-8.

[33] Gruber F, Peharda V, Kaštelan M, Brajac I. Occupational skin diseases caused by UV radiation. Acta Dermatovenerol Croat 2007; 15(3)

[34] Dupont E, Gomez J, Bilodeau D. Beyond UV radiation: A skin under challenge. Int J Cosmet Sci 2013; 35(3): 224-32.

[http://dx.doi.org/10.1111/ics.12036] [PMID: 23406155]

[35] Del Bino S, Duval C, Bernerd F. Clinical and biological characterization of skin pigmentation diversity and its consequences on UV impact. Int J Mol Sci 2018; 19(9): 2668. [http://dx.doi.org/10.3390/ijms19092668] [PMID: 30205563]

[36] Christensen L, Suggs A, Baron E. Ultraviolet photobiology in dermatology. Ultraviolet Light in Human Health, Diseases and Environment. 2017:89-104.

[37] Salminen A, Kaarniranta K, Kauppinen A. Photoaging: UV radiation-induced inflammation and immunosuppression accelerate the aging process in the skin. Inflamm Res 2022; 71(7-8): 817-31. [http://dx.doi.org/10.1007/s00011-022-01598-8] [PMID: 35748903]

[38] Krutmann J, Gilchrest BA. Photoaging of skin. Skin Aging 2006; 33-43. [http://dx.doi.org/10.1007/3-540-32953-6_4]

[39] de Gruijl FR. Skin cancer and solar UV radiation. Eur J Cancer 1999; 35(14): 2003-9. [http://dx.doi.org/10.1016/S0959-8049(99)00283-X] [PMID: 10711242]

[40] Mason S, Reichrath J. Sunlight vitamin D and skin cancer. Anti-Cancer Agents in Medicinal Chemistry (Formerly Current Medicinal Chemistry-Anti-Cancer Agents) 2013; 13(1): 83-97.

[41] Matsumura Y, Ananthaswamy HN. Short-term and long-term cellular and molecular events following UV irradiation of skin: implications for molecular medicine. Expert Rev Mol Med 2002; 4(26): 1-22. [http://dx.doi.org/10.1017/S146239940200532X] [PMID: 14585163]

[42] Coelho SG, Choi W, Brenner M, *et al.* Short-and long-term effects of UV radiation on the pigmentation of human skin. Journal of Investigative Dermatology Symposium Proceedings. 14(1): 32-5. [http://dx.doi.org/10.1038/jidsymp.2009.10]

[43] MacKie RM. Long-term health risk to the skin of ultraviolet radiation. Prog Biophys Mol Biol 2006; 92(1): 92-6. [http://dx.doi.org/10.1016/j.pbiomolbio.2006.02.008] [PMID: 16616325]

[44] Morganroth PA, Lim HW, Burnett CT. Ultraviolet radiation and the skin: an in-depth review. Am J Lifestyle Med 2013; 7(3): 168-81. [http://dx.doi.org/10.1177/1559827612460499]

[45] Grovies GA. Sunburn and its prevention. Australas J Dermatol 1980; 21(3): 115-41. [http://dx.doi.org/10.1111/j.1440-0960.1980.tb00156.x] [PMID: 7016109]

[46] Sivamani RK, Crane LA, Dellavalle RP. The benefits and risks of ultraviolet tanning and its alternatives: the role of prudent sun exposure. Dermatol Clin 2009; 27(2): 149-154, vi. [http://dx.doi.org/10.1016/j.det.2008.11.008] [PMID: 19254658]

[47] Saraiya M, Glanz K, Briss PA, *et al.* Interventions to prevent skin cancer by reducing exposure to ultraviolet radiation. Am J Prev Med 2004; 27(5): 422-66. [http://dx.doi.org/10.1016/j.amepre.2004.08.009] [PMID: 15556744]

[48] Krutmann J, Schalka S, Watson REB, Wei L, Morita A. Daily photoprotection to prevent photoaging. Photodermatol Photoimmunol Photomed 2021; 37(6): 482-9. [http://dx.doi.org/10.1111/phpp.12688] [PMID: 33896049]

[49] Piérard-Franchimont C, Uhoda I, Saint-Léger D, Piérard GE. Androgenic alopecia and stress-induced premature senescence by cumulative ultraviolet light exposure. Exogenous Dermatology 2002; 1(4): 203-6. [http://dx.doi.org/10.1159/000066146]

[50] Gracia-Cazaña T, Aguilera J, Navarro-Bielsa A, González S, Lim HW, Gilaberte Y. New trends on personalized sunscreens. Photodermatol Photoimmunol Photomed 2024; 40(3): 12967. [http://dx.doi.org/10.1111/phpp.12967] [PMID: 38616500]

[51] Hart PH, Gorman S, Finlay-Jones JJ. Modulation of the immune system by UV radiation: more than

just the effects of vitamin D?. Nat Rev Immunol 2011; 11(9): 584-96. [http://dx.doi.org/10.1038/nri3045] [PMID: 21852793]

[52] Desai SR. Hyperpigmentation therapy: a review. J Clin Aesthet Dermatol 2014; 7(8): 13-7. [PMID: 25161755]

[53] Lou Z, Wang L, Shen G. Recent advances in smart wearable sensing systems. Adv Mater Technol 2018; 3(12): 1800444. [http://dx.doi.org/10.1002/admt.201800444]

[54] Natarajan VT, Ganju P, Ramkumar A, Grover R, Gokhale RS. Multifaceted pathways protect human skin from UV radiation. Nat Chem Biol 2014; 10(7): 542-51. [http://dx.doi.org/10.1038/nchembio.1548] [PMID: 24937072]

[55] Baeg KJ, Binda M, Natali D, Caironi M, Noh YY. Organic light detectors: photodiodes and phototransistors. Adv Mater 2013; 25(31): 4267-95. [http://dx.doi.org/10.1002/adma.201204979] [PMID: 23483718]

[56] Mamun MAA, Yuce MR. Sensors and systems for wearable environmental monitoring toward IoT-enabled applications: A review. IEEE Sens J 2019; 19(18): 7771-88. [http://dx.doi.org/10.1109/JSEN.2019.2919352]

[57] Wilson DJ, Martín-Martínez FJ, Deravi LF. Wearable light sensors are based on the unique features of a natural biochrome. ACS Sens 2022; 7(2): 523-33. [http://dx.doi.org/10.1021/acssensors.1c02342] [PMID: 35138085]

[58] Damulira E, Yusoff MNS, Omar AF, Mohd Taib NH. A review: photonic devices used for dosimetry in medical radiation. Sensors (Basel) 2019; 19(10): 2226. [http://dx.doi.org/10.3390/s19102226] [PMID: 31091779]

[59] Yagura T, Makita K, Yamamoto H, Menck CFM, Schuch AP. Biological sensors for solar ultraviolet radiation. Sensors (Basel) 2011; 11(4): 4277-94. [http://dx.doi.org/10.3390/s110404277] [PMID: 22163847]

[60] Fioletov V, Kerr JB, Fergusson A. The UV index: definition, distribution and factors affecting it. Can J Public Health 2010; 101(4): I5-9. [http://dx.doi.org/10.1007/BF03405303] [PMID: 21033538]

[61] Snyder A, Valdebran M, Terrero D, Amber KT, Kelly KM. Solar ultraviolet exposure in individuals who perform outdoor sports activities. Sports Med Open 2020; 6(1): 42. [http://dx.doi.org/10.1186/s40798-020-00272-9] [PMID: 32880767]

[62] Hammond V, Reeder AI, Gray A. Patterns of real-time occupational ultraviolet radiation exposure among a sample of outdoor workers in New Zealand. Public Health 2009; 123(2): 182-7. [http://dx.doi.org/10.1016/j.puhe.2008.12.007] [PMID: 19181351]

[63] Ali SM, Ali U. An approach to design a wristwatch for the protection of the human skin damage induced by ultraviolet and infrared radiations. Photodermatol Photoimmunol Photomed 2020; 36(4): 278-89. [http://dx.doi.org/10.1111/phpp.12551] [PMID: 32187717]

[64] Chiou WL. Prevention of skin cancer: healthy sun exposure and no sunscreen for intense intermittent exposure; photoaging theories questioned and new strategies. Journal of Dermatology Research 2022; 3(3): 1-16. [http://dx.doi.org/10.46889/JDR.2022.3304]

[65] Wright CY, Reeder AI. Youth solar ultraviolet radiation exposure, concurrent activities and sun-protective practices: a review. Photochem Photobiol 2005; 81(6): 1331-42. [http://dx.doi.org/10.1562/2005-8-19-IR-655] [PMID: 16354111]

[66] Lawler S, Spathonis K, Eakin E, Gallois C, Leslie E, Owen N. Sun exposure and sun protection behaviours among young adult sport competitors. Aust N Z J Public Health 2007; 31(3): 230-4. [http://dx.doi.org/10.1111/j.1467-842X.2007.00053.x] [PMID: 17679240]

[67] Kazanskiy NL, Butt MA, Khonina SN. Recent advances in wearable optical sensor automation powered by battery *versus* skin-like battery-free devices for personal healthcare—A review. Nanomaterials (Basel) 2022; 12(3): 334.
[http://dx.doi.org/10.3390/nano12030334] [PMID: 35159679]

[68] Samon SM, Hammel SC, Stapleton HM, Anderson KA. Silicone wristbands as personal passive sampling devices: Current knowledge, recommendations for use, and future directions. Environ Int 2022; 169: 107339.
[http://dx.doi.org/10.1016/j.envint.2022.107339] [PMID: 36116363]

[69] Idris SA, Lazam NA, Izhar LI, Azman DB, Way LJ, Aida I. Smart health monitoring wristband with auto-alert function. 2022 IEEE 5th International Symposium in Robotics and Manufacturing Automation (ROMA). 1-7.
[http://dx.doi.org/10.1109/ROMA55875.2022.9915677]

[70] Kowshik MR, Narayan A, Nagarajan PM, Gopalan S. Dynamic dual-function safety wristband: A simulation-driven design for enhancing women's security and personal safety. Procedia Comput Sci 2025; 259: 386-97.
[http://dx.doi.org/10.1016/j.procs.2025.03.340]

[71] Seçkin M, Seçkin AÇ, Gençer Ç. Biomedical sensors and applications of wearable technologies on arm and hand. Biomed Mater Devices 2023; 1(1): 443-55.
[http://dx.doi.org/10.1007/s44174-022-00002-7]

[72] Kim JH, Park SY, Kim MK, *et al.* Long-term UV detecting wearable patches enabled by III-N compound semiconductor-based microphotodetectors. Adv Opt Mater 2023; 11(13): 2203083.
[http://dx.doi.org/10.1002/adom.202203083]

[73] Lee HJ, Hong WG, Yang HY, Ha DH, Jun Y, Yun YJ. A wearable patch based on flexible porous reduced graphene oxide paper sensor for real-time and continuous ultraviolet radiation monitoring. Adv Mater Technol 2022; 7(3): 2100709.
[http://dx.doi.org/10.1002/admt.202100709]

[74] Barajas-Carmona JG, Francisco-Aldana L, Morales-Narváez E. Wearable nanoplasmonic patch detecting sun/UV exposure. Anal Chem 2017; 89(24): 13589-95.
[http://dx.doi.org/10.1021/acs.analchem.7b04066] [PMID: 29155557]

[75] Shi Y, Manco M, Moyal D, *et al.* Soft, stretchable, epidermal sensor with integrated electronics and photochemistry for measuring personal UV exposures. PLoS One 2018; 13(1): 0190233.
[http://dx.doi.org/10.1371/journal.pone.0190233] [PMID: 29293664]

[76] Soutar A, Semple S, Aitken RJ, Robertson A. Use of patches and whole body sampling for the assessment of dermal exposure. Ann Occup Hyg 2000; 44(7): 511-8.
[http://dx.doi.org/10.1016/S0003-4878(00)00043-0] [PMID: 11042252]

[77] Takebira UM, Mohibullah AT, Mehbub A, Islam MM, Pervez MN, Mondal MI. Wearable smart textiles—recent development and applications. Smart Textiles from Natural Resources 2024; 395-442.

[78] Lee H, Baek K. Developing a smart multifunctional outdoor jacket with wearable sensing technology for user health and safety. Multimedia Tools Appl 2021; 80(21-23): 32273-310.
[http://dx.doi.org/10.1007/s11042-021-11166-7]

[79] Ahsan M, Teay SH, Sayem ASM, Albarbar A. Smart clothing framework for health monitoring applications. Signals (Basel) 2022; 3(1): 113-45.
[http://dx.doi.org/10.3390/signals3010009]

[80] Khan A, Nazir A, Rehman A, *et al.* A review of UV radiation protection on humans by textiles and clothing. Int J Cloth Sci Technol 2020; 32(6): 869-90.
[http://dx.doi.org/10.1108/IJCST-10-2019-0153]

[81] Sharma A, Singh A, Gupta V, Arya S. Advancements and future prospects of wearable sensing technology for healthcare applications. Sens Diagn 2022; 1(3): 387-404.

[http://dx.doi.org/10.1039/D2SD00005A]

[82] Guk K, Han G, Lim J, *et al.* Evolution of wearable devices with real-time disease monitoring for personalized healthcare. Nanomaterials (Basel) 2019; 9(6): 813. [http://dx.doi.org/10.3390/nano9060813] [PMID: 31146479]

[83] Kanellis VG. Ultraviolet radiation sensors: a review. Biophys Rev 2019; 11(6): 895-9. [http://dx.doi.org/10.1007/s12551-019-00556-9] [PMID: 31230215]

[84] Benavides NR, Rutkey HE, DiDomenico CM, *et al.* A wearable mobile-app-controlled device for continuous monitoring of UV exposure and hydration levels. 2021 IEEE 11th Annual Computing and Communication Workshop and Conference (CCWC). 1167-72. [http://dx.doi.org/10.1109/CCWC51732.2021.9376109]

[85] Virginia Anikwe C, Friday Nweke H, Chukwu Ikegwu A, *et al.* Mobile and wearable sensors for data-driven health monitoring system: State-of-the-art and future prospect. Expert Syst Appl 2022; 202: 117362. [http://dx.doi.org/10.1016/j.eswa.2022.117362]

[86] Banerjee S, Hoch eg, Kaplan PD, Dumont EL. A comparative study of wearable ultraviolet radiometers. 2017 IEEE Life Sciences Conference (LSC). 9-12. [http://dx.doi.org/10.1109/LSC.2017.8268131]

[87] Shakeriaski F, Ghodrat M. Challenges and limitation of wearable sensors used in firefighters' protective clothing. J Fire Sci 2022; 40(3): 214-45. [http://dx.doi.org/10.1177/07349041221079004]

[88] Heikenfeld J, Jajack A, Rogers J, *et al.* Wearable sensors: modalities, challenges, and prospects. Lab Chip 2018; 18(2): 217-48. [http://dx.doi.org/10.1039/C7LC00914C] [PMID: 29182185]

[89] Nassar JM. Affordable and scalable manufacturing of wearable multi-functional sensory "Skin" for internet of everything applications

[90] Yu Z, Xu J, Gong H, *et al.* Bioinspired self-powered piezoresistive sensors for simultaneous monitoring of human health and outdoor UV light intensity. ACS Appl Mater Interfaces 2022; 14(4): 5101-11. [http://dx.doi.org/10.1021/acsami.1c23604] [PMID: 35050572]

[91] Kantheti RB, Kantheti KR. Smart watch to track the levels of vitamin D. Int Res J Eng Technol 2020; 7: 4880-3.

[92] Mei B, Li R, Cheng W, Yu J, Cheng X. Ultraviolet radiation measurement *via* smart devices. IEEE Internet Things J 2017; 4(4): 934-44. [http://dx.doi.org/10.1109/JIOT.2017.2717845]

[93] Black TA, George M, Rousseau MA, Rashid RM. Smart watches lack skin smarts: Current and future dermatologic applications in device metrics. Cureus 2024; 16(2): 55273. [http://dx.doi.org/10.7759/cureus.55273] [PMID: 38558692]

[94] Nelson EE, Rousseau MA, Black TA, George MN, Rashid RM. Smartwatch technology in medicine: A call for future dermatologic research. JMIR Dermatol 2023; 6(1): 47252. [http://dx.doi.org/10.2196/47252] [PMID: 37843896]

[95] Behera A, Behera A. Chromogenic materials. Advanced materials: An introduction to modern materials science 2022; 157(91). [http://dx.doi.org/10.1007/978-3-030-80359-9_5]

[96] Eppig T, Speck A, Gillner M, Nagengast D, Langenbucher A. Photochromic dynamics of ophthalmic lenses. Appl Opt 2012; 51(2): 133-8. [http://dx.doi.org/10.1364/AO.51.000133] [PMID: 22270510]

[97] Yimyai T, Crespy D, Pena-Francesch A. Self-healing photochromic elastomer composites for

wearable UV-sensors. Adv Funct Mater 2023; 33(20): 2213717. [http://dx.doi.org/10.1002/adfm.202213717]

[98] Morsümbül S, Akçakoca Kumbasar EP, Alır Kıyak S, Alemdar IG. A new approach to photochromic nanofiber-based ultraviolet sensors with grayscale adaptation. Polym Eng Sci 2024; 64(9): 4246-57. [http://dx.doi.org/10.1002/pen.26844]

[99] Viková M, Vik M. Description of photochromic textile properties in selected color spaces. Text Res J 2015; 85(6): 609-20. [http://dx.doi.org/10.1177/0040517514549988]

[100] Pardo R, Zayat M, Levy D. Photochromic organic–inorganic hybrid materials. Chem Soc Rev 2011; 40(2): 672-87. [http://dx.doi.org/10.1039/c0cs00065e] [PMID: 21229130]

[101] McGrath MJ, Scanaill CN. Sensor technologies: healthcare, wellness, and environmental applications. Springer Nature 2013. [http://dx.doi.org/10.1007/978-1-4302-6014-1]

[102] Islam T, Mukhopadhyay SC, Suryadevara NK. Smart sensors and internet of things: A postgraduate paper. IEEE Sens J 2017; 17(3): 577-84. [http://dx.doi.org/10.1109/JSEN.2016.2630124]

[103] Abusultan A, Abunahla H, Halawani Y, Mohammad B, Alamoodi N, Alazzam A. Artificial Intelligence-aided low cost and flexible graphene oxide-based paper sensor for ultraviolet and sunlight monitoring. Nanoscale Res Lett 2022; 17(1): 89. [http://dx.doi.org/10.1186/s11671-022-03727-y] [PMID: 36094698]

[104] Vu CC, Kim SJ, Kim J. Flexible wearable sensors - an update in view of touch-sensing. Sci Technol Adv Mater 2021; 22(1): 26-36. [http://dx.doi.org/10.1080/14686996.2020.1862629] [PMID: 33854405]

[105] Tang X, Yang T, Yu D, Xiong H, Zhang S. Current insights and future perspectives of ultraviolet radiation (UV) exposure: Friends and foes to the skin and beyond the skin. Environ Int 2024; 185: 108535. [http://dx.doi.org/10.1016/j.envint.2024.108535] [PMID: 38428192]

[106] Dey S, Sahoo S, Agrawal H, Mondal A, Bhowmik T, Tiwari VN. Personalized cumulative UV tracking on mobiles & wearables. 2017 39th Annual International Conference of the IEEE Engineering in Medicine and Biology Society (EMBC). 2341-4. [http://dx.doi.org/10.1109/EMBC.2017.8037325]

[107] Buller DB, Berwick M, Lantz K, *et al.* Smartphone mobile application delivering personalized, real-time sun protection advice: a randomized clinical trial. JAMA Dermatol 2015; 151(5): 497-504. [http://dx.doi.org/10.1001/jamadermatol.2014.3889] [PMID: 25629710]

[108] Stock ML, Gerrard M, Gibbons FX, *et al.* Sun protection intervention for highway workers: long-term efficacy of UV photography and skin cancer information on men's protective cognitions and behavior. Ann Behav Med 2009; 38(3): 225-36. [http://dx.doi.org/10.1007/s12160-009-9151-2] [PMID: 20049658]

[109] Li H, Colantonio S, Dawson A, Lin X, Beecker J. Sunscreen application, safety, and sun protection: the evidence. J Cutan Med Surg 2019; 23(4): 357-69. [http://dx.doi.org/10.1177/1203475419856611] [PMID: 31219707]

[110] Buller DB, Berwick M, Shane J, Kane I, Lantz K, Buller MK. User-centered development of a smart phone mobile application delivering personalized real-time advice on sun protection. Transl Behav Med 2013; 3(3): 326-34. [http://dx.doi.org/10.1007/s13142-013-0208-1] [PMID: 24058385]

[111] Turner J, Igoe D, Parisi AV, McGonigle AJ, Amar A, Wainwright L. A review on the ability of smartphones to detect ultraviolet (UV) radiation and their potential to be used in UV research and for

public education purposes. Sci Total Environ 2020; 706: 135873. [http://dx.doi.org/10.1016/j.scitotenv.2019.135873] [PMID: 31862595]

[112] Bernasconi S, Angelucci A, Aliverti A. A scoping review on wearable devices for environmental monitoring and their application for health and wellness. Sensors (Basel) 2022; 22(16): 5994. [http://dx.doi.org/10.3390/s22165994] [PMID: 36015755]

[113] Panahi O. Wearable sensors and personalized sustainability: Monitoring health and environmental exposures in real-time. Eur J Innov Stud Sustain 2025; 1(2): 11-9. [http://dx.doi.org/10.59324/ejiss.2025.1(2).02]

[114] Glanz K, Mayer JA. Reducing ultraviolet radiation exposure to prevent skin cancer methodology and measurement. Am J Prev Med 2005; 29(2): 131-42. [http://dx.doi.org/10.1016/j.amepre.2005.04.007] [PMID: 16005810]

[115] Hussain MS, Nicholson BD, Freyne J. Tune your sun right: persuasive app towards healthy & safe sun exposure. Proceedings of the 29th Australian Conference on Computer-Human Interaction. 361-5. [http://dx.doi.org/10.1145/3152771.3156137]

[116] Lucas R, Repacholi MH, McMichael AJ. Is the current public health message on UV exposure correct?. Bull World Health Organ 2006; 84(6): 485-91. [http://dx.doi.org/10.2471/BLT.05.026559] [PMID: 16799733]

[117] Mahler HIM, Kulik JA, Gerrard M, Gibbons FX. Long-term effects of appearance-based interventions on sun protection behaviors. Health Psychol 2007; 26(3): 350-60. [http://dx.doi.org/10.1037/0278-6133.26.3.350] [PMID: 17500622]

[118] Zhang X, Xu W, Huang MC, Amini N, Ren F. See UV on your skin: an ultraviolet sensing and visualization system. Proceedings of the 8th International Conference on Body Area Networks. 22-8. [http://dx.doi.org/10.4108/icst.bodynets.2013.253701]

[119] Watson M, Garnett E, Guy GP, Holman DM. The surgeon general's call to action to prevent skin cancer. International Journal of Cancer Research and Prevention 2015; 8(1): 55.

[120] Robinson JK, Durst DA, Gray E, *et al.* Sun exposure reduction by melanoma survivors with wearable sensor providing real-time UV exposure and daily text messages with structured goal setting. Arch Dermatol Res 2021; 313(8): 685-94. [http://dx.doi.org/10.1007/s00403-020-02163-1] [PMID: 33185716]

SUBJECT INDEX

A

B

C

Akhil Sharma, Shaweta Sharma, Shivkanya Fuloria & Sudhir Kumar (Eds.)

D

E

F

G

H

I

K

L

M

N

O

P

R

S

T

U

V

W

www.ingramcontent.com/pod-product-compliance
Lightning Source LLC
LaVergne TN
LVHW070946210926
848482LV00002B/109